Vascular Cognitive Impairment in Clinical Practice

Vascular Cognitive Impairment in Clinical Practice

Edited by

Lars-Olof Wahlund

Timo Erkinjuntti

Serge Gauthier

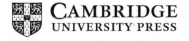

CAMBRIDGE UNIVERSITY PRESS

CAMBRIDGE UNIVERSITY PRESS
Cambridge, New York, Melbourne, Madrid, Cape Town, Singapore, São Paulo, Delhi

Cambridge University Press
The Edinburgh Building, Cambridge CB2 8RU, UK

Published in the United States of America by Cambridge University Press, New York

www.cambridge.org
Information on this title: www.cambridge.org/9780521875370

© Cambridge University Press 2009

First published 2009

Printed in the United Kingdom at the University Press, Cambridge

A catalog record for this publication is available from the British Library

Library of Congress Cataloguing in Publication data
Vascular cognitive impairment in clinical practice / [edited by]
Lars-Olof Wahlund, Timo Erkinjuntti, Serge Gauthier.
    p. ; cm.
  Includes bibliographical references and index.
  ISBN 978-0-521-87537-0 (hardback)
  1. Cerebrovascular disease – Complications. 2. Dementia. 3. Cognitive disorders. I. Wahlund, Lars-Olof.
  II. Erkinjuntti, Timo. III. Gauthier, Serge, 1950–
  [DNLM: 1. Dementia, Vascular. 2. Cognition Disorders. WM 220 V33055 2009]
  RC388.5.V3653 2009
  616.8′1–dc22   2008039237

ISBN 978-0-521-87537-0 hardback

Contents

Color plates are found between pp. 84 and 85.

Contributors

Rimma Axelsson, MD, PhD
CLINTEC, Division of Radiology, Karolinska Institutet, Karolinska University Hospital Huddinge, Stockholm, Sweden

Lars Bäckman, PhD
Aging Research Center, Department of Neurobiology, Care Sciences and Society, Karolinska Institutet, Stockholm, Sweden

Frederik Barkhof, MD, PhD
Professor of Neuroradiology
Alzheimer Center and Department of Diagnostic Radiology, VU University Medical Center, Amsterdam, the Netherlands

Emelia J. Benjamin, MD, ScM
National Heart, Lung and Blood Institute's Framingham Heart Study, Framingham. Department of Preventive Medicine and Whitaker Cardiovascular Institute, School of Medicine, and Department of Epidemiology, School of Public Health, Boston University, Boston, USA

Lena Borell, PhD, OT (reg)
Professor of Occupational Therapy, Department of Neurobiology, Care Sciences and Society, Karolinska Institutet, Stockholm, Sweden

Alistair Burns, FRCP, FRCPysch, MD
Professor of Old Age Psychiatry, University of Manchester, Wythenshawe Hospital, Manchester, UK

Catherine Cole, MRCPsych
Specialist Registrar in Old Age Psychiatry, University of Manchester, Wythenshawe Hospital, Manchester, UK

Charles DeCarli, MD, PhD
Professor of Neurology and Director, Alzheimer's Disease Center and Imaging of Dementia and Aging (IDeA) Laboratory, Department of Neurology and Center for Neuroscience, University of California at Davis, Sacramento, USA

Christian Enzinger, MD
Department of Neurology and Department of Radiology, Division of Neuroradiology, Medical University, Graz, Austria

Timo Erkinjuntti, MD, PhD
Department of Neurology, University of Helsinki, Helsinki, Finland

Franz Fazekas, MD, PhD
Department of Neurology, Medical University, Graz, Austria

Wiesje M. van der Flier, PhD
Assistant Professor, Alzheimer Center and Department of Neurology, VU University Medical Center, Amsterdam, the Netherlands

Laura Fratiglioni, MD, PhD
Aging Research Center, Department of Neurobiology, Care Sciences and Society, Karolinska Institutet, and Stockholm Gerontology Research Center, Stockholm, Sweden

Serge Gauthier, MD, PhD
Alzheimer's Disease and Related Disorders Research Unit, McGill Centre for Studies on Aging, Douglas Mental Health University Institute, Montre?al, Que?bec, Canada

Jorge Ghiso, PhD
Associate Professor, Departments of Pathology and Psychiatry, NYU School of Medicine, New York, USA

Deborah Gustafson, MS, PhD
Associate Professor, NeuroPsychiatric Epidemiology Unit, Institute of Neuroscience and Physiology, Department of Psychiatry and Neurochemistry, Sahlgrenska Academy, University of Gothenburg, Gothenburg, Sweden, Rush University Medical Center, Chicago, USA, Medical College of Wisconsin, Milwankee, USA

Angela L. Jefferson, PhD
Department of Neurology and Alzheimer's Disease Center, Boston University School of Medicine, Boston, USA

Raj N. Kalaria, MD, PhD
Wolfson Research Centre, Institute for Ageing and Health, Newcastle General Hospital, Newcastle upon Tyne, UK

Sari Karlsson, PhD
Aging Research Center, Department of Neurobiology, Care Sciences and Society, Karolinska Institutet, and Department of Clinical Neuroscience, Karolinska Institutet, Karolinska Hospital, Stockholm, Sweden

Miia Kivipelto, MD, PhD
Aging Research Center, Department of Neurobiology, Caring Sciences and Society (NVS), Karolinska Institutet, Stockholm, Sweden, and Department of Neuroscience and Neurology, University of Kuopio, Finland

Erika J. Laukka, PhD
Aging Research Center, Department of Neurobiology, Care Sciences and Society, Karolinska Institutet, Stockholm, Sweden

Oscar L. Lopez, MD
Departments of Neurology and Psychiatry, Alzheimer's Disease Research Center, University of Pittsburgh School of Medicine, Pittsburgh, USA

Stuart W. S. MacDonald, PhD
Aging Research Center, Department of Neurobiology, Care Sciences and Society, Karolinska Institutet,

Stockholm, Sweden, and Department of Psychology, University of Victoria, Victoria, Canada

Adriane Mayda, BS
Imaging of Dementia and Aging (IDeA) Laboratory, Center for Neuroscience, University of California at Davis, Sacramento, USA

Tiia Ngandu, PhD
Aging Research Center, Department of Neurobiology, Caring Sciences and Society (NVS), Karolinska Institutet, Stockholm, Sweden, and Department of Neuroscience and Neurology, University of Kuopio, Finland

Leonardo Pantoni, MD, PhD
Department of Neurological and Psychiatric Sciences, University of Florence, Florence, Italy

Francesca Pescini, MD
Department of Neurological and Psychiatric Sciences, University of Florence, Florence, Italy

Tuula Pirttilä, MD, PhD
Neurology Unit, Department of Clinical Science, University of Kuopio, Kuopio, Finland

Anna Poggesi, MD
Department of Neurological and Psychiatric Sciences, University of Florence, Florence, Italy

Chengxuan Qiu, PhD
Aging Research Center, Department of Neurobiology Care Science and Society, Karolinska Institutet, Stockholm, Sweden

Stefan Ropele, PhD
Department of Neurology, Medical University, Graz, Austria

Agueda Rostagno, PhD
Associate Professor, Department of Pathology, NYU School of Medicine, New York, USA

Philip Scheltens, MD, PhD
Professor of Cognitive Neurology, Alzheimer Center and Department of Neurology, VU University Medical Center, Amsterdam, the Netherlands

Reinhold Schmidt, MD, PhD
Department of Neurology and Department of Radiology, Division of Neuroradiology, Medical University, Graz, Austria

Ingmar Skoog, MD, PhD
NeuroPsychiatric Epidemiology Unit, Institute of Neuroscience and Physiology, Section of Psychiatry and Neurochemistry, Sahlgrenska Academy, University of Gothenburg, Gothenburg, Sweden

Alina Solomon
Aging Research Center, Department of Neurobiology, Caring Sciences and Society, Karolinska Institutet, Stockholm, Sweden, and Department of Neuroscience and Neurology, University of Kuopio, Finland

Salka S. Staekenborg, MD
Alzheimer Center and Department of Neurology, VU University Medical Center, Amsterdam, the Netherlands

Lars-Olof Wahlund, MD, PhD
Department of Neurobiology Care Science and Society, Section for Clinical Geriatrics, Karolinska Institutet, Karolinska University Hospital Huddinge, Stockholm

Anders Wallin, MD, PhD
Section of Psychiatry and Neurochemistry, Sahlgrenska Academy, University of Gothenburg, Göteborg, Sweden

David A. Wolk, MD
Assistant Professor, Department of Neurology, University of Pennsylvania, Philadelphia, USA

Preface

The concepts of vascular cognitive impairment and vascular dementia have recently been discussed assiduously both in the clinical and research worlds. Vascular dementia is regarded as being the second most common dementia disease, second only to Alzheimer's disease. Knowledge of how changes in the blood vessels induce a change in our cognitive capacity and constitute a cause of dementia has increased considerably in recent years.

A discussion is underway as to whether changes in the vascular functions of the brain can, to some extent, form the background to neurodegenerative diseases such as Alzheimer's. This thinking is reinforced by the increasing amount of data which suggest that the risk factors we link to cardiovascular diseases are also those linked to Alzheimer's disease.

The purpose of this book is, from a broad clinical perspective, to compile the very latest findings within clinical research on vascular dementia and vascular cognitive impairment. This will create a foundation for the implementation of good clinical dementia care. The book is divided into three parts. The first deals with definitions of vascular dementia and the concept of vascular cognitive impairment, diagnostics by reviewing neuropsychological methods, imaging and neurochemical analysis.

The second part addresses the underlying histopathological and pathophysiological mechanisms influencing the onset of vascular cognitive impairment as well as the cerebral and cardiovascular risk factors. This also includes a section on genetically influenced vascular conditions.

Finally, a section on treatment from a somewhat broader perspective – a review of the pharmacological treatment of cognitive symptoms, the pharmacological treatment and care of secondary symptoms, as well as non-pharmacological measures applied to enhance the daily lives of patients with vascular dementia. Finally, the possibility of primary preventive measures to decrease the risk of falling victim to vascular cognitive impairment is discussed.

The book is intended primarily for those interested in, and clinically active specialists within the sphere of dementia, for example, geriatricians, neurologists, internal medics, and the general practitioner. It proposes to present a profound background to what we today regard as being state-of-the-art within the field of vascular dementia, and clinically applicable facts. In this respect, the book also offers a degree of practical application.

It is written by some of the world's most prominent researchers within their fields.

We would particularly like to thank Anette Eidehall for her excellent editorial contribution during the writing of the book. Drs Maria Kristoffersen Wiberg and Bertil Leidner are specifically acknowledged for providing the MRI and CT images for the cover.

Diagnosis

Diagnosing vascular cognitive impairment and dementia: concepts and controversies

Timo Erkinjuntti and Serge Gauthier

Introduction

Vascular cognitive impairment, the recent modification of the terminology related to vascular burden of the brain, reflects the all-encompassing effects of vascular disease or lesions on cognition. It incorporates the complex interactions between vascular etiologies, risk factors and cellular changes within the brain and cognition. The concept covers the frequent post-stroke cognitive impairment and dementia, as well as cerebrovascular disease (CVD) as the second most common factor related to dementia.

Post-stroke cognitive impairment and dementia are more frequent than traditionally recognized (Pohjasvaara et al., 1997). Further CVD is the second most common cause of dementia (Lobo et al., 2000; Rockwood et al., 2000). CVD as well as vascular risk factors including arterial hypertension, history of high cholesterol, diabetes, and forms of heart disease are independently associated with increased risk of cognitive impairment and dementia (Kivpelto et al., 2006). In addition to these vascular factors, CVD, infarcts and white matter lesions may trigger and modify progression of Alzheimer's disease (AD) as the most common cause of neurodegenerative dementia (Roman et al., 2006; Snowdon et al., 1997). Whilst CVD is preventable and treatable it clearly is a major factor in the prevalence of cognitive impairment in the elderly world-wide (Hachinski, 1992; O'Brien et al., 2003).

Concepts on vascular burden of the brain

During the 1980s and the early 1990s, almost all cerebrovascular injury leading to dementia was ascribed to large cortical and subcortical infarcts, so called multi-infarct dementia (MID) (Erkinjuntti and Hachinski, 1993). The concept of vascular dementia (VaD) was introduced to further refine the description of dementias caused by infarcts of varying sizes, including the smaller lacunar and microinfarcts (Roman et al., 1993). VaD appropriately defined a group of heterogeneous syndromes of vascular origin of which subcortical vascular disease was considered an important subtype (Roman et al., 2002). Although this was an important step forward, it was not adequate to describe the vascular causes of early cognitive impairments, which might lead to a spectrum of dementing illnesses. In addition, the impact of CVD and vascular risk in AD has prompted reconsideration of the broad implications of vascular disease on cognitive function (de la Torre, 2004; DeCarli, 2004; Skoog et al., 1999).

Vascular cognitive impairment (VCI) is currently considered the most recent modification of the

Vascular Cognitive Impairment in Clinical Practice, ed. Lars-Olof Wahlund, Timo Erkinjuntti and Serge Gauthier. Published by Cambridge University Press. © Cambridge University Press 2009.

terminology to reflect the all-encompassing effects of vascular disease or lesions on cognition and incorporates the complex interactions between vascular etiologies, risk factors and cellular changes within the brain and cognition (Roman *et al.*, 2004; O'Brien *et al.*, 2003).

Vascular cognitive concept

The recognition of AD as the commonest cause of dementia led to the development of operational criteria for the diagnosis of dementia in general. The criteria included early and prominent memory loss, progressive cognitive impairment, evidence of irreversibility, and presence of cognitive impairment sufficient to affect normal activities of daily living (ADL). Other definitions of dementia required variable combinations of impairment in different domains of cognition, including executive dysfunction (Erkinjutti *et al.*, 1997). These definitions could, however, result in markedly different prevalence estimates and, therefore consequences for health care planning.

The characteristic episodic memory impairment apparent in AD is attributed to atrophy of the medial temporal lobe. In contrast, cerebrovascular lesions do not necessarily have the same regional predilection. The emphasis of the current dementia criteria limited to episodic memory underestimates the vascular burden on cognition as well as potentially losing sight of effective prevention and treatment strategies. Accordingly, it has been suggested that the "Alzheimerized" dementia concept should be abandoned in the setting of CVD, and indeed this was one of the motives behind the development of the broader category of VCI (Bowler *et al.*, 1999; O'Brien *et al.*, 2003).

VCI refers to all etiologies of CVD including vascular risks which can result in brain damage leading to cognitive impairment. The impairment encompasses all levels of cognitive decline, from the earliest deficits to a severe and broad dementia-like cognitive syndrome (Bowler *et al.*, 1999; O'Brien *et al.*, 2003). VCI cases that do not meet the criteria for dementia can also be labeled as VCI with no dementia or vascular cognitive impairment no dementia (vascular CIND) (Rockwood *et al.*, 2000). These patients have also been labeled as vascular mild cognitive impairment similar to that of amnestic mild cognitive impairment (MCI) for AD (Petersen *et al.*, 2002).

VCI may include cases with cognitive impairment related to hypertension, diabetes or atherosclerosis, transient ischemic attacks, multiple cortico-subcortical infarcts, silent infarcts, strategic infarcts, small vessel disease with white matter lesions (WMLs) and lacunae, as well as AD pathology with co-existing CVD (Kalaria *et al.*, 2004). VCI can also encompass those patients who survive intracerebral and other intracranial hemorrhages but are left with residual cognitive impairment. The concept and definition of VCI or vascular CIND are still evolving (Roman *et al.*, 2004), but it seems clear that the diagnosis should not be confined to a single etiology comparable to the traditional "pure AD" concept. The two main factors to be defined in VCI are the severity of cognitive impairment, and the pattern of affected cognitive domains (O'Brien *et al.*, 2003).

Vascular burden of the brain: size of the problem

Estimates of the population distribution of VCI and its outcomes is influenced by the variety of definitions used (Lobo *et al.*, 2000). For example, if AD with CVD or the previously defined VaD with AD pathology is included, then VCI would most certainly be the most common cause of chronic progressive cognitive impairment in elderly people (Rockwood *et al.*, 2000). In a Canadian study, the prevalence of VCI has been estimated at 5% in people over age 65–90 years. These included patients with CIND. The prevalence of vascular CIND, however, was 2.4%; that of AD with CVD was 0.9%, and of VaD alone was 1.5%. By comparison, the prevalence of AD without a vascular component, at all ages up to age 85 years, was 5.1%, and was determined to be less common than VCI (Rockwood *et al.*, 2000). The Canadian studies also emphasize that failure to consider VCI without dementia (i.e. vascular CIND) underestimates the prevalence of impairment and risk for adverse outcomes associated with VCI.

Post-stroke cognitive impairment

Post-stroke cognitive impairment is frequent, although it has been a neglected consequence of stroke. An example of a detailed clinical study is the Helsinki Stroke Ageing study (Pohjasvaara et al., 1997). Cognitive impairment 3 months after ischemic stroke was present in one domain in 62% and in two domains in 35% of the patients aged 55–85 years. The cognitive domains affected included short-term memory (31%), long-term memory (23%), constructive and visuospatial functions (37%), executive functions (25%), and aphasia (14%) (Pohjasvaara et al., 1997).

Post-stroke dementia

The frequency of post-stroke dementia varies from 12 to 32% within 3 months to 1 year after stroke (Leys et al., 2005). In the Helsinki study, the frequency was 25% 3 months after incident stroke, and the frequency increased with increasing age: 19% among those aged 55–64 years, and 32% in those aged 75–85 years (Pohjasvaara et al., 1997). The incidence of post-stroke dementia increases with a longer follow-up time from 10 at 1 year to 32% after 5 years (Leys et al., 2005). A history of stroke increases the risk of subsequent dementia by a factor of 5 (Leys et al., 2005; Linden et al., 2004).

Determinants of post-stroke dementia include, among others, high age, low education, pre-stroke dependency and cognitive impairment (Leys et al., 2005). Risk factors of incident post-stroke dementia include epileptic seizures, sepsis, cardiac arrhythmias and congestive heart failure (Leys et al., 2005; Moroney et al., 1996). In one large cohort study, the independent clinical correlates of post-stroke dementia included dysphasia, major dominant stroke syndrome, history of prior CVD and low education (Pohjasvaara et al., 1998). Brain lesion correlates of post-stroke dementia include a combination of infarct features (volume, site), the presence of white matter lesions (extent, location), as well as brain atrophy (Leys et al., 2005; Pohjasvaara et al., 2000). Important critical locations include dominant hemisphere and lesions affecting the prefrontal–subcortical circuit. Lesions mediating executive dysfunction are critical (Vataja et al., 2003). Concomitant behavioral problems and depression relate to dependency (Vataja et al., 2005).

Vascular dementia

Vascular dementia, defined as the subset of VCI patients who fulfill the traditional Alzheimer-type dementia criteria, is considered the second most common cause of dementia accounting for 10–50% of the cases, but this depends on the geographic location, patient population, and use of clinical methods (Lobo et al., 2000). The prevalence of VaD had been reported to range from 1.2 to 4.2% in persons aged 65 years and older (Helsert and Brayne, 1995). Using population-based identification of persons aged 65 years and above, the European collaborative study reported that the age-standardized prevalence of dementia was 6.4% (all causes), 4.4% for AD and 1.6% for VaD (Lobo et al., 2000). In this study, 15.8% of all the cases had VaD and 53.7% AD (Lobo et al., 2000). However, these studies have not estimated the size of the AD with CVD population in more detail. The incidence of VaD increases with increasing age, without any substantial difference between men and women (Fratiglioni et al., 2000). The reported incidence estimates of VaD vary between 6 and 12 cases per year in 1000 persons aged 70 years and older (Hebert and Brayne, 1995).

Risk factors of cognitive impairment and dementia

It is now apparent that the traditional vascular risk factors and stroke are also independent factors for the clinical presentation of mild cognitive impairment and AD (Skoog et al., 1999). The important independent mid-life risk factors of clinical AD include arterial hypertension, high cholesterol, diabetes, obesity, and reduced physical activity, among others (Kivpelto *et al.*, 2006; Skoog *et al.*, 1999).

Risk factors associated with VCI include risks for CVD, stroke, infarcts and ischemic white matter lesions. Besides completed clinically symptomatic infarcts, also called silent infarcts, the presence of white matter lesions also relates to higher dementia risk (Prins *et al.*, 2004; Vermeer *et al.*, 2003). Similarly to AD, the risks for VCI may be considered under demographic (e.g. age, education), vascular (e.g. arterial hypertension, atrial fibrillation, myocardial infarction, coronary heart disease, diabetes, generalized atherosclerosis, lipid abnormalities, smoking), genetic (e.g. family history and specific genetic features), and ischemic lesion-related (e.g. type of CVD, site and size of stroke) variables (Gorelick, 1997; Skoog, 1998). Hypoxic ischemic events (cardiac arrhythmias, congestive heart failure, myocardial infarction, seizures, pneumonia) giving rise to global cerebrovascular insufficiency are important risk factors for incident dementia in patients with stroke (Moroney *et al.*, 1997). Increasing evidence also suggests that reducing the burden of vascular risk decreases the prevalence of dementia (DeCarli, 2004; O'Brien *et al.*, 2003; Skoog *et al.*, 1999).

Subtypes of vascular dementias

VaD, as well as VCI, encompasses many clinical features which themselves reflect a variety of vascular mechanisms and changes in the brain, with different causes and neurological outcomes. The pathophysiology is attributed to interactions between vascular etiologies (CVD and vascular risk factors), changes in the brain (infarcts, WMLs, atrophy), and host factors (age, education) (Chiu, 1989, 1998; Desmond, 1996; Erkirjuntti and Hachinski, 1993; Roman *et al.*, 1993; Tatemichi, 1990).

The main subtypes of previously defined VaD included in current classifications are cortical VaD or MID, also referred to as post-stroke VaD, subcortical ischemic vascular disease and dementia,

(SIVD) or small vessel dementia, and strategic infarct dementia. Hypoperfusion dementia resulting from global cerebrovascular insufficiency is also included. Further subtypes include hemorrhagic dementia, hereditary vascular dementia (e.g. Cerebral autosomal dominant arteriopathy with subcortical infarcts and leukoencephalopathy (CADASIL)), and AD with CVD.

Cortical VaD or multi-infarct dementia

Cortical VaD (MID, post-stroke VaD) has been traditionally characterized by a relatively abrupt onset (days to weeks), a step-wise deterioration (some recovery after worsening), and a fluctuating course (e.g. difference between days) of cognitive functions (Chui *et al.*, 1992; Erkinjuntti, 1987; Erkinjuntti and Machinski, 1993; Roman *et al.*, 1993). Cortical VaD relates predominantly to large vessel disease and cardiac embolic events. It is a syndrome, not a disease entity, related to strokes, and rarely fulfills current criteria modeled on Alzheimer-type dementia. It is characterized by predominantly cortical and cortico-subcortical arterial territorial and distal field (watershed) infarcts. The early cognitive syndrome of cortical VaD includes some memory impairment, which may be mild, and some heteromodal cortical symptom(s) such as aphasia, apraxia, agnosia and visuospatial or constructional difficulty. In addition, most patients have some degree of dysexecutive syndrome (Mahler and Cummings, 1991). Due to the multiple cortico-subcortical infarcts, patients with cortical VaD often have additional neurological symptoms, such as visual field deficits, lower facial weakness, lateralized sensorimotor changes and gait impairment (Erkinjuntti, 1987).

Subcortical VaD

Subcortical ischemic vascular disease and dementia (SIVD) or small vessel dementia incorporates two entities: "the lacunar state" and "Binswanger's disease" (Roman *et al.*, 2002). Whether the SIVD syndrome can be considered as a distinct disease is debatable. However, as a syndrome it may be readily confused with AD in view of the neuronal loss and co-existing vascular factors. The onset is variable, as reported by Babikian and Ropper (1987): 60% of the patients had a slow onset, and only 30% an acute onset of cognitive symptoms. The course was gradual without (40%) and with (40%) acute deficits, and fluctuating in only 20% (Babikian and Ropper, 1987). There is often a clinical history of "prolonged (transient ischemic attack) TIA" or "multiple TIAs", which are mostly small strokes without residual symptoms and with only mild focal findings (e.g. drift, reflex asymmetry, gait disturbance).

SIVD is attributed to small vessel disease and is characterized by lacunar infarcts, focal and diffuse ischemic WMLs, and incomplete ischemic injury (Erkinjuntti, 1987; Roman et al., 2002; Wallin et al., 2003). The infarcts and WMLs are expected consequences of small vessel disease. A subcortical cognitive syndrome is the cardinal clinical manifestation in SIVD attributed to preferential damage to the prefrontal–subcortical circuits (Cummings, 1993; Erkinjuntti et al., 2000). Clinically, small vessel dementia is characterized by the subcortical cognitive syndrome plus pure motor hemiparesis, bulbar signs and dysarthria, gait disorder, variable depressive illness, emotional lability, and deficits in executive functioning. Neuroimaging patients with SIVD reveals multiple lacunaes and extensive WMLs, supporting the importance of imaging in the diagnostic criteria (Erkinjuntti et al., 2000).

The early cognitive syndrome of SIVD is characterized by a dysexecutive syndrome with slowed information processing, usually mild memory deficit and behavioral symptoms. The dysexecutive syndrome in SIVD includes impairment in goal formulation, initiation, planning, organizing, sequencing, executing, set-shifting and set maintenance, as well as in abstraction (Cummings, 1994). The memory deficit in SIVD is usually milder than in AD, and is characterized by impaired recall, relative intact recognition, less severe forgetting and better benefit from cues. Behavioral and psychological symptoms in SIVD include depression, personality change, emotional lability and incontinence, as well as inertia, emotional bluntness, and psychomotor retardation.

Earlier phases of SIVD may include episodes of mild upper motor neuron signs (drift, reflex asymmetry, incoordination), gait disorder (apractic–atactic or small-stepped), imbalance and falls, urinary frequency and incontinence, dysarthria, dysphagia as well as extrapyramidal signs such as hypokinesia and rigidity (Roman et al., 2002). However, these focal neurological signs are often subtle.

Strategic infarct dementia

Depending on the precise location, the time course and clinical features of strategic infarct dementia are highly variable. Strategic infarct dementia is characterized by focal, often small, ischemic lesions involving specific sites critical for higher cortical functions. The cortical sites include the hippocampal formation, angular gyrus and cingulate gyrus. The subcortical sites leading to impairment are the thalamus, fornix, basal forebrain, caudate, globus pallidus and the genu or anterior limb of the internal capsule (Erkinjuntti and Hachinski, 1993; Tatemichi, 1990).

Diagnostic criteria

Clinical criteria

The most widely used criteria for VaD include DSM-IV, ICD-10, the ADDTC criteria (Chui et al., 1992) and the NINDS-AIREN criteria (Roman et al., 1993).

The NINDS-AIREN criteria have been the most widely used criteria in randomized clinical trials. They:
- emphasize the heterogeneity of VaD syndromes and pathological subtypes, including not only ischemic stroke but other causes of CVD such as cerebral hypoxic ischemic events, white matter lesions and hemorrhagic strokes;
- recognize the variability in clinical course, which may be static, remitting or progressive;

- highlight the question of the location of ischemic lesions and the need to establish a causal relationship between vascular brain lesions and cognition;
- recognize the need to establish a temporal relationship between stroke and dementia onset;
- include specific findings early in the course that support a vascular rather than a degenerative cause;
- emphasize the importance of brain imaging to support clinical findings; and
- recognize the value of neuropsychological testing in documenting impairments in multiple cognitive domains.

Sensitivity of the criteria: the NINDS-AIREN criteria treat VaD as a syndrome with different causes and different clinical manifestations, not as a single entity, and list possible subtypes to be used in research studies. The focus is on consequences of CVD, but different causes are also taken into account. The criteria incorporate different levels of certainty of the clinical diagnosis (possible, probable, definite).

In a neuropathological series, sensitivity of the criteria for probable and possible VaD was 58% and specificity 80% (Gold *et al.*, 1997). The criteria succesfully excluded AD in 91% of cases, and the proportion of combined cases misclassified as probable VaD was 29%. Compared with the ADDTC criteria, the NINDS-AIREN criteria were more specific and they excluded combined cases better (54% vs. 29%). In a more recent series, the sensitivity of NINDS-AIREN criteria for probable VaD was 20% and specificity 93%; the corresponding figures for probable ADDTC were 25% and 91% (Gold *et al.*, 2002). The inter-rater reliability of the criteria is moderate to substantial (*k* 0.46–0.72) (Lopez *et al.*, 1994).

Alzheimer's disease with CVD

AD and CVD co-exist in a large proportion of patients (Kalaria and Ballard, 1999). Such patients may present clinically either as AD with evidence of cerebrovascular lesions on brain imaging, or with features of both AD and VCI (Rockwood *et al.*, 1999). It remains a major clinical undertaking to distinguish dementia due to AD from that arising from CVD in view of the considerable overlap. Both result in cognitive, functional and behavioral impairments. There are also shared pathophysiological mechanisms (e.g. WMLs, delayed neuronal death and apoptosis) (Pantoni Garcia, 1997; Skoog *et al.*, 1999; Snowdon *et al.*, 1997), associated risk factors (e.g. age, education, arterial hypertension) (DeCarli, 2004; Skoog *et al.*, 1999) and neurochemical deficits including cholinergic neuronal dysfunction (Roman and Kalaria, 2006; Wallin *et al.*, 2002). Based on the findings from the Nun Study (Snowdon *et al.*, 1997), it has been further suggested that CVD may play an important role in determining the presence and severity of clinical symptoms of AD. Either way, the prevalence of AD with CVD appears grossly underestimated (Kalaria and Ballard, 1999; Langa *et al.*, 2004).

The diagnosis of mixed AD and CVD is a challenge. Accumulating evidence shows that different vascular factors, including hypertension and stroke, increase the risk of AD, and frequently CVD co-exists with AD (de la Torre, 2004; DeCarli, 2004; Kalaria and Ballard, 1999; Skoog *et al.*, 1999). This overlap is increasingly important in the oldest (>85 years of age) populations. Clinical recognition of patients with AD and CVD is problematic as is evident from the neuropathological series of Moroney *et al.* (1997) and others (Neuropathology Group, 2001). These patients exhibit a history of vascular risk and a sign of CVD providing a clinical picture that is close to VaD. However, fluctuating course (Odd ratio; OR=0.2) and history of strokes (OR=0.1) were the only items differentiating AD from AD with CVD.

Some of the challenging clinical scenarios include the developing AD in patients with post-stroke dementia, and VaD patients with an insidious onset or a slow progressive course. AD with CVD can present clinically either as AD with evidence of vascular lesions upon brain imaging, or with clinical features of both AD and VaD (Rockwood *et al.*, 1999). In a Canadian study, typical AD presentations with one or more features pointing to "vascular aspects" derived from the Hachenski Ischemic Scale (HIS) were used successfully to diagnose AD plus CVD in combination with the neuroimaging of ischemic lesions (Rockwood *et al.*, 2000). Vascular risk factors and focal neurological signs were present more often in AD with CVD than in "pure" AD. Other clinical clues for a diagnosis of AD with CVD were gained from analyses of disease course characteristics and presentations of patchy cognitive deficits, early onset of seizures, and gait disorder.

A better solution to recognizing patients with AD plus CVD would be to discover reliable biological markers of clinical AD. Other potential markers include early prominent episodic memory impairment, early and significant medial temporal lobe atrophy on MRI, bilateral parietal hypoperfusion on single photon emission computed tomography, and low concentrations of CSF Aβ peptides with high tau-protein.

REFERENCES

Babikian V, Ropper AH. Binswanger's disease: a review. *Stroke* 1987; **18**: 2–12.

Bowler JV, Steenhuis R, Hachinski V. Conceptual background of vascular cognitive impairment. *Alzheimer Dis Assoc Disord* 1999; **13**: S30–7.

Chui HC. Dementia: a review emphasizing clinicopathologic correlation and brain–behavior relationships. *Arch Neurol* 1989; **46**: 806–14.

Chui HC. Rethinking vascular dementia: moving from myth to mechanism. In: Growdon JH, Rossor MN, eds. *The Dementias*. Boston: Butterworth-Heinemann. 1998; 377–401.

Chui HC. Victoroff JI, Margolin D, Jagust W, Shankle R, Katzman R. Criteria for the diagnosis of ischemic vascular dementia proposed by the State of California Alzheimer's Disease Diagnostic and Treatment Centers. *Neurology* 1992; **42**; 473–80.

Chui HC. Mack W, Jackson JE, *et al.* Clinical criteria for the diagnosis of vascular dementia. *Arch Neurol* 2000; **57**: 191–6.

Cummings JL. Fronto-subcortical circuits and human behavior. *Arch Neurol* 1993; **50**: 873–80.
Vascular subcortical dementias: clinical aspects. *Dementia* 1994; **5**: 177–80.

de la Torre JC. Alzheimer's disease is a vasocognopathy: a new term to describe its nature. *Neurol Res* 2004; **26**: 517–24.

DeCarli C. Vascular factors in dementia: an overview. *J Neurol Sci* 2004; **226**: 19–23.

Desmond DW. Vascular dementia: a construct in evolution. *Cerebrovasc Brain Metab Rev* 1996; **8**: 96–325.

Erkinjuntti T. Types of multi-infarct dementia. *Acta Neurol Scand* 1987; **75**: 391–9.

Erkinjuntti T. Hachinski VC. Rethinking vascular dementia. *Cerebrovasc Dis* 1993; **3**: 3–23.

Erkinjuntti T. Ostbye T, Steenhuis R, Hachinski V. The effect of different diagnostic criteria on the prevalence of dementia. *N Engl J Med* 1997; **337**: 1667–74.

Erkinjuntti T. Inzitari D, Pantoni L, *et al.* Research criteria for subcortical vascular dementia in clinical trials. *J Neural Transam* 2000; **59**: 23–30.

Fratiglioni L, Launer LJ, Andersen K, *et al.* Incidence of dementia and major subtypes in Europe: a collaborative study of population-based cohorts. *Neurology* 2000; **54**: S10–15.

Gold G, Giannakopoulos P, Montes-Paixao JC, *et al.* Sensitivity and specificity of newly proposed clinical criteria for possible vascular dementia. *Neurology* 1997 **49**: 690–4.

Gold G, Bouras C, Canuto A, *et al.* Clinicopathological validation study of four sets of clinical criteria for vascular dementia. *Am J Psychiatry* 2002; **159**: 82–7.

Gorelick PB. Status of risk factors for dementia associated with stroke. *Stroke* 1997; **28**: 459–63.

Hachinski V. Preventable senility: a call for action against the vascular dementias. *J Am Ger Soc* 1992; **340**: 645–8.

Hebert R, Brayne C. Epidemiology of vascular dementia. [Review] [75 refs]. *Neuroepidemiology* 1995; **14**: 240–57.

Kalaria RN, Ballard C. Overlap between pathology of Alzheimer disease and vascular dementia. *Alzheimer Dis Assoc Disord* 1999; **13**: S115–23.

Kenny RA, Ballard CG, Perry R, Ince P, Polvikoski T. Towards defining the neuropathological substrates of vascular dementia. *J Neurol Sci* 2004; **226**: 75–80.

Kivpelto M, Ngandu T, Laatikainen T, Winblad B, Soininen H, Tuomilehto J. Risk score for the prediction of dementia risk in 20 years among middle aged people: a longitudinal, population-based study. *Lancet Neurol* 2006; **5**: 735–41.

Langa KM, Forster NL, Larson EB. Mixed dementia: emerging concepts and therapeutic implications. *JAMA* 2004; **292**: 2901–08.

Leys D, Henon H, Mackowiak-Cordoliani M-A, Pasquier F. Poststroke dementia. *Lancet Neurol* 2005; **4**: 752–9.

Linden T, Skoog I, Fagerber B, Steen B, Blomstrand C. Cognitive impairment and dementia 20 months after stroke. *Neuroepidemiology* 2004; **23**: 45–52.

Lobo A, Launer LJ, Fratiglioni L, *et al.* Prevalence of dementia and major subtypes in Europe: A collaborative study of population-based cohorts. *Neurology* 2000; **54**: S4–S9.

Lopez OL, Larumbe MR, Becker JT, *et al.* Reliability of NINDS-AIREN clinical criteria for the diagnosis of vascular dementia. *Neurology* 1994; **44**: 1240–5.

Mahler ME, Cummings JL. The behavioural neurology of multi-infarct dementia. *Alzheimer Dis Assoc Disord* 1991; **5**: 122–30.

Moroney JT, Bagiella E, Desmond DW, Paik MC, Stern Y, Tatemichi TK. Risk factors for incident dementia after stroke. Role of hypoxic and ischemic disorders. *Stroke* 1996; **27**: 1283–9.

Moroney JT, Bagiella E, Desmond DW, Paik MC, Stern Y, Tatemichi TK. Cerebral hypoxia and ischemia in the pathogenesis of dementia after stroke. *Ann NY Acad Sci* 1997; **826**: 433–6.

Moroney JT, Bagiella E, Desmond DW, *et al.* Meta-analysis of the Hachinski Ischemic Score in pathologically verified dementias. *Neurology* 1997; **49**: 1096–105.

Neuropathology Group. Medical Research Council Cognitive Function and Aging Study. Pathological correlates of late-onset dementia in a multicentre, community-based population in England and Wales. Neuropathology Group of the Medical Research Council Cognitive Function and Ageing Study (MRC CFAS). *J Am Ger Soc* 2001; **357**: 169–75.

O'Brien JT, Erkinjuntti T, Reisberg B, *et al.* Vascular cognitive impairment. *Lancet Neurology* 2003; **2**: 89–98.

Pantoni L, Garcia JH. Pathogenesis of leukoaraiosis: a review. *Stroke* 1997; **28**: 652–9.

Petersen RC, Doody R, Kurz A, *et al.* Current concepts in mild cognitive impairment. *Arch Neurol* 2002; **58**: 1985–92.

Pohjasvaara T, Erkinjuntti T, Vataja R, Kaste M. Dementia three months after stroke. Baseline frequency and effect of different definitions of dementia in the Helsinki Stroke Aging Memory Study (SAM) cohort. *Stroke* 1997; **28**: 785–92.

Pohjasvaara T, Erkinjuntti T, Ylikoski R, Hietanen M, Vataja R, Kaste M. Clinical determinants of poststroke dementia. *Stroke* 1998; **29**: 75–81.

Pohjasvaara T, Mäntylä R, Salonen O, *et al.* How complex interactions of ischemic brain infarcts, white matter lesions and atrophy relate to posstroke dementia. *Arch Neurol* 2000; **57**: 1295–300.

Prins ND, van Dijk EJ, den Heijer T, *et al.* Cerebral white matter lesions and the risk of dementia. *Arch Neurol* 2004; **61**: 1503–04.

Rockwood K, Wenzel C, Hachinski V, Hogan DB, MacKnight C, McDowell I. Prevalence and outcomes of vascular cognitive impairment. *Neurology* 2000; **54**: 447–51.

Rockwood K, Howard K, MacKnight C, Darvesh S. Spectrum of disease in vascular cognitive impairment. *Neuroepidemiology* 1999; **18**: 248–54.

Roman GC, Kalaria RN. Vascular determinants of cholinergic deficits in Alzheimer disease and vascular dementia. *Neurobiol Aging* 2006; **27**: 1769–85.

Roman GC, Tatemichi TK, Erkinjuntti T, *et al.* Vascular dementia: diagnostic criteria for research studies. Report of the NINDS-AIREN International Work Group. *Neurology* 1993; **43**: 250–60.

Roman GC, Erkinjuntti T, Wallin A, Pantoni L, Chui HC. Subcortical ischemic vascular dementia. *Lancet Neurol* 2002; **1**: 426–36.

Roman GC, Sachdev P, Royall DR, *et al.* Vascular cognitive disorder: a new diagnostic category updating vascular cognitive impairment and vascular dementia. *J Neurol Sci* 2004; **226**: 81–7.

Skoog I. Status of risk factors for vascular dementia. [Review] [89 refs]. *Neuroepidemiology* 1998; **17**: 2–9.

Skoog I, Kalaria RN, Breteler MMB. Vascular factors and Alzheimer's disease. *Alzheimer Dis Assoc Disord* 1999; **13**: S106–14.

Snowdon DA, Greiner LH, Mortimer JA, Riley KP, Greiner PA, Markesbery WR. Brain infarction and the clinical expression of Alzheimer disease. The Nun Study. *JAMA* 1997; **277**: 813–17.

Tatemichi TK. How acute brain failure becomes chronic. A view of the mechanisms and syndromes of dementia related to stroke. *Neurology* 1990; **40**: 1652–9.

Vataja R, Pohjasvaara T, Mäntylä R, *et al.* MRI correlates of executive dysfunction in patients with ischemic stroke. *Eur J Neurol* 2003; **10**: 625–631.

Vataja R, Pohjasvaara T, Mäntylä R, *et al.* Depressio-executive dysfunction syndrome in stroke patients. *Am J Ger Psychiatry* 2005; **13**: 99–107.

Vermeer SE, Prins ND, den Heijer T, Hofman A, Kloudstaal PJ, Breteler MM. Silent brain infarcts and the risk of dementia and cognitive decline. *N Engl J Med* 2003; **348**: 1215–22.

Wallin A, Milos V, Sjögren M, Pantoni L, Erkinjuntti T. Classification and subtypes of vascular dementia. *Int Psychoger* 2003; **15**: 27.

Wallin A, Blennow K, Gottfries CG. Neurochemical abnormalities in vascular dementia. *Dementia* 2002; **1**: 120–30.

2

Vascular cognitive impairment: prodrome to VaD?

Adriane Mayda and Charles DeCarli

Introduction

Dementia is a public health problem, particularly affecting those over age 80 (Evans *et al.*, 1989; Hebet *et al.*, 2001). While Alzheimer's disease (AD) is the most common cause for dementia among older individuals (Evans *et al.*, 1989; Sayetta 1986), the lifetime risk for stroke equals and may exceed the risk of AD in some circumstances (Seshadri *et al.*, 2006). In addition, MRI evidence of asymptomatic cerebrovascular disease (CVD) occurs in one-third of older individuals (DeCarli *et al.*, 2005). It is, therefore, not surprising that concurrent CVD is often seen in older dementia patients even though they may have a slowly progressive dementing illness most consistent with AD (Mungas *et al.*, 2001b). Although research in this area is ongoing, the impact of clinically silent CVD on cognition and the interaction between CVD and AD processes remains incompletely understood. In this chapter, we discuss the potential role that vascular risk factors and asymptomatic CVD may have on lifetime risk for dementia. In particular, we hypothesize that asymptomatic CVD – in contrast to stroke or other forms of symptomatic CVD – acts as a susceptibility factor for the expression of dementia, most commonly due to AD.

Vascular cognitive impairment defined

As our understanding of the relationship between vascular disease and cognition continues to evolve, so does our terminology. In this light, vascular dementia (VaD) is now considered to be the extreme end of a spectrum of syndromes of vascular cognitive impairment (VCI) (Hachinski, 1992). As such, the concept of VCI encompasses all forms of cognitive impairment associated with CVD, ranging from subtle impairments in otherwise cognitively normal individuals through mild cognitive impairment to dementia (O'Brien *et al.*, 2003). VCI also encompasses dementias where both CVD and AD processes are thought to co-occur (O'Brien *et al.*, 2003). Finally, it is important to stress the difference between VCI and VaD. For the diagnosis of VaD, CVD is assumed to be the sole cause for the dementia. Although VaD may result from many forms of CVD, VaD is most clearly delineated by the presence of symptomatic CVD, usually due to stroke, in association with stepwise declines in cognition (Roman *et al.*, 1993) or evidence of multiple, bilateral gray matter infarcts (Knopman *et al.*, 2003). In contrast, VCI is a term used mostly for individuals who do not fulfill all the specified criteria for dementia and for whom the

Vascular Cognitive Impairment in Clinical Practice, ed. Lars-Olof Wahlund, Timo Erkinjuntti and Serge Gauthier. Published by Cambridge University Press. © Cambridge University Press 2009.

presence of CVD is asymptomatic and usually detected by brain imaging.

The goal of this chapter is to examine evidence regarding the extent and character by which VCI influences cognition and by what mechanism VCI may contribute to incident dementia whether the dementia syndrome results from AD, VaD or a mixed dementia.

Spectrum of cerebrovascular disease

CVD can take many forms. In this section, we describe the spectrum of brain-related injury from CVD as a prelude to our discussion of VCI. Stroke or symptoms of transient brain ischemia have long been viewed as the hallmark expression of CVD. Multiple studies conclusively show that the two most significant risk factors for stroke – advancing age and hypertension – are also the most common risk factors for cardiovascular and peripheral vascular disease, suggesting that these disorders share a common mechanism of vascular injury (Antikainen *et al.*, 1998; Cooper *et al.*, 2000; Gillom, 1996; Papademetriou *et al.*, 1998; Weber, 1996; Zheng *et al.*, 1997). With improving medical imaging methods, more attention has been paid to the possible spectrum of clinically silent brain injury resulting from hypertension or other vascular risk factors. For example, early work showed that a considerable number of cerebral infarcts are clinically silent although they shared the same risk factors as clinically apparent stroke (Boon *et al.*, 1994; Brott *et al.*, 1994; Ezekowite *et al.*, 1995; Jørgensen *et al.*, 1994; Kase *et al.*, 1989; Shinkawa *et al.*, 1995). In addition, the hallmark observations of Hachinski and colleagues relating abnormalities of cerebral white matter to vascular factors (Hachinski *et al.*, 1986, 1987; Steingart *et al.*, 1986, 1987) have been confirmed and extended (DeCarli *et al.*, 1999; Jeerakathi *et al.*, 2004; Liao *et al.*, 1996, 1997; Manolio *et al.*, 1994; Miyao *et al.*, 1992; Ott *et al.*, 1999; Swan *et al.*, 1998; Yue *et al.*, 1997). The fact that white matter hyperintensities (WMH) significantly predict future stroke (Miyao *et al.*, 1992) and mortality (Sreifler

et al., 1999) and are associated with evidence of carotid (Manolio *et al.*, 1994) and other end organ systems disease (DeCarli *et al.*, 1999; de Leeuw *et al.*, 2000; Swan *et al.*, 1998) lends further support to the notion that WMH are part of a spectrum of vascular-related brain injury (DeCarli *et al.*, 1999). Finally, vascular risk factors are also significantly associated with cerebral atrophy in humans (Salecno *et al.*, 1992; Seshadri *et al.*, 2004; Strassburger *et al.*, 1997; Swan *et al.*, 2000) and animal models (Gesztelyi *et al.*, 1993; Tajima *et al.*, 1993), and at least one hypothesis suggests that atrophy results from an ischemic process (Mentis *et al.*, 1994).

In conclusion, it appears that vascular factors lead to a spectrum of asymptomatic brain injury. This spectrum can be viewed as a hierarchy of potential pathologies with stroke at the peak. As discussed in later sections, we believe these various forms of brain injury also affect behavior in a variety of ways, contributing to our notion that VCI includes asymptomatic brain injury.

Time course of CVD

While there is growing evidence that the AD process may begin years before clinical symptoms are evident (Monis and Price, 2001; Price and Monis, 1999), the time course of CVD has been less well studied. As noted in the previous section, vascular factors can impact on the brain in a variety of ways, even in the absence of clinical symptoms. Associations between these various MRI measures and vascular factors, therefore, may give indication of the time course related to CVD.

Data from one longitudinal study suggest that midlife blood pressure (DeCarli *et al.*, 1999) and the lifetime pattern of blood pressure (Swan *et al.*, 1998) strongly predict the extent of cerebral atrophy and WMH. These MRI changes were also strongly associated with the presence of other clinically relevant vascular diseases. Modest reductions in cognitive performance, particularly affecting speeded cognitive processes, accompany these MRI changes (Swam *et al.*, 2000).

A second study, from a younger group of individuals, suggests that the pernicious effects of CVD may occur relatively early in life in individuals who were free of clinically detectable cognitive impairment or stroke (Seshadri *et al.*, 2004). In this study, a global measure of stroke risk, the Framingham Stroke Risk Scale (D'Agostino *et al.*, 1994; Wolf *et al.*, 1991), was strongly related to brain volume. Importantly, further analyses found that this effect was unchanged when examining individuals less than 55 years of age. Brain volume also correlated strongly with cognitive measures of speeded processing and attention, similar to the previous study (Swan *et al.*, 2000). These data are further supported by a third study of relatively young individuals that found a significant association between diabetes and impairments in cognitive function (Kuopman *et al.*, 2001).

From this brief review, it is clear that vascular risk factors can have a pernicious effect on brain structure and function that may begin during middle age (Launer, 2005). The total impact of vascular risk factors, therefore, may include a prolonged duration of effect. Not only do these data suggest that the time course of vascular risk factors may be long, but they may also have substantial public health implications. For example, it may be that aggressive treatment of vascular factors during early life not only translates into immediate health benefits, but could also convey substantially increased likelihood of better health in later life (Dufail *et al.*, 2005; Hanon and Forette, 2004; Ratnasabapathy *et al.*, 2003). Studies of late life cognitive impairment rarely account for the duration and severity of associated medical illnesses, particularly as they may relate to vascular risk factors. Absence of a clear understanding regarding the time course of CVD as it impacts on brain function may explain some of the conflicting results reported regarding vascular risk factors and cognition (Monis *et al.*, 2002), and clearly deserves further study.

Importantly, most asymptomatic brain injury affects subcortical white or strategic gray matter structures. In the next section, we discuss the understudied role of cerebral white matter as it relates to widely dispersed cognitive systems.

Functional anatomy of cerebral white matter

Research on brain–behavior relationships has historically stressed the importance of the cerebral cortex and subcortical gray matter for cognitive processing. Recent evidence, however, indicates that, as an essential component of extended neural networks in the brain, white matter is also critical for many higher-order cognitive processes including attention, executive functioning, non-verbal/visual–spatial processing, and generalized processing speed (Gunning-Dixon and Raz, 2000). Though the relationship between cerebral white matter and cognition has yet to be fully explored, Geschwind's seminal paper linked disconnection of the cerebral white matter to a variety of neurobehavioral disorders over four decades ago (Geschwind, 1965b). Clinical evidence of the effects of white matter disconnection can be observed in patients with conduction aphasia, in which a lesion of the arcuate fasciculus uncouples Broca's area and Wernicke's area, leading to poor verbal repetition skills (Geschwind, 1965a). Although data from these patients clearly support white matter disconnection leading to dysfunction, recent evidence suggests that even asymptomatic disruption of the white matter may lead to subtle cognitive impairments. The advent of MRI has facilitated the investigation of detailed functional specialization of cerebral white matter and advanced our understanding considerably of the importance of distributed neural systems.

In recent years, the way we think about the brain mechanisms underlying complex cognitive, behavioral, and even motor processes has moved from a localization approach, attempting to attribute one function to one locus, to a more global circuits approach, investigating the contribution of distributed neural networks to function (Goldman-Rakic, 1988; Mesulam, 1990). This paradigm shift includes the realization that disconnection of white matter tracts may be just as effective in producing functional impairment as lesions in the gray matter. Functions attributable to the frontal lobes may be of particular importance in this disconnection hypothesis because of the extensive reciprocal connections of the frontal lobe to subcortical areas as well as the parietal, temporal, and occipital lobes (Miller and Asaad, 2002).

Of particular interest are the behavioral effects of disruption of frontal–subcortical circuits thought to be involved in executive function, especially the dorso-lateral prefrontal circuit (Alexander *et al.*, 1986). Five parallel frontal–subcortical circuits form closed anatomical loops, originating and ending in the frontal cortex and traveling through the caudate nucleus, globus pallidus, and thalamus (Cummings, 1995, 1998). Disruption of this circuit at any point can result in behavioral deficits associated with dorsolateral prefrontal cortex (DLPFC) dysfunction. In a recent study by Aizenstein and colleagues (2006), elderly adults showed reduced striatal (putamen) activation in an implicit learning task relative to young controls, supporting the theory that a change in a network of regions, including the prefrontal cortex and striatum, is related to cognitive aging. Another potentially important circuit that may be disrupted by white matter abnormalities is the prefrontal–parietal circuit described by Goldman-Rakic (1987). Reciprocal anatomical connections between prefrontal cortex and posterior parietal cortex are thought to play a role in visuospatial processing, attending to selective stimuli, and holding visuospatial information online, therefore disruption of this circuit could potentially affect working memory and visual processing. Research on the anatomic specificity of white matter abnormalities is ongoing, but white matter hyperintensity frequency mapping and diffusion tensor imaging have the potential to increase our understanding of the particular areas of white matter that are affected by normal and abnormal aging.

Further understanding of the role of white matter connections that subserve widely distributed cognitive systems may affect our concepts of how asymptomatic vascular brain injury may adversely impact cognitive function. It is, however, equally important to fully understand these cognitive systems, particularly in relation to complex processes such as memory. In the next section, we review the basic principles of memory systems in order to reconcile evolving data that attribute impaired memory performance to CVD.

Human memory systems: a brief review

Human memory is the process by which information is received, encoded, stored and retrieved. Milner et al. (1998) have further defined memory as explicit (declarative) and implicit (non-declarative). Explicit memory is denoted as memory of people, places and things. Implicit memory is denoted as memory of reflexive or motor skills. Clinically relevant memory impairment such as amnestic mild cognitive impairment (aMCI) involves deficits in explicit memory (Petersen *et al.*, 1999). Explicit memory can be further subdivided into semantic memory (memory of facts) and episodic memory (memory of recent events) (Tulving, 1987). Episodic memory is the form of explicit memory most affected in aMCI (Petersen *et al.*, 1999). Successful explicit memory function is believed to involve a number of separate processes that includes encoding, storage and retrieval. Encoding is the function by which cerebral resources are directed through the use of attentional mechanisms to the processing of information. Memory encoding is believed to be a function of working memory processes that have specific anatomic localization within frontal, parietal and temporal cortices (Baddeley, 2003). Results from neuroimaging studies show that the DLPFC implements processes critical for organizing items in working memory (Blumenfeld and Ranganath, 2006) and that DLPFC connections to the hippocampus are important for long-term memory storage (Ranganath, 2006). Conversely, the hippocampus is believed to be responsible for memory consolidation (Gold *et al.*, 2006), although the exact role of the hippocampus in memory post-consolidation remains controversial (Moscovitch *et al.*, 2006; Squire, 2004; Squire *et al.*, 2004). Since memory function is the consequence of widely distributed neural systems involving parietal, frontal and hippocampal cortices, it is clearly possible that impairments in episodic memory may result from injury to any of these brain regions, or, importantly, the axons which join these various neuronal populations to an integrated system.

CVD and cognition

In the previous sections, we reviewed the concept of VCI, discussed the spectrum and potentially long time course of vascular-related brain injury, and the potentially important role of cerebral white matter in relation to widely distributed cognitive processes such as memory. In the following sections, we begin to address cognitive changes associated with aging, the potential role of asymptomatic vascular brain injury in these processes, the identification of clinically relevant episodic memory impairment (aMCI) due solely to presumed brain vascular disease, and finally the role of CVD as a risk factor for dementia.

Cognitive aging

The process of normal aging has profound effects on brain anatomy, neurochemistry, and physiology. The universal signs of aging as seen by neuroimaging include cortical atrophy, ventricular enlargement, expanded sulci, and WMH (Yue *et al.*, 1997). In addition to these changes in brain structure, elderly individuals exhibit age-related cognitive decline (Wilson *et al.*, 1999, 2002), though individuals vary considerably in their degree of functional loss (Rapp and Amaral, 1992). Behavioral studies indicate that even normal healthy adults show declines in performance on many cognitive tasks such as those that tap working memory, episodic memory, prospective memory, and executive

functions (Grady and Craik, 2000). This constellation of frontally based functions, including working memory, problem-solving, attention, and other executive functions, seem particularly vulnerable to the effects of age. This has lead to the theory that age-related cognitive deficits are mediated by pre frontal cortex dysfunction (West, 1996). Volumetric studies indicate that the prefrontal cortex is selectively decreased in elderly individuals (Raz *et al.*, 1997). Functional neuroimaging evidence also suggests that successful cognitive performance in elderly individuals is associated with increased prefrontal activation indicative of compensatory processes. For example, Cabeza (2002) has reported that under similar conditions, prefrontal activity during cognitive processes tends to be less lateralized in older adults than younger adults. Moreover, retained cognitive performance is associated with increased bilateral involvement in older adults. Thus a pattern of increased bilateral activation is seen in high-performing older adults, but not in young adults or low-performing older adults consistent with some type of cognitive compensation. Interestingly, it has been hypothesized that slight compromise of white matter circuits may facilitate compensatory bilateral recruitment by attenuating inter-hemispheric inhibition, whereas more serious disruption may hinder this additional recruitment (Buckner, 2004). In the next section, we present evidence to support the hypothesis that white matter injury may influence compensatory processes that facilitate retention of cognitive function with advancing age.

Impact of CVD on cognition in normal individuals

A number of epidemiological studies show strong associations between elevations in middle life blood pressure and the prevalence of later life cognitive impairment and dementia (Elias *et al.*, 1993, 1995a, 1995b, 2004; Launer *et al.*, 1995). The mechanisms by which CVD leads to cognitive impairment remain unclear, but a number of cross-sectional epidemiological studies as well as longitudinal prospective studies suggest that CVD-related brain changes are associated with these cognitive changes.

As we noted previously, clinically asymptomatic cerebral infarction is common to older individuals (DeCarli et al., 2005; Longstreth et al., 1998). Two studies from the Cardiovascular Health Study have examined the relation between cognitive impairment and clinically silent cerebral infarction (Longstreth et al., 1998; Price et al., 1997). While Price et al. (1997) focused primarily on the neurological manifestations of silent cerebral infarcts, they did note a significant increase in the number of individuals with a history of memory loss amongst those with silent cerebral infarction. Longstreth et al. (1998) examined cognitive function in more detail and noted a significant association between silent cerebral infarctions and diminished performances on the modified Mini-Mental State Examination (MMSE) and the Digit–Symbol Substitution Test (DSS). These findings are remarkably similar to their previously reported effect of WMH on cognition (Longstreth et al., 1996). These initial observations have been extended by the Rotterdam study, where silent cerebral infarctions were associated with accelerated cognitive decline and incident dementia (Vermeer et al., 2002, 2003).

Large epidemiological studies, while sometimes limited in the extent of cognitive testing available, also consistently show moderate associations between brain atrophy or white matter hyperintensity (WMH) volumes and diminished cognitive impairment (Au et al., 2006; Breteler, 2000; de Groot et al., 1998, 2000; de Leeuw et al., 2001; Longstreth et al., 1996, 2000; Ott et al., 1996). A number of smaller, cross-sectional studies consistently suggest deficits in tests of attention and mental processing (Boone et al., 1992; Breteler et al., 1994; DeCarli et al., 1995; Gunning-Dixar and Raz, 2000; Schmidt et al., 1995a), although impairments in memory and general intelligence are also seen (Breteler et al., 1994; DeCarli et al., 1995). There is evidence for a threshold effect as well, where extensive amounts of WMH are necessary before cognitive impairments are seen (Boone et al., 1992; DeCarli et al., 1995; Schmidt et al., 1995).

Unfortunately, the previously discussed studies did not examine the impact of lifetime cerebrovascular risk factors (CVRFs) on brain structure and cognition. Results from the National Heart Lung and Blood Institute (NHLBI) Twin Study, however, confirm the suspected link between CVRFs, brain injury and decline in cognitive performance over time (Swan et al., 1998). Lifetime patterns of systolic blood pressure were significantly associated with differences in brain atrophy, WMH volume and 10-year changes in MMSE and DSS scores (Swan et al., 1998). Importantly, however, even after correcting for age, education, baseline cognitive performance and incident CVD, there were strongly significant associations between WMH volume, DSS, Benton Visual Retention Test (BVRT) and a Verbal Fluency Test (VFT). Significant associations between brain volume and 10-year differences in MMSE, DSS and VFT were also found. These results suggest that the cognitive changes associated with elevations in midlife blood pressure may be mediated by the brain injury induced by prolonged elevations of blood pressure (and possibly other CVRFs). A follow-up study of the same subjects explored the pattern of cognitive changes in association with midlife blood pressure patterns more carefully (Swan et al., 2000). Cognitive tests selected for this study fell into the two broad functional categories of memory and psychomotor speed. Subjects with combined brain atrophy and WMH were significantly older and had a higher prevalence of CVRFs (Swan et al., 2000) and performed more poorly on all tests of psychomotor speed even after correcting for age, educational achievement and incident CVD, whereas group differences on memory tests were small. These results confirm the notion that the cognitive changes associated with CVRFs generally impact frontal executive functioning (Swan et al., 2000).

Longitudinal studies offer the advantage of examining lifetime CVRF influences on brain–behavior relations. Unfortunately, these studies have generally focused on older individuals (Swan et al., 1998, 2000), while epidemiological studies show that the impact of CVRFs – especially diabetes and hypertension – may occur at a considerably younger age (Knopman *et al.*, 2001). Seshadri *et al.* (2004) examined the relation between stroke risk factors, brain volume and cognition in a younger group of individuals with an average age of 62 years. Age-corrected differences in brain volume were significantly and positively associated with performance on tests of attention and executive function (e.g. Trails A and B), new learning (e.g. Paired Associates), and visuospatial function (e.g. delayed visual reproduction and Hooper visual organization test), but not with performance on tests of verbal memory or naming. While these results are consistent with those of Swan *et al.* (2000), they suggest that the impact of CVRFs on brain structure and function may begin shortly after midlife. A follow-up study examining the impact of WMH on the same cohort had similar findings (Au *et al.*, 2006).

In summary, subtle cognitive deficits in community-dwelling essentially normal individuals are associated with CVRFs and appear to be mediated by CVD-related brain injury. This process begins relatively early in life, as cognitive impairment and brain injury are present to some degree even in individuals 60 years of age or younger. The frontal lobe mediated cognitive domains of attention, concentration, and psychomotor speed are most affected in subjects free of dementia or stroke (Au *et al.*, 2006). Evidence of frontal lobe dysfunction is supported by positron emission tomography (PET) imaging, which finds reduced frontal metabolism in association with vascular-related brain injury, particularly WMH (DeCarli *et al.*, 1995; Tullberg *et al.*, 2004), as well as significant associations between frontal lobe metabolism, memory impairment and future cognitive decline in patients with dementia and WMH (Reed *et al.*, 2000, 2001).

Recently, more direct evidence for frontal dysfunction associated with WMH has been revealed. An fMRI study of healthy elderly adults found that increasing WMH burden was associated with a decrease in prefrontal cortex activations during episodic retrieval and verbal working memory tasks, suggesting disruption of white matter tracts as a mechanism for age-related prefrontal cortex dysfunction (Nordahl *et al.*, 2001).

Subjects for this study consisted of 15 cognitively normal individuals (4 male, 11 female) over the age of 65 (range: 66–86). Importantly, individuals in this study were not pre-selected for presence or absence of WMH, but were selected on the basis of normal cognitive ability. In this respect, this sample is comparable to samples used in other functional neuroimaging studies of normal aging. The subjects performed the episodic memory and the verbal maintenance task as previously reported (Nordahl *et al.*, 2005).

All subjects performed at a high level of accuracy on the cognitive tasks (generally greater than 80% correct). Total WMH volume was not significantly correlated with memory performance; however, frontal WMH volume was significantly associated with immediate memory recall, and there was a trend toward a significant relationship between total WMH and high load verbal maintenance task. This association between cognitive performance and WMH volumes suggests subtly impaired working memory function even for a group of cognitively normal individuals performing at a very high level of accuracy.

Results of the fMRI study revealed a strong relationship between increased global WMH volume and decreased prefrontal cortex (PFC) activity during both episodic and working memory performance. Dorsal PFC WMH volume was also strongly correlated with decreased PFC activity, as well as with decreased medial temporal and anterior cingulate activity during episodic memory and posterior parietal and anterior cingulate during working memory. Importantly, WMH volume was not correlated with visual cortex activity during a simple visual task, suggesting that nonspecific vascular changes associated with WMH did not fundamentally alter the BOLD signal.

These results strongly suggest that WMH disrupt the functional integrity of a widely distributed memory system involving parietal, dorsal lateral prefrontal, anterior cingulate and hippocampal regions (Baddeley, 2003). Although the exact pathophysiology by which WMH may affect this system requires further research, it is clear that disruption of specific pathways must be involved. As noted above, these might include connections between the dorsolateral prefrontal cortex and their subcortical targets (Alexander *et al.*, 1986), the long cortico-cortical connections between prefrontal and posterior parietal cortex (Burruss *et al.*, 2000; Cavada *et al.*, 1989a, 1989b; Cummings, 1993; Selemon and Goldman-Rakic, 1988; Tekin and Cummings, 2002), or the prefrontal, retrosplenial, hippocampal circuit (Monis *et al.*, 1999; Petrides and Pandya, 1999). Current research in the laboratory is systematically exploring these various pathways using diffusion tensor imaging. We hypothesize that those pathways directly involved in memory system dysfunction by WMH will show reduced fractional anisotropy (FA) that is more highly correlated with memory task performance and cognitive activation than regional WMH, indicating the specificity of the identified white matter bundles. This study suggests that adequate integrity of white matter circuits is necessary to engage supplemental neural sites for compensatory bilateral recruitment (Sullivan and Pfefferbaum, 2006).

These data illustrate that the relationship between frontal lobe impairments in normal aging and CVD related brain injury has yet to be fully explored. Unfortunately, many studies of cognitive aging do not take into account the effect of white matter abnormalities. It is important to consider this effect as a contributing factor, considering that CVD as measured by WMH may have a significant effect on cognition and is highly prevalent in the elderly population. Commonly held beliefs related to aging and cognition, therefore, may be contaminated by studies that included individuals with varying degrees of (and sometimes extreme) white matter lesions. Some studies have attempted to control for white matter lesions by excluding subjects with cerebrovascular risk factors (Rosen *et al.*, 2002) or those on any type of prescription medication (Rypma and D'Esposito, 2000), but this may not be an exhaustive exclusion and is certainly not a representative sample of the aging population. Therefore, more studies are needed that take into account the effect of white matter abnormalities on cognitive aging.

The anatomic specificity of white matter tract disruption in cognitive impairment associated with aging remains unclear. Frontal white matter appears to be selectively compromised in older individuals in studies that use diffusion tensor imaging (DTI) to measure the integrity of white matter fiber tracts (O'Sullivan *et al.*, 2004). As we note from the Nordahl study (Nordahl *et al.*, 2005), there are several lines of evidence that implicate specific white matter tracts including the dorsolateral–prefrontal circuit and prefrontal–parietal circuits. Disruption of the DLPFC circuit at any point can result in behavioral deficits associated with DLPFC dysfunction (Cummings, 1998). Since WMH correlate with deficits in DLPFC function and are associated with disruption of white matter tracts, the mechanism of impairment may be related to disruption of this circuit. Other potentially important circuits that may be disrupted by WMH are prefrontal–parietal circuits described by Goldman-Rakic, as disruption of this circuit could potentially affect working memory and visual processing (1987). Both of these white matter circuits are part of the larger memory system discussed earlier in this chapter. The potential exists, therefore, that extensive injury to these white matter circuits could led to clinically relevant memory impairment. In the next section, we describe data from our laboratory giving evidence for the existence of a vascular form of aMCI.

Evidence for vascular aMCI

WMH have been associated with increased risk for MCI in a few studies (DeCarli *et al.*, 2001; Lopez *et al.*, 2003). More recently, Nordahl et al. (2005) used WMH as a marker for small vessel CVD severity to identify and contrast two groups of subjects with aMCI. In this study, the authors proposed that WMH related to small vessel CVD might play a role in the episodic memory impairment characteristic of aMCI. The authors predicted that WMH might compromise executive control processes that are critical for working memory, which in turn may lead to episodic memory deficits and a diagnosis of aMCI. As discussed above, this theory is based on the preposition that if information cannot be actively maintained and manipulated at an immediate or short-term level, impairments in consolidation and retrieval could occur. Thus, whereas hippocampal dysfunction may be associated with isolated episodic memory impairments, small vessel CVD may lead to a distinct pattern of deficits that includes both episodic memory impairment and deficits in executive control processes.

To test their hypothesis, the authors examined a group of individuals who were clinically diagnosed with aMCI and used MRI to stratify the subjects into two subgroups: (1) those with severe WMH without hippocampal atrophy (MCI-WMH), and (2) those with severe hippocampal atrophy without extensive WMH (MCI-HA). Cognitive performance for each of these groups was compared to a group of age-matched control subjects. Importantly, these specific subgroups of aMCI subjects were selected to isolate the different mechanisms by which WMH and HA may lead to episodic memory impairment in MCI. Although cerebrovascular disease and AD pathology often co-occur, the nature of the interaction is unclear and complex to study due to the difficulty of disentangling the two in standard clinical samples. Thus, a highly selected sample was studied in order to investigate the separate roles that each type of brain lesion may play in producing memory impairment.

The study was divided into two parts. First, the authors compared performance of aMCI patients and controls on the neuropsychological tests that were used to diagnose aMCI according to standard criteria (Petersen *et al.*, 1999). This explored whether standard neuropsychological tests used widely in clinical practice would differ between the two MCI groups. Second, the authors compared the performance of these subjects on a battery of behavioral tasks used widely in the cognitive neuroscience literature. This second series of tasks was designed to explore the different cognitive mechanisms that underlie memory loss in aMCI. The battery included an episodic memory task, two working memory tasks, and a version of the continuous performance test (CPT) (see Nordahl *et al.*, 2005 for complete details). The authors predicted that both groups of MCI participants would show deficits on the episodic memory task, but that the MCI-WMH group would show additional impairments on the working memory tasks and on the CPT consistent with the hypothesized deficits in frontal function associated with WMH.

Results showed that – by design – MCI-HA individuals had significantly smaller hippocampi than MCI-WMH, whereas MCI-WMH did not differ from healthy controls with regard to hippocampal volume. Conversely, MCI-WMH had significantly higher WMH volumes than MCI-HA, which also did not differ from control volumes. The two MCI groups were equally impaired on all episodic memory tests relative to controls: WMS-R Logical Memory I & II, and MAS List Learning, Immediate Recall and Delayed Recall (Nordahl *et al.*, 2005). The two MCI groups did not differ from each other or controls on other neuropsychological tasks such as the Digit Span or Boston Naming. There were, however, striking differences in performance on all of the working memory tasks, including the n-back and verbal and spatial variants of the item recognition task, where the MCI-HA group performed similar to normal controls, but the MCI-WMH performed significantly more poorly. Further testing of executive control using the CPT revealed that MCI-WMH subjects had poorer attention and committed more impulsive errors that MCI-HA or normal controls.

This study was designed to test the hypothesis that among individuals diagnosed with aMCI, small vessel CVD and hippocampal dysfunction give rise to different profiles of cognitive deficits (Nordahl *et al.*, 2005). Results revealed that, although these two groups were virtually indistinguishable on standard neuropsychological tests administered at the time of diagnosis of MCI, more detailed testing revealed reliable differences between the two subgroups of MCI subjects. Whereas MCI-HA patients exhibited relatively specific episodic memory impairment, MCI-WMH patients exhibited deficits on episodic memory, working memory, and attentional control tasks. These findings suggest that MCI-WMH subjects, in contrast to MCI-HA subjects, suffered from impaired executive control processes that affect a wide variety of cognitive domains.

Although episodic memory has historically been linked to the hippocampus and surrounding cortices, as noted above, evidence from neuropsychological and neuroimaging studies suggests that the prefrontal cortex plays a critical role in implementing executive control processes that contribute to normal episodic memory functioning (Ranganath et al., 2003). In this study, MCI-WMH subjects were impaired not only on episodic memory tasks, but also on a battery of working memory tasks in both verbal and spatial domains as well as an attentional control task. The authors' interpretation of the data was that episodic memory failure in MCI-WMH subjects was secondary to a more general impairment in executive control processes.

The authors conclude by hypothesizing that WMH may reflect disruption of the white matter tracts that connect the DLPFC with its targets. Disruption of these neural circuits could lead to deficits in executive control processes that impact a wide range of cognitive domains, including episodic memory. The anatomy of this pathological process is unclear, as multiple neural circuits exist that, if disrupted, might lead to the findings described above. For example, lesions affecting connections between the DLPFC and its subcortical targets (Alexander et al., 1986), or lesions affecting the long cortico-cortical connections between the prefrontal and posterior parietal cortices (Cavada et al., 1989a, 1989b; Selemon and Goldman-Rakic, 1988) would be expected to result in impaired working memory and executive control processes (Burruss et al., 2000; Cummings, 1993; Tekin and Cummings, 2002). Disconnection of the prefrontal, retrosplenial, hippocampal circuit may

also give rise to deficits observed (Morris et al., 1999; Petrides and Pandya, 1999).

Does VCI lead to vascular dementia?

In the previous sections, we reviewed evidence that CVD-related brain injury leads to subtle cognitive impairments in otherwise healthy older individuals and, when sufficient, may even lead to clinically significant cognitive impairment, such as aMCI. In this section, we critically review available data relating the role of CVD to progression of cognitive impairment to clinical dementia. It is important to remind the reader that we are focusing our review on asymptomatic CVD common to advancing age, and will not directly address the issue of repeated stroke commonly believed to underlie the multi-infarct dementia (MID) form of VaD.

The relative impact of CVD on dementia occurrence has a long and debatable history (Brust, 1988; O'Brien, 1988). While there is a well-developed literature with regard to dementia after stroke (Henon et al., 2001; Moroney et al., 1996, 1997a, 1997b; Tatemici, 1990; Tatemici et al., 1990, 1992, 1995a, 1995b), it remains quite common to identify individuals who have a slowly progressive dementing illness, multiple vascular risk factors and extensive WMH or lacunar infarction detected by brain imaging. The impact of this asymptomatic cerebrovascular brain injury on dementia incidence remains unclear, but accumulating evidence suggests that CVD-related brain injury may significantly increase the likelihood of developing dementia, possibly through an additive interaction with AD (Esiri et al., 1999; Jagust, 2001; Schneider et al., 2003, 2004; Snowdon et al., 1997).

As we have summarized in previous sections, it is clear that CVD can influence cognition through clinically silent brain injury, such as asymptomatic brain infarction and WMH. It is unclear, however, why some individuals with apparently minor amounts of cerebrovascular injury in the absence of stroke develop dementia whereas others do not. Recent data from neuroimaging studies suggest common anatomical brain changes in individuals with CVD and dementia that may offer possible explanations.

Silent cerebral infarctions, commonly seen on MRI (DeCarli *et al.*, 2005), offer the opportunity to evaluate the role of discrete neural systems and dementia incidence. For example, clinical stroke involving the thalamus is recognized to cause profound cognitive impairment (Van der Werf *et al.*, 2003). A number of studies suggest that asymptomatic signal abnormalities in the thalamus also result in cognitive impairment and increase the risk for dementia (Longstreth *et al.*, 1988; Swartz and Black, 2006; Vermeer *et al.*, 2003). In the Swartz and Black study (2006), thalamic lesions were significantly more frequent among individuals with clinically defined vascular dementia. Moreover, it was noted that while large lesions (> 55 mm^3) were independently associated with cognitive impairment, smaller lesions were only accompanied with cognitive impairment in association with medial temporal lobe atrophy (Swartz and Black, 2006). Similarly, in the Vermeer *et al.* study (2003), baseline thalamic infarcts were associated with memory deficits whereas infarcts in other brain regions were most strongly associated with psychomotor speed. Importantly, in this non-demented group, future cognitive decline was only significantly associated with new infarction seen on repeat MRI, suggesting that repeated or multiple vascular events were necessary for cognitive decline. Unfortunately, the extent of medial temporal atrophy was not measured in this study. In summary, these data suggest that strategic brain infarction, even in the absence of stroke or abrupt change in cognition, can be associated with increased risk of substantial cognitive decline and dementia. As we will discuss in greater detail below, however, the extent to which these factors independently contribute to future dementia remains debatable, particularly when multiple and quantitative measures of brain structure are analyzed simultaneously.

While MRI evidence of cerebral infarction can be both localized and quantified, spatial localization and, hence, the significance of WMH poses a greater challenge. Increased WMH burden is found in both MCI (DeCarli *et al.*, 2001; Lopez *et al.*, 2003) and dementia (Barber *et al.*, 1999; Fazekas *et al.*, 1996; McDonald *et al.*, 1991; Mirsen *et al.*, 1991; Scheltens *et al.*, 1992, 1995; Waldemar *et al.*, 1994). In addition, while some studies find significant relationships between WMH and certain cognitive functions or dementia severity (Bondareff *et al.*, 1988, 1990; Diaz *et al.*, 1991; Harrell *et al.*, 1991; Kertesz *et al.*, 1990; Ott *et al.*, 1997; Stout *et al.*, 1996), other studies (Barber *et al.*, 1999; Benrett *et al.*, 1992, 1994; Brilliant *et al.*, 1995; DeCarli *et al.*, 1995; Doody *et al.*, 1998; Fazetas *et al.*, 1987, 1996; Kozachuk *et al.*, 1990; Leys *et al.*, 1990; Lopez *et al.*, 1992, 1995; Marder *et al.*, 1995; McDonald *et al.*, 1991; Mirsen *et al.*, 1991; Schelten *et al.*, 1992, 1995; Schmidt, 1992; Starkstein *et al.*, 1997; Teipel *et al.*, 1998; Wahlund *et al.*, 1994) do not. Differences in study populations and the heterogeneity of white matter changes may explain the inconsistency amongst these studies. For example, selection of AD patients without vascular risk factors may result in excluding individuals with extensive WMH (Kozachuk *et al.*, 1990), thereby minimizing their effects. In patients with CVD and dementia, small subcortical infarcts also frequently accompany WMH (Caplan, 1995; Roman, 1987) 'obscuring the independent effects that WMH confer to the dementia (Bennett *et al.*, 1994). Recently, new methods have been developed that allow for anatomical mapping of WMH (DeCarli *et al.*, 2005; Wen and Sachdev, 2004). One study using this technology (Yoshita *et al.*, 2006) evaluated the anatomical distribution of WMH amongst a group of cognitively normal, MCI and AD patients. A total of 87 individuals were studied, nearly equally divided amongst the three cognitive groups. The prevalence of vascular risk factors, such as hypertension, was also determined. The results found a significant rostral to caudal progression of WMH in association with cognitive ability with all three groups having WMH in the anterior periventricular areas, but MCI extending to the mid-portion of the periventricular region and AD patients having significantly more WMH posteriorly. Post-hoc analyses revealed two patterns of WMH distribution. Among individuals with vascular risk factors, periventricular WMH was significantly increased, whereas there was a localized increase of WMH in posterior regions in association with increasing cognitive impairment. Multiple regression analysis found these two spatial distributions to be independent, although both were more prevalent in the demented group. These findings raised the possibility that WMH may result from both degenerative and vascular processes, and both may contribute to the cognitive disability associated with dementia. These data suggest, like the pathological literature (Schneider *et al.*, 2003, 2004), that CVD may serve as a risk factor for expressed dementia in association with AD.

Can asymptomatic CVD as evidenced by infarction and WMH independently lead to dementia? This answer can be pursued in two ways. The first is to identify a group of younger individuals with subcortical CVD. Individuals with cerebral autosomal dominant arteriopathy with subcortical infarcts and leukoencephalopathy (CADASIL) are ideal for such a study. CADASIL is a Notch 3 mutation associated with a progressive small vessel vasculopathy (Dichgans, 2003) (see also p. 47). Nearly 80% of individuals with CADASIL have cognitive impairment before the age of 60. Typical imaging findings include multiple lacunar infarctions and extensive WMH with characteristic involvement of the anterior temporal lobes (Aver *et al.*, 2001; Peters *et al.*, 2005). One study of 62 subjects examined the impact of lacunar infarcts and WMH on cognition in CADASIL (Liem *et al.*, 2007). Most infarcts were symptomatic and were only found in individuals with cognitive impairment or other symptoms of CADASIL. The number of infarcts correlated significantly with most cognitive tasks, even after correcting for the effect of age on cognitive performance. WMH also correlated strongly with cognitive tasks, but the relationship was substantially weakened after correcting for subject age. In a multivariate model, the number of lacunar infarcts remained the strongest predictor of cognitive ability. The authors noted that a number of other publications have suggested a strong role for WMH in the cognitive impairment of CADASIL (Dichgans *et al.*, 1999; Yousry *et al.*, 1999), but noted that neither study corrected for age-related differences in cognitive ability, nor included the extent of lacunar infarction. Unfortunately, this study (Liem *et al.*, 2007) did not discuss the anatomic location of the lacunar infarctions, nor did it examine the potential impact of medial temporal atrophy (if present). These results strongly suggest that extensive small vessel disease with symptomatic infarction can result in dementia. Clinical studies of individuals with CADASIL reveal a general progression from normal cognition to cognitive impairment short of dementia and then onto dementia, supporting the notion that in some cases VCI can lead to a dementia syndrome consistent with VaD. CADASIL, however, is a very rare disorder, with a pathophysiology that does not apply to the general population.

In a second series of experiments from the Ischemic Vascular Dementia program project, Chui *et al.* (2006) set out to understand the role of subcortical ischemic vascular disease (SIVD) on cognition. This study was designed to investigate the impact of asymptomatic CVD brain injury on cognition in a group of individuals primarily seen through memory disorder clinics. SIVD was operationally defined as the presence of one or more subcortical infarctions with or without concurrent presence of extensive WMH. Importantly, individuals with and without subcortical infarctions were recruited with cognitive ability ranging from normal, MCI and dementia (Chui *et al.*, 2006). In contrast to the CADASIL subjects (Liem *et al.*, 2007), greater than 50% of these subjects were asymptomatic for subcortical infarctions. In a detailed pathological study, evidence for vascular brain injury of multiple types was used to create a CVD pathological score and was combined with measures of AD pathology to assess the extent of independent and additive effects on neuropsychological measures and clinical syndromes (Chui *et al.*, 2006). In multiple regression analyses treating each of the pathological measures as continuous measures, AD pathology was the sole significant predictor of both cognition and clinical syndrome. Further analyses, however, revealed that when AD pathology was minimal, CVD pathological scores contributed significantly to clinical syndrome. The highest tertile of CVD pathological scores contributed most strongly to clinical status irrespective of AD pathological score. Hippocampal sclerosis was quite prevalent in this series (18%), double in prevalence among those with high CVD pathology scores, and independently contributed to cognition when AD pathology was mild. The authors (Chui et al., 2006) conclude from this convenience sample taken mostly from memory disorder clinics that AD pathology generally overwhelms the effects of CVD and is the major determinant of dementia in patients with subcortical vascular disease. They note, however, that the impact of symptomatic or large-vessel stroke may make stronger contributions to the dementia syndrome, even in the presence of AD pathology, and deserves further investigation.

A series of MRI studies from the same clinical cohort of the IVD program project (Mungas et al., 2001a, 2002, 2005) showed that the volumes of cortical gray matter and hippocampus were the strongest predictors of cognitive impairment and cognitive decline as compared to quantitative measures of infarct volume or WMH. Another study of the same cohort also showed that memory impairment and hippocampal volume were the strongest predictors of progression from MCI to dementia (DeCarli et al., 2004). These results support the pathological study, although two MRI studies from this group (Du et al., 2005; Fein et al., 2000) found significant associations between the extent of WMH and cerebral atrophy that may be an independent mediator of cognitive impairment (Fein et al., 2000), consistent with a longitudinal study of atrophy and cognition in CADASIL patients (Peters et al., 2006).

These data suggest that, in a cohort of individuals recruited through memory disorder clinics, even if allowed to have evidence of subcortical vascular brain injury, AD pathology remains the predominate etiology of cognitive impairment. These results contrast somewhat with epidemiological studies

(Kuller et al., 2003; Vermeer et al., 2003; Wu et al., 2002) where WMH and brain infarction are significantly associated with dementia, sometimes in an additive fashion (Wu et al., 2002). Such differences could result from differences in methodology (most MRI analyses of large cohorts are qualitative) or sample selection as these cohorts are unselected and, therefore, may have higher degrees of CVD or less AD pathology. The relative roles of AD and CVD pathologies in dementia, therefore, require further detailed study. Newer imaging tools, such as brain amyloid imaging (Mathis et al., 2005), may prove extremely helpful in determining the extent of concurrent AD pathology, thereby allowing for accurate estimation of the relative contributions of both CVD and AD pathologies to cognition across the spectrum of cognitive ability.

Conclusion

In this chapter we set out to critically review the literature as it relates to evidence supporting VCI as a prodrome to VaD. We operationally defined VCI in the most broad of terms, although we emphasized the potential role of clinically asymptomatic CVD as opposed to evaluating the impact of stroke on cognition. We noted that in CVD there is a spectrum of related brain injury that includes silent brain infarction, WMH and even cerebral atrophy. We also noted that CVD might affect brain structure and function over a prolonged time course. Careful studies of individuals with auspiciously normal cognition and amnestic MCI conclusively show that both clinically asymptomatic infarction and WMH can impair cognitive abilities. We further postulate that impairment of executive control function is at least one possible mechanism for these findings. The data relating subcortical infarction and extensive WMH to either progression from MCI to dementia or directly associated with the dementia syndrome is less clear. Evidence from patients with CADASIL conclusively proves that subcortical infarction and WMH are sufficient for dementia. Data from a group of older individuals with subcortical infarctions and

WMH, however, suggest that AD is the major factor for the dementia syndrome and progression of MCI to dementia. The major differences between these two dementia groups appears to be the generally younger age of the CADASIL group (hence a lower prevalence of AD) and more severe CVD pathology with 100% of the CADASIL subjects having clinical strokes (often multiple) and extensive WMH. How, then, do we reconcile these apparent discrepancies? First, as suggested by the pathological literature (Schneider *et al.*, 2004), CVD may have the greatest effect on cognition when concurrent AD pathology is minimal. Our own data (DeCarli *et al.*, 1995; Nordahl *et al.*, 2005, 2006) would suggest that the independent cognitive effects of asymptomatic CVD are most easily detectable when the syndrome of cognitive impairment is mild or nearly normal. We further note that CVD, particularly as represented by WMH, may impact frontal subcortical circuits (DeCarli *et al.*, 2007; Nordahl *et al.*, 2005), leading to deficits in executive control (Nordahl *et al.*, 2005). Such deficits are likely to be independent of AD pathology for individuals who are either cognitively normal or have only MCI. We conclude, therefore, that even asymptomatic CVD-related brain injury is likely to serve as a risk factor for future cognitive impairment among older individuals through an additive and independent effect on executive control. Although we believe that older individuals with extensive CVRFs and stroke, particularly repeated strokes, can move from normal cognition to MCI and onto dementia, for most older individuals where CVD is prevalent but asymptomatic, there is sufficient evidence to state that this degree of CVD is sufficient to cause VCI, but that degenerative pathologies such as AD are the most likely etiology of dementia. For the vast majority of individuals, therefore, VCI does not lead to VaD, but increases an individual's susceptibility to expressing dementia due to AD.

Significance

From this review, it is apparent that the relationship between age-related cognitive impairment and CVD has yet to be fully elucidated. Given that cerebrovascular risk factors, subcortical infarctions and WMH are so prevalent and play a significant role in producing cognitive impairment, understanding their role in the aging brain and future risk for late life dementia is essential. This is especially vital given that the presence of WMH and subcortical infarctions are often undetected. Because the CVRFs contributing to subcortical infarction and WMH are treatable by changes in lifestyle or medication, understanding these mechanisms could lead to interventions that serve to slow age-related cognitive changes potentially leading to dementia. Cognitive impairment, CVD and their effects on health and well-being will continue to be a major public health concern as the elderly population continues to become an ever-increasing proportion of the population.

REFERENCES

Aizenstein HJ, Butters MA, Clark KA, *et al.* Prefrontal and striatal activation in elderly subjects during concurrent implicit and explicit sequence learning. *Neurobiol Aging* 2006; **27**: 741–51.

Alexander GE, DeLong MR, Strick PL. Parallel organization of functionally segregated circuits linking basal ganglia and cortex. *Ann Rev Neurosci* 1986; **9**: 357–81.

Antikainen R, Jousilahti P, Tuomilehto J. Systolic blood pressure, isolated systolic hypertension and risk of coronary heart disease, strokes, cardiovascular disease and all-cause mortality in the middle-aged population. *J Hypertens* 1998; **16**: 577–83.

Au R, Massaro JM, Wolf PA, *et al.* Association of white matter hyperintensity volume with decreased cognitive functioning: the Framingham Heart Study. *Arch Neurol* 2006; **63**: 246–50.

Auer DP, Putz B, Gossl C, Elbel G, Gasser T, Dichgans M. Differential lesion patterns in CADASIL and sporadic subcortical arteriosclerotic encephalopathy: MR imaging study with statistical parametric group comparison. *Radiology* 2001; **218**: 443–51.

Baddeley A. Working memory: looking back and looking forward. *Nat Rev Neurosci* 2003; **4**: 829–39.

Barber R, Scheltens P, Gholkar A, *et al.* White matter lesions on magnetic resonance imaging in dementia with Lewy bodies, Alzheimer's disease, vascular dementia, and normal aging. *J Neurol Neurosurg Psychiatry* 1999; **67**: 66–72.

Bennett DA, Gilley DW, Wilson RS, Huckman MS, Fox JH. Clinical correlates of high signal lesions on magnetic resonance imaging in Alzheimer's disease. *J Neurol* 1992; **239**: 186–90.

Bennett DA, Gilley DW, Lee S, Cochran EJ. White matter changes: neurobehavioral manifestations of Binswanger's disease and clinical correlates in Alzheimer's disease. *Dementia* 1994; **5**: 148–52.

Blumenfeld RS, Ranganath C. Dorsolateral prefrontal cortex promotes long-term memory formation through its role in working memory organization. *J Neurosci* 2006; **26**: 916–25.

Bondareff W, Raval J, Colletti PM, Hauser DL. Quantitative magnetic resonance imaging and the severity of dementia in Alzheimer's disease. *Am J Psychiatry* 1988; **145**: 853–6.

Bondareff W, Raval J, Woo B, Hauser DL, Colletti PM. Magnetic resonance imaging and the severity of dementia in older adults. *Arch Gen Psychiatry* 1990; **47**: 47–51.

Boon A, Lodder J, Heuts-van Raak L, Kessels F. Silent brain infarcts in 755 consecutive patients with a first-ever supratentorial ischemic stroke. Relationship with index-stroke subtype, vascular risk factors, and mortality. *Stroke* 1994; **25**: 2384–90.

Boone KB, Miller BL, Lesser IM, Mehringer CM, Hill E, Berman N. Cognitive deficits with white-matter lesions in healthy elderly. *Arch Neurol* 1992; **49**: 549–54.

Breteler MM. Vascular involvement in cognitive decline and dementia. Epidemiologic evidence from the Rotterdam Study and the Rotterdam Scan Study. *Ann NY Acad Sci* 2000; **903**: 457–65.

Breteler MM, van Amerongen NM, van Swieten JC *et al*. Cognitive correlates of ventricular enlargement and cerebral white matter lesions on MRI: the Rotterdam Study. *Stroke* 1994; **25**: 1109–15.

Brilliant M, Hughes L, Anderson D, Ghobrial M, Elble R. Rarefied white matter in patients with Alzheimer disease. *Alzheimer Dis Assoc Disord* 1995; **9**: 39–46.

Brott T, Tomsick T, Feinberg W, *et al*. Baseline silent cerebral infarction in the Asymptomatic Carotid Atherosclerosis Study. *Stroke* 1994; **25**: 1122–9.

Brust JCM. Vascular dementia is overdiagnosed. *Arch Neurol* 1988; **45**: 799–801.

Buckner RL. Memory and executive function in aging and AD: multiple factors that cause decline and reserve factors that compensate. *Neuron* 2004; **44**: 195–208.

Burruss JW, Hurley RA, Taber KH, Rauch RA, Norton RE, Hayman LA. Functional neuroanatomy of the frontal lobe circuits. *Radiology* 2000; **214**: 227–30.

Cabeza R. Hemispheric asymmetry reduction in older adults: the HAROLD model. *Psychol Aging* 2002; **17**: 85–100.

Caplan LR. Binswanger's disease – revisited. *Neurology* 1995; **45**: 626–33.

Cavada C, Goldman-Rakic PS. Posterior parietal cortex in rhesus monkey: I. Parcellation of areas based on distinctive limbic and sensory corticocortical connections. *J Comp Neurol* 1989a; **287**: 393–421.

Cavada C, Goldman-Rakic PS. Posterior parietal cortex in rhesus monkey: II. Evidence for segregated corticocortical networks linking sensory and limbic areas with the frontal lobe. *J Comp Neurol* 1989b; **287**: 422–45.

Chui HC, Zarow C, Mack WJ, *et al*. Cognitive impact of subcortical vascular and Alzheimer's disease pathology. *Ann Neurol* 2006; **60**: 677–87.

Cooper R, Cutler J, Desvigne-Nickens P, *et al*. Trends and disparities in coronary heart disease, stroke, and other cardiovascular diseases in the United States: findings of the national conference on cardiovascular disease prevention. *Circulation* 2000; **102**: 3137–47.

Cummings JL. Frontal–subcortical circuits and human behavior. *Arch Neurol* 1993; **50**: 873–80.

Cummings JL. Anatomic and behavioral aspects of frontal–subcortical circuits. In: Grafman J, Holyoak KJ, eds. *Annals of the New York Academy of Sciences*. New York: The New York Academy of Sciences, 1995: 1–13.

Cummings JL. Frontal–subcortical circuits and human behavior. *J Psychosom Res* 1998; **44**: 627–8.

D'Agostino RB, Wolf PA, Belanger AJ, Kannel WB. Stroke risk profile: adjustment for antihypertensive medication. The Framingham Study. *Stroke* 1994; **25**: 40–3.

de Groot JC, de Leeuw FE, Breteler MM. Cognitive correlates of cerebral white matter changes. *J Neural Transm Supplementum* 1998; **53**: 41–67.

de Groot JC, de Leeuw FE, Oudkerk M, *et al*. Cerebral white matter lesions and cognitive function: the Rotterdam Scan Study . *Ann Neurol* 2000; **47**: 145–51.

de Leeuw FE, Cees De Groot J, Oudkerk M, *et al*. Aortic atherosclerosis at middle age predicts cerebral white matter lesions in the elderly. *Stroke* 2000; **31**: 425–9.

de Leeuw FE, de Groot JC, Achten E, *et al*. Prevalence of cerebral white matter lesions in elderly people: a population based magnetic resonance imaging study. The Rotterdam Scan Study. *J Neurol Neurosurg Psychiatry* 2001; **70**: 9–14.

DeCarli C, Murphy DG, Tranh M, *et al*. The effect of white matter hyperintensity volume on brain structure, cognitive performance, and cerebral metabolism of glucose in 51 healthy adults. *Neurology* 1995; **45**: 2077–84.

DeCarli C, Miller BL, Swan GE, *et al*. Predictors of brain morphology for the men of the NHLBI twin study. *Stroke* 1999; **30**: 529–36.

DeCarli C, Miller BL, Swan GE, Reed T, Wolf PA, Carmelli D. Cerebrovascular and brain morphologic correlates of mild cognitive impairment in the National Heart, Lung, and Blood Institute Twin Study. *Arch Neurol* 2001; **58**: 643–7.

DeCarli C, Mungas D, Harvey D, *et al*. Memory impairment, but not cerebrovascular disease, predicts progression of MCI to dementia. *Neurology* 2004; **63**: 220–7.

DeCarli C, Fletcher E, Ramey V, Harvey D, Jagust WJ. Anatomical mapping of white matter hyperintensities (WMH): exploring the relationships between periventricular WMH, deep WMH, and total WMH burden. *Stroke* 2005; **36**: 50–5.

DeCarli C, Massaro J, Harvey D, *et al*. Measures of brain morphology and infarction in the Framingham heart study: establishing what is normal. *Neurobiol Aging* 2005b; **26**: 491–510.

Diaz JF, Merskey H, Hachinski VC, *et al*. Improved recognition of leukoaraiosis and cognitive impairment in Alzheimer's disease. *Arch Neurol* 1991; **48**: 1022–5.

Dichgans M. Monogenic causes of stroke. *Int Psychoger* 2003; **15** Suppl 1: 15–22.

Dichgans M., Filippi M, Bruning R, *et al*. Quantitative MRI in CADASIL: correlation with disability and cognitive performance. *Neurology* 1999; **52**: 1361–7.

Doody RS, Massman PJ, Mawad M, Nance M. Cognitive consequences of subcortical magnetic resonance imaging changes in Alzheimer's disease: comparison to small vessel ischemic vascular dementia. *Neuropsychiatry Neuropsychol Behav Neurol* 1998; **11**: 191–9.

Du AT, Schuff N, Chao LL, *et al*. White matter lesions are associated with cortical atrophy more than entorhinal and hippocampal atrophy. *Neurobiol Aging* 2005; **26**: 553–9.

Dufouil C, Chalmers J, Coskun O, *et al*. Effects of blood pressure lowering on cerebral white matter hyperintensities in patients with stroke: the PROGRESS (Perindopril Protection Against Recurrent Stroke Study) Magnetic Resonance Imaging Substudy. *Circulation* 2005; **112**: 1644–50.

Elias MF, Wolf PA, D'Agostino RB, Cobb J, White LR. Untreated blood pressure level is inversely related to cognitive functioning: the Framingham Study. *Am J Epidemiol* 1993; **138**: 353–64.

Elias MF, Sullivan LM, D'Agostino RB, *et al*. Framingham stroke risk profile and lowered cognitive performance. *Stroke* 2004; **35**: 404–09.

Elias MF, D'Agostino RB, Elias PK, Wolf PA. Neuropsychological test performance, cognitive functioning, blood pressure, and age: the Framingham Heart Study. *Exp Aging Res* 1995a; **21**: 369–91.

Elias MF, D'Agostino RB, Elias MF, Wolf PA. Blood pressure, hypertension, and age as risk factors for poor cognitive performance. *Exp Aging Res* 1995b; **21**: 393–417.

Esiri MM, Nagy Z, Smith MZ, Barnetson L, Smith AD. Cerebrovascular disease and threshold for dementia in the early stages of Alzheimer's disease. *Lancet* 1999; **354**: 919–20.

Evans DA, Funkenstein HH, Albert MS, *et al*. Prevalence of Alzheimer's disease in a community population of older persons. Higher than previously reported. *JAMA* 1989; **262**: 2551–6.

Ezekowitz MD, James KE, Nazarian SM, *et al*. Silent cerebral infarction in patients with nonrheumatic atrial fibrillation. The Veterans Affairs Stroke Prevention in Nonrheumatic Atrial Fibrillation Investigators. *Circulation* 1995; **92**: 2178–82.

Fazekas F, Chawluk JB, Alavi A, Hurtig HI, Zimmerman RA. MR signal abnormalities at 1.5 T in Alzheimer's dementia and normal aging. *Am J Neuroradiol* 1987; **8**: 421–6.

Fazekas F, Kapeller P, Schmidt R, Offenbacher H, Payer F, Fazekas G. The relation of cerebral magnetic resonance signal hyperintensities to Alzheimer's disease. *J Neurol Sci* 1996; **142**: 121–5.

Fein G, Di Sclafani V, Tanabe J, *et al*. Hippocampal and cortical atrophy predict dementia in subcortical ischemic vascular disease. *Neurology* 2000; **55**: 1626–35.

Geschwind N. Disconnexion syndromes in animals and man. I. *Brain* 1965a; **88**: 237–94.

Geschwind N, Disconnexion syndromes in animals and man. II. *Brain* 1965b; **88**: 585–644.

Gesztelyi G, Finnegan W, DeMaro JA, Wang JY, Chen JL, Fenstermacher J. Parenchymal microvascular systems and cerebral atrophy in spontaneously hypertensive rats. *Brain Res* 1993; **611**: 249–57.

Gillum RF. Coronary heart disease, stroke, and hypertension in a U.S. national cohort: the NHANES I

Epidemiologic Follow-up Study. National Health and Nutrition Examination Survey. *Ann Epidemiol* 1996; **6**: 259–62.

Gold JJ, Hopkins RO, Squire LR. Single-item memory, associative memory, and the human hippocampus. *Learn Mem* 2006; **13**: 644–9.

Goldman-Rakic PS. Circuitry of the frontal association cortex and its relevance to dementia. *Arch Gerontol Geriatr* 1987; **6**: 299–309.

Goldman-Rakic PS, Topography of cognition: parallel distributed networks in primate association cortex. *Ann Rev Neurosci* 1988; **11**: 137–56.

Grady CL, Craik FI. Changes in memory processing with age. *Curr Opin Neurobiol* 2000; **10**: 224–31.

Gunning-Dixon FM, Raz N. The cognitive correlates of white matter abnormalities in normal aging: a quantitative review. *Neuropsychology* 2000; **14**: 224–32.

Hachinski V. Preventable senility: a call for action against the vascular dementias. *Lancet* 1992; **340**: 645–8.

Hachinski V, Potter P, Merskey H. Leuko-araiosis: an ancient term for a new problem. *Can J Neurol Sci* 1986; **13**: 533–4.

Hachinski V, Potter P, Merskey H. Leuko-araiosis. *Arch Neurol* 1987; **44**: 21–3.

Hanon O, Forette F. Prevention of dementia: lessons from SYST-EUR and PROGRESS. *J Neurol Sci* 2004; **226**: 71–4.

Hanon O, Seux ML, Lenoir H, Rigaud AS, Forette F. Prevention of dementia and cerebroprotection with anti-hypertensive drugs. *Curr Hypertens Rep* 2004; **6**: 201–07.

Harrell LE, Duvall E, Folks DG, *et al.* The relationship of high intensity signals on magnetic resonance images to cognitive and psychiatric state in Alzheimer's disease. *Arch Neurol* 1991; **48**: 1136–40.

Hebert LE, Beckett LA, Scherr PA, Evans DA. Annual incidence of Alzheimer disease in the United States projected to the years 2000 through 2050. *Alzheimer Dis Assoc Disord* 2001; **15**: 169–73.

Henon H, Durieu I, Guerouaou D, Lebert F, Pasquier F, Leys D. Poststroke dementia: incidence and relationship to prestroke cognitive decline. *Neurology* 2001; **57**: 1216–22.

Jagust W. Untangling vascular dementia. *Lancet* 2001; **358**: 2097–8.

Jeerakathil T, Wolf PA, Beiser A, *et al.* Stroke risk profile predicts white matter hyperintensity volume: the Framingham Study. *Stroke* 2004; **35**: 1857–61.

Jørgensen HS, Nakayama H, Raaschou HO, Gam J, Olsen TS. Silent infarction in acute stroke patients. Prevalence, localization, risk factors, and clinical significance: the Copenhagen Stroke Study. *Stroke* 1994; **25**: 97–104.

Kase CS, Wolf PA, Chodosh EH, et al. Prevalence of silent stroke in patients presenting with initial stroke: the Framingham Study. *Stroke* 1989; **20**: 850–2.

Kertesz A, Polk M, Carr T. Cognition and white matter changes on magnetic resonance imaging in dementia. *Arch Neurol* 1990; **47**: 387–91.

Knopman D, Boland LL, Mosley T, *et al.* Cardiovascular risk factors and cognitive decline in middle-aged adults. *Neurology* 2001; **56**: 42–8.

Knopman D, Parisi JE, Boeve BF, *et al.* Vascular dementia in a population-based autopsy study. *Arch Neurol* 2003; **60**: 569–75.

Kozachuk WE, DeCarli C, Schapiro MB, Wagner EE, Rapoport SI, Horwitz B. White matter hyperintensities in dementia of Alzheimer's type and in healthy subjects without cerebrovascular risk factors: a magnetic resonance imaging study. *Arch Neurol* 1990; **47**: 1306–10.

Kuller LH, Lopez OL, Newman A, *et al.* Risk factors for dementia in the cardiovascular health cognition study. *Neuroepidemiology* 2003; **22**: 13–22.

Launer LJ. The epidemiologic study of dementia: a life-long quest? *Neurobiol Aging* 2005; **26**: 335–40.

Launer LJ, Masaki K, Petrovich H, Foley D, Havlik, RJ. The association between mid-life blood pressure levels and late-life cognitive function. The Honolulu–Asia Aging Study. *JAMA* 1995; 274.

Leys D, Soetaert G, Petit H, Fauquette A, Pruvo JP, Steinling M. Periventricular and white matter magnetic resonance imaging hyperintensities do not differ between Alzheimer's disease and normal aging. *Arch Neurol* 1990; **47**: 524–7.

Liao D, Cooper L, Cai J, *et al.* Presence and severity of cerebral white matter lesions and hypertension, its treatment, and its control. The ARIC Study. Atherosclerosis Risk in Communities Study. *Stroke* 1996; **27**: 2262–70.

Liao D, Cooper L, Cai J, *et al.* The prevalence and severity of white matter lesions, their relationship with age, ethnicity, gender, and cardiovascular disease risk factors: the ARIC Study. *Neuroepidemiology* 1997; **16**: 149–62.

Liem MK, van der Grond J, Haan J, *et al.* Lacunar infarcts are the main correlate with cognitive dysfunction in CADASIL. *Stroke* 2007; **38**: 923–8.

Longstreth WT, Jr., Manolio TA, Arnold A, *et al.* Clinical correlates of white matter findings on cranial magnetic resonance imaging of 3301 elderly people. The Cardiovascular Health Study. *Stroke* 1996; **27**: 1274–82.

Longstreth WT, Jr., Bernick C, Manolio TA, Bryan N, Jungreis CA, Price TR. Lacunar infarcts defined by magnetic resonance imaging of 3660 elderly people: the Cardiovascular Health Study. *Arch Neurol* 1998; **55**: 1217–25.

Longstreth WT, Jr., Arnold AM, Manolio TA, *et al.* Clinical correlates of ventricular and sulcal size on cranial magnetic resonance imaging of 3,301 elderly people. The Cardiovascular Health Study. Collaborative Research Group. *Neuroepidemiology* 2000; **19**: 30–42.

Lopez OL, Becker JT, Rezek D, *et al.* Neuropsychiatric correlates of cerebral white-matter radiolucencies in probable Alzheimer's disease. *Arch Neurol* 1992; **49**: 828–34.

Lopez OL, Becker JT, Jungreis CA, *et al.* Computed tomography – but not magnetic resonance imaging – identified periventricular white-matter lesions predict symptomatic cerebrovascular disease in probable Alzheimer's disease. *Arch Neurol* 1995; **52**: 659–64.

Lopez OL, Jagust WJ, Dulberg C, *et al.* Risk factors for mild cognitive impairment in the cardiovascular health study cognition study: part 2. *Arch Neurol* 2003; **60**: 1394–9.

Manolio TA, Kronmal RA, Burke GL *et al.*, Magnetic resonance abnormalities and cardiovascular disease in older adults: the Cardiovascular Health Study. *Stroke* 1994; **25**: 318–27.

Manolio TA, Burke GL, O'Leary DH, *et al.* Relationships of cerebral MRI findings to ultrasonographic carotid atherosclerosis in older adults: the Cardiovascular Health Study. CHS Collaborative Research Group. *Arterioscler Thromb Vasc Biol* 1999; **19**: 356–65.

Marder K, Richards M, Bello J, *et al.* Clinical correlates of Alzheimer's disease with and without silent radiographic abnormalities. *Arch Neurol* 1995; **52**: 146–51.

Mader K, Mathis CA, Klunk WE, Price JC, DeKosky ST. Imaging technology for neurodegenerative diseases: progress toward detection of specific pathologies. *Arch Neurol* 2005; **62**: 196–200.

McDonald WM, Krishnan KR, Doraiswamy PM, *et al.* Magnetic resonance findings in patients with early-onset Alzheimer's disease. *Biol Psychiatry* 1991; **29**: 799–810.

Mentis MJ, Salerno J, Horwitz B, *et al.* Reduction of functional neuronal connectivity in long-term treated hypertension. *Stroke* 1994; **25**: 601–7.

Mesulam MM. Large-scale neurocognitive networks and distributed processing for attention, language, and memory. *Ann Neurol* 1990; **28**: 597–613.

Miller EK, Asaad WF. The prefrontal cortex, conjunction and cognition. In: Grafman J, ed. Handbook of Neuropsychology. St. Louis: Elsevier, 2002.

Milner B, Squire LR, Kandel ER. Cognitive neuroscience and the study of memory. *Neuron* 1998; **20**: 445–68.

Mirsen TR, Lee DH, Wong CJ, *et al.* Clinical correlates of white-matter changes on magnetic resonance imaging scans of the brain. *Arch Neurol* 1991; **48**: 1015–21.

Miyao S, Takano A, Teramoto J, Takahashi A. Leukoaraiosis in relation to prognosis for patients with lacunar infarction. *Stroke* 1992; **23**: 1434–8.

Moroney JT, Bagiella E, Desmond DW, Paik MC, Stern Y, Tatemichi TK. Risk factors for incident dementia after stroke. Role of hypoxic and ischemic disorders. *Stroke* 1996; **27**: 1283–9.

Moroney JT, Bagiella E, Desmond DW, Paik MC, Stern Y, Tatemichi TK. Cerebral hypoxia and ischemia in the pathogenesis of dementia after stroke. *Ann NY Acad Sci* 1997a; **826**: 433–6.

Lopez OLBagiella E, Tatemichi TK, Paik MC, Stern Y, Desmond DW. Dementia after stroke increases the risk of long-term stroke recurrence. *Neurology* 1997b; **48**: 1317–25.

Morris JC, Price AL. Pathologic correlates of nondemented aging, mild cognitive impairment, and early-stage Alzheimer's disease. *J Mol Neurosci* 2001; **17**: 101–118.

Morris JC, Scherr PA, Hebert LE, *et al.* Association between blood pressure and cognitive function in a biracial community population of older persons. *Neuroepidemiology* 2002; **21**: 123–30.

Morris R, Pandya DN, Petrides M. Fiber system linking the mid-dorsolateral frontal cortex with the retrosplenial/presubicular region in the rhesus monkey. *J Comp Neurol* 1999; **407**: 183–92.

Moscovitch M, Nadel L, Winocur G, Gilboa A, Rosenbaum RS. The cognitive neuroscience of remote episodic, semantic and spatial memory. *Curr Opin Neurobiol* 2006; **16**: 179–90.

Moscovitch M, Jagust WJ, Reed BR, *et al.* MRI predictors of cognition in subcortical ischemic vascular disease and Alzheimer's disease. *Neurology* 2001a; **57**: 2229–35.

Moscovitch M, Reed B, Ellis WG, Jagust WJ. The effects of age on rate of progression of Alzheimer disease and dementia with associated cerebrovascular disease. *Arch Neurol* 2001b; **58**: 1243–7.

Mungas D, Reed BR, Jagust WJ, *et al.* Volumetric MRI predicts rate of cognitive decline related to AD and cerebrovascular disease. *Neurology* 2002; **59**: 867–73.

Mungas D, Harvey D, Reed BR, *et al.* Longitudinal volumetric MRI change and rate of cognitive decline. *Neurology* 2005; **65**: 565–71.

Nordahl CW, Ranganath C, Yonelinas AP, DeCarli C, Reed BR, Jagust WJ. Different mechanisms of episodic memory failure in mild cognitive impairment. *Neuropsychologia* 2005; **43**: 1688–97.

Nordahl CW, Ranganath C, Yonelinas AP, DeCarli C, Fletcher E, Jagust WJ. White matter changes compromise prefrontal cortex function in healthy elderly individuals. *J Cogn Neurosci* 2006; **18**: 418–29.

O'Brien JT, Erkinjuntti T, Reisberg B, *et al.* Vascular cognitive impairment. *Lancet Neurol* 2003; **2**: 89–98.

O'Brien JT. Vascular dementia is underdiagnosed. *Arch Neurol* 1988; **45**: 797–8.

O'Sullivan M, Morris RG, Huckstep B, Jones DK, Williams SC, Markus HS. Diffusion tensor MRI correlates with executive dysfunction in patients with ischaemic leukoaraiosis. *J Neurol Neurosurg Psychiatry* 2004; **75**: 441–7.

Ott A, Stolk RP, Hofman A, van Harskamp F, Grobbee DE, Breteler MM. Association of diabetes mellitus and dementia: the Rotterdam Study. *Diabetologia* 1996; **39**: 1392–7.

Ott A, Stolk RP, van Harskamp F, Pols HA, Hofman A, Breteler MM. Diabetes mellitus and the risk of dementia: the Rotterdam Study. *Neurology* 1999; **53**: 1937–42.

Ott BR, Faberman RS, Noto RB, *et al.* A SPECT imaging study of MRI white matter hyperintensity in patients with degenerative dementia. *Dement Geriatr Cogn Disord* 1997; **8**: 348–54.

Papademetriou V, Narayan P, Rubins H, Collins D, Robins S. Influence of risk factors on peripheral and cerebrovascular disease in men with coronary artery disease, low high-density lipoprotein cholesterol levels, and desirable low-density lipoprotein cholesterol levels. HIT Investigators. Department of Veterans Affairs HDL Intervention Trial. *Am Heart J* 1998; **136**: 734–40.

Peters N, Opherk C, Danek A, Ballard C, Herzog J, Dichgans M. The pattern of cognitive performance in CADASIL: a monogenic condition leading to subcortical ischemic vascular dementia. *Am J Psychiatry* 2005; **162**: 2078–85.

Peters N, Holtmannspotter M, Opherk C, *et al.* Brain volume changes in CADASIL: a serial MRI study in pure subcortical ischemic vascular disease. *Neurology* 2006; **66**: 1517–22.

Petersen RC, Smith GE, Waring SC, Ivnik RJ, Tangalos EG, Kokmen E. Mild cognitive impairment: clinical characterization and outcome. *Arch Neurol* 1999; **56**: 303–08.

Petrides M, Pandya DN. Dorsolateral prefrontal cortex: comparative cytoarchitectonic analysis in the human and the macaque brain and corticocortical connection patterns. *Eur J Neurosci* 1999; **11**: 1011–36.

Price JL, Morris JC. Tangles and plaques in nondemented aging and "preclinical" Alzheimer's disease. *Ann Neurol* 1999; **45**: 358–68.

Price TR, Manolio TA, Kronmal RA, *et al.* Silent brain infarction on magnetic resonance imaging and neurological abnormalities in community-dwelling older adults. The Cardiovascular Health Study. CHS Collaborative Research Group. *Stroke* 1997; **28**: 1158–64.

Ranganath C. Working memory for visual objects: complementary roles of inferior temporal, medial temporal, and prefrontal cortex. *Neuroscience* 2006; **139**: 277–89.

Ranganath C, Johnson MK, D'Esposito M. Prefrontal activity associated with working memory and episodic long-term memory. *Neuropsychologia* 2003; **41**: 378–89.

Rapp PR, Amaral DG. Individual differences in the cognitive and neurobiological consequences of normal aging. *Trends Neurosci* 1992; **15**: 340–5.

Ratnasabapathy Y, Lawes CM, Anderson CS. The Perindopril Protection Against Recurrent Stroke Study (PROGRESS): clinical implications for older patients with cerebrovascular disease. *Drugs Aging* 2003; **20**: 241–51.

Raz N, Gunning FM, Head D, *et al.* Selective aging of the human cerebral cortex observed in vivo: differential vulnerability of the prefrontal gray matter. *Cerebral Cortex* 1997; **7**: 268–82.

Reed BR, Eberling JL, Mungas D, Weiner MW, Jagust WJ. Memory failure has different mechanisms in subcortical stroke and Alzheimer's disease. *Ann Neurol* 2000; **48**: 275–84.

Reed BR, Eberling JL, Mungas D, Weiner M, Jagust WJ. Frontal lobe hypometabolism predicts cognitive decline in patients with lacunar infarcts. *Arch Neurol* 2001; **58**: 493–7.

Roman GC. Senile dementia of the Binswanger type: a vascular form of dementia in the elderly. *JAMA* 1987; **258**: 1782–8.

Roman GC, Tatemichi TK, Erkinjuntti T, *et al.* Vascular dementia: diagnostic criteria for research studies. Report of the NINDS-AIREN International Workshop. *Neurology* 1993; **43**: 250–60.

Rosen AC, Prull MW, O'Hara R, *et al.* Variable effects of aging on frontal lobe contributions to memory. *Neuroreport* 2002; **13**: 2425–8.

Rypma B, D'Esposito M. Isolating the neural mechanisms of age-related changes in human working memory. *Nat Neurosci* 2000; **3**: 509–15.

Salerno JA, Murphy DG, Horwitz B, *et al.* Brain atrophy in hypertension. A volumetric magnetic resonance imaging study. *Hypertension* 1992; **20**: 340–8.

Sayetta RB. Rates of senile dementia, Alzheimer's type, in the Baltimore Longitudinal Study. *J Chronic Dis* 1986; **39**: 271–86.

Scheltens P, Barkhof F, Valk J, *et al.* White matter lesions on magnetic resonance imaging in clinically diagnosed Alzheimer's disease: evidence for heterogeneity. *Brain* 1992; **115**: 735–48.

Scheltens P, Barkhof F, Leys D, Wolters EC, Ravid R, Kamphorst W. Histopathologic correlates of white matter changes on MRI in Alzheimer's disease and normal aging. *Neurology* 1995; **45**: 883–8.

Schmidt R. Comparison of magnetic resonance imaging in Alzheimer's disease, vascular dementia and normal aging. *Eur Neurol* 1992; **32**: 164–9.

Schmidt R, Fazekas F, Koch M, *et al.* Magnetic resonance imaging cerebral abnormalities and neuropsychologic test performance in elderly hypertensive subjects. A case-control study. *Arch Neurol* 1995; **52**: 905–10.

Schneider JA, Wilson RS, Cochran EJ, *et al.* Relation of cerebral infarctions to dementia and cognitive function in older persons. *Neurology* 2003; **60**: 1082–8.

Schneider JA, Wilson RS, Bienias JL, Evans DA, Bennett DA. Cerebral infarctions and the likelihood of dementia from Alzheimer disease pathology. *Neurology* 2004; **62**: 1148–55.

Selemon LD, Goldman-Rakic PS. Common cortical and subcortical targets of the dorsolateral prefrontal and posterior parietal cortices in the rhesus monkey: evidence for a distributed neural network subserving spatially guided behavior. *J Neurosci* 1988; **8**: 4049–68.

Seshadri S, Wolf PA, Beiser A, *et al.* Stroke risk profile, brain volume, and cognitive function: the Framingham Offspring Study. *Neurology* 2004; **63**: 1591–9.

Seshadri S, Beiser A, Kelly-Hayes M, *et al.* The lifetime risk of stroke: estimates from the Framingham Study. *Stroke* 2006; **37**: 345–50.

Shinkawa A, Ueda K, Kiyohara Y, *et al.* Silent cerebral infarction in a community-based autopsy series in Japan. The Hisayama Study. *Stroke* 1995; **26**: 380–5.

Snowdon DA, Greiner LH, Mortimer JA, Riley KP, Greiner PA, Markesbery WR. Brain infarction and the clinical expression of Alzheimer disease. The Nun Study. *JAMA* 1997; 77.

Squire LR. Memory systems of the brain: a brief history and current perspective. *Neurobiol Learn Mem* 2004; **82**: 171–7.

Squire LR, Stark CE, Clark RE. The medial temporal lobe. *Ann Rev Neurosci* 2004; **27**: 279–306.

Starkstein SE, Sabe L, Vazquez S, *et al.* Neuropsychological, psychiatric, and cerebral perfusion correlates of leukoaraiosis in Alzheimer's disease. *J Neurol Neurosurg Psychiatry* 1997; **63**: 66–73.

Steingart A, Lau K, Fox A, *et al.* The significance of white matter lucencies on CT scan in relation to cognitive impairment. *Can J Neurol Sci* 1986; **13**: 383–4.

Steingart A, Hachinski VC, Lau C, *et al.* Cognitive and neurologic findings in subjects with diffuse white matter lucencies on computed tomographic scan (leuko-araiosis). *Arch Neurol* 1987; **44**: 32–5.

Stout JC, Jernigan TL, Archibald SL, Salmon DP. Association of dementia severity with cortical gray matter and abnormal white matter volumes in dementia of the Alzheimer type. *Arch Neurol* 1996:742–9.

Strassburger TL, Lee HC, Daly EM, *et al.* Interactive effects of age and hypertension on volumes of brain structures. *Stroke* 1997; **28**: 1410–7.

Streifler JY, Eliasziw M, Fox AJ, *et al.* Prognostic importance of leukoaraiosis in patients with ischemic events and carotid artery disease. *Stroke* 1999; **30**: 254.

Sullivan EV, Pfefferbaum A. Diffusion tensor imaging and aging. *Neurosci Biobehav Rev* 2006; **30**: 749–61.

Swan GE, DeCarli C, Miller BL, *et al.* Association of midlife blood pressure to late-life cognitive decline and brain morphology. *Neurology* 1998; **51**: 986–93.

Swan GE, DeCarli C, Miller BL, Reed T, Wolf PA, Carmelli D. Biobehavioral characteristics of nondemented older adults with subclinical brain atrophy. *Neurology* 2000; **54**: 2108–14.

Swartz RH, Black SE. Anterior–medial thalamic lesions in dementia: frequent, and volume dependently associated with sudden cognitive decline. *J Neurol Neurosurg Psychiatry* 2006; **77**: 1307–12.

Tajima A, Hans FJ, Livingstone D, *et al.* Smaller local brain volumes and cerebral atrophy in spontaneously hypertensive rats. *Hypertension* 1993; **21**: 105–11.

Tatemichi TK. How acute brain failure becomes chronic: a view of the mechanisms of dementia related to stroke. *Neurology* 1990; **40**: 1652–9.

Tatemichi TK, Foulkes MA, Mohr JP, *et al*. Dementia in stroke survivors in the stroke data bank cohort. Prevalence, incidence, risk factors, and computed tomographic findings. *Stroke* 1990; **21**: 858–66.

Tatemichi TK, Desmond DW, Mayeux R, *et al*. Dementia after stroke: baseline frequency, risks, and clinical features in a hospitalized cohort. *Neurology* 1992; **42**: 1185–93.

Tatemichi TK, Desmond DW, Prohovnik I. Strategic infarcts in vascular dementia. A clinical and brain imaging experience. *Arzneimittel-Forschung* 1995a; **45**: 371–85.

Tatemichi TK, Desmond DW, Prohovnik I, Eidelberg D. Dementia associated with bilateral carotid occlusions: neuropsychological and haemodynamic course after extracranial to intracranial bypass surgery. *J Neurol Neurosurg Psychiatry* 1995b; **58**: 633–6.

Teipel SJ, Hampel H, Alexander GE, *et al*. Dissociation between corpus callosum atrophy and white matter pathology in Alzheimer's disease. *Neurology* 1998; **51**: 1381–5.

Tekin S, Cummings JL. Frontal–subcortical neuronal circuits and clinical neuropsychiatry: an update. *J Psychosom Res* 2002; **53**: 647–54.

Tullberg M, Fletcher E, DeCarli C, *et al*. White matter lesions impair frontal lobe function regardless of their location. *Neurology* 2004; **63**: 246–53.

Tulving E. Multiple memory systems and consciousness. *Hum Neurobiol* 1987; **6**: 67–80.

Van der Werf VD, Scheltens P, Lindeboom J, Witter MP, Uylings HB, Jolles J. Deficits of memory, executive functioning and attention following infarction in the thalamus; a study of 22 cases with localised lesions. *Neuropsychologia* 2003; **41**: 1330–44.

Vermeer SE, Koudstaal PJ, Oudkerk M, Hofman A, Breteler MM. Prevalence and risk factors of silent brain infarcts in the population-based Rotterdam Scan Study. *Stroke* 2002; **33**: 21–5.

Vermeer SE, Prins ND, den Heijer T, Hofman A, Koudstaal PJ, Breteler MM. Silent brain infarcts and the risk of dementia and cognitive decline. *N Engl J Med* 2003; **348**: 1215–22.

Wahlund LO, Basun H, Almkvist O, Andersson-Lundman G, Julin P, Saaf J. White matter hyperintensities in dementia: does it matter? *Magn Res Imag* 1994; **12**: 387–94.

Waldemar G, Christiansen P, Larsson HB, *et al*. White matter magnetic resonance hyperintensities in dementia of the Alzheimer type: morphological and regional cerebral blood flow correlates. *J Neurol Neurosurg Psychiatry* 1994; **57**: 1458–65.

Weber MA. Role of hypertension in coronary artery disease. *Am J Nephrol* 1996; **16**: 210–16.

Wen W, Sachdev P. The topography of white matter hyperintensities on brain MRI in healthy 60- to 64-year-old individuals. *Neuroimage* 2004; **22**: 144–54.

West RL. An application of prefrontal cortex function theory to cognitive aging. *Psychol Bull* 1996; **120**: 272–92.

Wilson RS, Beckett LA, Bennett DA, Albert MS, Evans DA. Change in cognitive function in older persons from a community population: relation to age and Alzheimer disease. *Arch Neurol* 1999; **56**: 1274–9.

Wilson RS, Beckett LA, Barnes LL, *et al*. Individual differences in rates of change in cognitive abilities of older persons. *Psychol Aging* 2002; **17**: 179–93.

Wolf PA, D'Agostino RB, Belanger AJ, Kannel WB. Probability of stroke: a risk profile from the Framingham Study. *Stroke* 1991; **22**: 312–8.

Wu CC, Mungas D, Petkov CI, *et al*. Brain structure and cognition in a community sample of elderly Latinos. *Neurology* 2002; **59**: 383–91.

Yoshita M, Fletcher E, Harvey D, *et al*. Extent and distribution of white matter hyperintensities in normal aging, MCI, and AD. *Neurology* 2006; **67**: 2192–8.

Yousry TA, Seelos K, Mayer M, *et al*. Characteristic MR lesion pattern and correlation of T1 and T2 lesion volume with neurologic and neuropsychological findings in cerebral autosomal dominant arteriopathy with subcortical infarcts and leukoencephalopathy (CADASIL). *Am J Neuroradiol* 1999; **20**: 91–100.

Yue NC, Arnold AM, Longstreth WT, Jr., *et al*. Sulcal, ventricular, and white matter changes at MR imaging in the aging brain: data from the cardiovascular health study. *Radiology* 1997; **202**: 33–9.

Zheng ZJ, Sharrett AR, Chambless LE, *et al*. Associations of ankle-brachial index with clinical coronary heart disease, stroke and preclinical carotid and popliteal atherosclerosis: the Atherosclerosis Risk in Communities (ARIC) Study. *Atherosclerosis* 1997; **131**: 115–25.

3

Clinical evaluation: a systematic but user-friendly approach

Oscar L. Lopez and David A. Wolk

Evolution of the concept of vascular dementia

The scientific literature has recognized that cerebrovascular disease (CVD) can cause severe cognitive deficits for several centuries (Willis, 1984). However, for most of the 1900s, the border zone between Alzheimer's disease (AD) and vascular dementia (VaD) was not clearly defined, and the use of the term "hardening of the arteries" for all dementia syndromes was common practice. A significant advance in the clinical characterization of VaD occurred in the 1970s when V. Hachinski described the term "multi-infarct dementia" (MID) (Hachinski and Lassen, 1974). The MID syndrome was supported by a history of clinical strokes with focal neurological signs and symptoms. Further diagnostic refinement has led classification of any type of dementia syndrome caused by vascular disease, either ischemic or hemorrhagic, single or multiple, under the term VaD (Chui *et al.*, 1992; Erkinjunnti *et al.*, 2000; Roman *et al.*, 1993).

Research and clinical criteria for the diagnosis of vascular dementia

Over the last two decades more specific diagnostic criteria have been developed for both research and clinical practice, but these criteria tend to have relatively poor sensitivity and modest specificity (Gold *et al.*, 2002; Knopman *et al.*, 2003). Further, there is often disagreement for classification of individual patients depending on the criteria used, as well as poor inter-rater reliability (Chui *et al.*, 2000). Evidence for these issues is exemplified by the vastly different prevalence and incidence data depending upon which criteria are applied. While neuroimaging has certainly improved diagnosis and awareness of "silent" CVD in aging, specific imaging criteria are also difficult to apply and contentious (van Straaten *et al.*, 2003).

Difficulties in the diagnosis of vascular dementia

A number of factors have contributed to difficulty in the development and implementation of diagnostic criteria for VaD. The most obvious is that current constructions of VaD include a heterogeneous population, which is due, in part, to the heterogeneity of CVD itself. Patients can have VaD after a single ischemic lesion, or after multiple lesions. In other cases, patients with progressive cognitive decline can have multiple ischemic lesions or severe white matter disease on

Vascular Cognitive Impairment in Clinical Practice, ed. Lars-Olof Wahlund, Timo Erkinjuntti and Serge Gauthier. Published by Cambridge University Press. © Cambridge University Press 2009.

neuroimaging studies without clinical strokes (Esiri et al., 1997; Hulette et al., 1997). The etiology of the strokes can also be varied and include thromboembolic disease, lipohyalinosis, cerebral amyloid angiopathy (CAA), and primary hemorrhagic stroke. Differences in etiology, of course, result in differences in pathology. Further, the topography of CNS injury producing the dementia syndrome can be quite varied, necessarily resulting in heterogeneous cognitive and neurological clinical profiles. Finding diagnostic criteria which encapsulate this clinical, pathological, and etiological diversity is challenging, if not impossible. Note that this is a more daunting task than for neurodegenerative dementias, in which there is a more homogeneous pathology and topographic distribution over time producing a more specific clinical presentation and progression.

A second major obstacle to accurate diagnosis of VaD is the frequent concomitant manifestation of AD and CVD. Because AD is the most frequent form of dementia in the elderly and can co-exist with severe CVD, it is often difficult to determine whether the cognitive deterioration is solely a consequence of vascular factors or underlying AD. Neuropathological series have shown that more than 50% of the cases with VaD had AD pathology (Chui et al., 2006; Galasko et al., 1994; Tomlinson et al., 1970; Zekry et al., 2003). Several studies have found that AD patients with CVD need less AD pathology to express their dementia syndrome (Petrovitch et al., 2005; Snowdon et al., 1997). For example, Snowdon and colleagues (1997) found that for a given dementia severity three times as many neurofibrillary tangles would need to be present in patients without CVD. Another example of the potential synergy between AD and CVD pathology is that patients with mesial temporal lobe atrophy, presumably due to AD, have increased risk of dementia after stroke compared to those without atrophy (Cordoliani-Mackowiak et al., 2003). Nonetheless, not all studies have found such a clear relationship (Schneider et al., 2003), and determining the impact of stroke on the pathogenesis and expression of AD remains

a fundamental area of research in the study of vascular cognitive impairment. Much of the work defining the cognitive profile of VaD does not include autopsy data and, thus, leaves to question whether there is a contribution of AD pathology or that of other neurodegenerative conditions.

An additional issue with regard to the overlap of AD with VaD is the relationship of CAA and vascular disease (Attems and Jellinger, 2004; Lopez and Claassen, 1991; Pfeifer et al., 2002). CAA involves the deposition of fibrillar amyloid in the media of vessel walls which can result in lobar hemorrhage. However, in addition to hemorrhage, such pathology may be associated with increased risk of cortical microinfarcts and subcortical ischemic disease (Attems and Jellinger, 2004). While CAA can occur in the absence of AD pathology, there is a high association between these processes, and it is unclear to what extent the degree of CAA and CVD impact the clinical expression of cases of AD.

A related and essential factor limiting the establishment of clear clinical criteria is the lack of a consensus on the required pathology for diagnosis of VaD. Outside of cortical infarcts it remains unclear what type of cerebrovascular pathology can be definitively related to cognitive symptoms. There is no current "gold standard" to determine the accuracy of the clinical diagnosis (Reed et al., 2004b). For example, it remains uncertain how much, in what distribution, and what type of white matter disease should constitute VaD.

Classification of vascular dementia

In order to appropriately diagnose VaD it is critical to define the different subtypes that fall within this rubric (see Chapter 1 for more detail). Briefly, the classification of VaD is usually based on its suspected neuropathological etiology, and it may be divided into the following subtypes:
- multi-infarct dementia (MID),
- strategically localized infarcts,
- small vessel disease,

- hemorrhagic lesions, and
- hypoperfusion type.

Another classification scheme is to broadly divide VaD into cortical and subcortical types. The concept of cortical and subcortical dementia was used to differentiate neurodegenerative processes that cause dementia (e.g. Huntington's disease vs. AD). However, it was felt that this concept could also be useful in differentiating and diagnosing different types of VaD, which appear to have different clinical profiles and, perhaps, pathogenesis.

Subcortical vascular dementia

Subcortical VaD is usually associated with lacunar infarcts and periventricular and/or subcortical white matter lesions (e.g. Binswanger's disease; De Reuck *et al.*, 1980; Roman, 1996). Microinfarcts and lacunes of the deep gray matter may also be present. The direct role of white matter lesions on cognition has been a source of significant debate. While it does appear that white matter disease increases the risk of dementia (Kuller *et al.*, 2005; Vermeer *et al.*, 2003), this evidence does not directly implicate the CVD as being causal. However, increasingly, more data support a direct correlation between white matter disease and performance on a number of cognitive measures (de Groot *et al.*, 2000; Prins *et al.*, 2004), including in autopsy cases free of AD pathology (Reed *et al.*, 2004b). Reports of individuals with significant white matter disease on MRI in the absence of significant cognitive deficits may be due to the type of white matter pathology and the presence of such other factors as microinfarcts and hypoperfusion (Selnes and Vinters, 2006). Imaging is presently not able to clearly make such distinctions.

The presentation and cognitive profile of subcortical vascular dementia may be distinguishable from cortical VaD and is perhaps more homogenous (Pohjasvaara *et al.*, 2003). Unlike classic MID, these patients tend to have a more gradual, progressive course. Sensory and motor deficits, gait disorders, extrapyramidal signs, dysarthria, pseudobulbar palsy, urinary incontinence, depressed mood,

apathy, and emotional lability all may be present. Neuropsychologically, they can present with executive function deficits, slowing of the mental processing, and set-shifting deficits (see below). It is worth noting that cognitive deficits due to subcortical disease, but that do not qualify as dementia, may be relatively common (Reed *et al.*, 2004a)

Cortical vascular dementia

Cortical VaD is more associated with the classic step-wise progression of MID in which there is a temporal relationship between a clinical stroke and the development of dementia. Nonetheless, the combination of subcortical and cortical lesions may be seen in many patients (Min *et al.*, 2000). Such patients may present with florid neuropsychological and behavioral symptoms with or without sensory motor deficits (Bogousslavsky *et al.*, 1996; Boiten and Lodder, 1992; Graham *et al.*, 2004; Groves *et al.*, 2000).

It is clear that large ischemic lesions can cause VaD, especially those localized in bilateral cortical temporal–parietal areas (Knopman *et al.*, 2003). However, there are isolated infarcts in "strategically" localized areas that, regardless of their size, can cause cognitive disorders (Benson *et al.*, 1982; Damasio and Damasio, 1983; Damasio *et al.*, 1985; Graff-Radford *et al.*, 1984; Katz *et al.*, 1987; Kumral *et al.*, 1999, 2001; Ott and Saver, 1993; Tatemichi *et al.*, 1992b). For example, subjects with angular gyrus damage can present with language disturbance, alexia with agraphia, and/or a Gerstmann's syndrome, which mimics AD.

Pre-stroke cognitive impairment appears to play an important modifying role in the risk of post-stroke dementia. Some studies have reported that pre-stroke deficits were a strong predictor of incident VaD (Henon *et al.*, 2001). Brain atrophy, including in the medial temporal lobes, portends a higher risk of VaD after stroke (Pohjasvaara *et al.*, 2000), which suggests that Alzheimer's pathology may have an influential role in the development of dementia in such patients. To better establish the link between the stroke and dementia, clinicians have generally agreed that the symptoms should appear within 3 months after the stroke (Tatemichi *et al.*, 1992a). This designation is reflected in some of the clinical criteria discussed below (but may not capture the more gradual course of subcortical VaD). However, this is an arbitrary time, and symptoms may develop after, or may disappear before, this time frame.

Current clinical criteria for VaD

One important advance in the study and diagnosis of cognitive disorders associated with CVD has been the development of several diagnostic criteria for VaD. These are particularly important not only as diagnostic tools in clinical practice, but also to establish prevalence and incidence in population studies, to determine risk factors, and to recruit homogenous cohorts for drug trials. There are classification/diagnostic and research/diagnostic criteria. The *Diagnostic and Statistical Manual of Mental Disorders*, 4th Edition (DSM-IV; APA, 1994), and the *International Classification of Diseases*, 10th Edition (ICD-10; WHO, 1993) are classification criteria which are used for administrative purposes, for tracking disease, and, in some cases, as diagnostic criteria. Both are very vague, and with no operational guidelines. The National Institute of Neurological Disorders and Stroke – the Association Internationale pour la Recherche et l'Enseignement en Neurosciences (NINDS-AIREN; Roman *et al.*, 1993), and the State of California Alzheimer's Disease Diagnostic and Treatment Centers (ADDTC; Chui *et al.*, 1992) criteria for VaD are research diagnostic instruments, which operationalized specific signs and symptoms of the VaD syndrome. More recently, there have been proposals for clinical criteria to capture subcortical VaD. This subgroup of cases has only subcortical ischemic lesions and appears to have a more homogenous clinical presentation than cortical VaD cases. Such a population may be more suitable for multicenter drug trials (Erkinjuntti *et al.*, 2000). The characteristics of the different criteria for VaD are discussed in Chapter 1.

As noted above, the classification of VaD using the current clinical criteria has proven to be extremely difficult (Chui *et al.*, 2000; Lopez *et al.*, 1994). For example, Verhey *et al.* (1996) compared 7 different criteria for VaD, and found that all criteria agreed in only 8 of the 124 dementia cases, with a better agreement for the Hachinski Ischemic Scale (HIS) than for the subcortical VaD criteria proposed by Erkinjuntti *et al.*, ADDTC, and NINDS-AIREN criteria. These studies indicated that the more liberal the definition of VaD (e.g. HIS, DSM-IV), the better the agreement. By contrast, clinicians had more difficulty with the more stringent criteria (e.g. NINDS-AIREN). Neuropathological studies confirm that the current criteria for VaD have low sensitivity with high specificity, suggesting that CVD can co-exist with other disease processes (Gold *et al.*, 2002; Hogervorst *et al.*, 2003; Holmes *et al.*, 1999; Knopman *et al.*, 2003). The retrospective application of these criteria to neuropathological series with heterogeneous clinical data may have accounted for the discrepancies seen in these studies. Lack of clear agreement on the neuropathological basis of VaD further obfuscates the picture.

Two critical factors in the diagnosis of vascular dementia

All diagnostic criteria have focused on the two most important issues in VaD: the presence of dementia, and the presence of vascular disease of sufficient severity to cause cognitive deficits. However, there is a great variability in their approach to these two core issues.

Definition of dementia

All the major criteria for VaD have different definitions of dementia, which has been reported as a major discrepancy among investigators in reliability studies (Lopez *et al.*, 1994). The DSM-IV criteria require memory deficits, and impairments in at least one other cognitive domain; the NINDS-AIREN criteria require memory deficits and cognitive impairments in two other domains (which is similar to the ICD-10 criteria); and the ADDTC criteria require a level of deterioration of cognitive deficits to interfere with the subject's activities of daily living, but did not emphasize the presence of specific cognitive domain deficits.

Dementia criteria based on memory deficits derived from the concept of dementia proposed for AD. However, these criteria may not be suitable for the identification of a dementia syndrome associated with CVD, where the mesial temporal lobe could be intact. While VaD subjects can have global cognitive deficits (Graham *et al.*, 2004), others can have relatively preserved memory functions (Benson *et al.*, 1982). Therefore, the DSM-IV and NINDS-AIREN criteria may capture the more advanced cases. In addition, the NINDS-AIREN criteria require that the memory disorder must be accompanied by deficits in two other cognitive domains. In contrast, the ADDTC criteria did not require any specific dementia criteria, and state that the cognitive deficits should not be confined to a single category, which gives these criteria the flexibility to use them with different approaches to the concept of dementia.

The definition of dementia is critical for the diagnosis of VaD, and approaches different from those used to characterize AD have been used successfully in referral clinics (Lopez *et al.*, 2000b) and population studies (Lopez *et al.*, 2003). For example, in the Cardiovascular Health Study, the diagnosis of dementia was based on a deficit in performance in two or more cognitive domains that were of sufficient severity to affect the subjects' activities of daily living, and history of normal cognition before the onset of the symptoms of dementia. Thus, a memory deficit was not required for the diagnosis of dementia (Lopez *et al.*, 2005).

Vascular disease

The second critical clinical determinant of VaD is determination of the relationship of cerebrovascular disease to cognitive symptoms. As an attempt to establish this relationship, there is some agreement among clinicians that symptoms should appear within 3 months after a stroke (Tatemichi *et al.*, 1992a). However, as mentioned above, this is an arbitrary time and symptoms may develop after this time frame. In addition, there are patients who do not have a clinical stroke, and severe CVD is evident only in neuroradiological studies. Clinico-pathological studies found that half of the subjects with radiological evidence of critical ischemic lesions had a history of clinical stroke or focal motor deficits (Knopman *et al.*, 2003).

The severity of CVD is also important to establish for diagnostic purposes. Although it has been proposed that there must be a threshold of tissue loss (e.g. 50–100 ml) above which VaD is more likely (del Ser *et al.*, 1990; Galasko *et al.*, 1994; Liu *et al.*, 1992; Tomlinson *et al.*, 1970), sometimes the size and number of the lesions do not explain the cognitive deficits. Therefore, the determination of CVD of sufficient severity to cause VaD is a major challenge, and the operationalization of specific radiological criteria for the clinical diagnosis of VaD is under debate. Studies conducted to test the reliability of the radiological part of the NINDS-AIREN criteria for VaD found that the overall agreement among neuroradiologists was poor, although there was a better agreement among the most experienced radiologists compared to those with less experience (van Straaten *et al.*, 2003).

Neuropsychological profile

Identification of a clear neuropsychological profile in VaD is hindered by the heterogeneity of the condition. Large-vessel, cortical CVD produces a pattern of impairment consistent with the localization of the strokes. Evaluation of neuroimaging for consistency with the nature of the cognitive impairment will usually be helpful in determining the role of infarcts in the patient's dementia.

While cortical VaD is likely to be variable in its presentation, there are accruing data that subcortical cognitive impairment may be associated with a specific pattern of impairment allowing for some ability to differentiate from AD. There is relatively consistent agreement that executive functioning and processing speed are most affected by subcortical ischemic pathology (Jokinen *et al.*, 2006; Selnes and Vinters, 2006). For example, Prins and colleagues (2005) found that radiologically determined evidence of small-vessel disease was related to global cognition, but most specifically tests of processing speed and executive function. In a review of the literature, Libon and colleagues (2004) argued that many of the cognitive difficulties of these patients are an expression of weakness in the establishment and maintenance of a mental set. Other work has suggested a broader distribution of cognitive deficits, including visual spatial and semantic memory impairment, as well as episodic memory (Graham *et al.*, 2004).

Numerous studies have supported the common presence of episodic memory impairment in VaD. This may be an artifact of the diagnostic criteria used, which, as noted above, often define dementia with the necessity of memory impairment. Nonetheless, it does appear that white matter disease itself may be associated with an episodic memory impairment (Nordahl *et al.*, 2005), but it might be differentiated from that of AD based upon its pattern. A number of studies have supported the notion that the memory deficit of VaD is one of retrieval while that of AD is related to encoding and retention impairment. This is manifested on testing by both groups showing impairment on tests involving free recall, but patients with VaD showing less impairment on recognition memory tasks, often with close to normal performance (Tierney *et al.*, 2001). However, it should be noted that VaD may be associated, in some patients, with hippocampal CA1 neuronal loss (Chui *et al.*, 2006), which may produce a pattern of memory impairment similar to that of AD.

Perhaps the strongest insight into the nature of the cognitive profile of subcortical vascular cognitive impairment comes from the study of patients with CADASIL (see also p.47). As this population is younger than typical VaD patients, the possibility of a concomitant neurodegenerative process

clouding the link between the vascular pathology and the cognitive profile is limited. Such patients appear to have most prominent deficits in processing speed, executive function, and attention (Buffon *et al.*, 2006; Peters *et al.*, 2004). Nonetheless, more diffuse impairments are often seen in these patients as their cognitive deficits progress.

A practical approach for the clinical diagnosis of VaD

While we have outlined a number of the obstacles to the diagnosis of VaD, there are some cases when the diagnosis is relatively straightforward. Additionally, in cases where it is less clear, we have provided some clues to help the clinician better determine the role of CVD in the clinical presentation of VaD. As a general rule, one should have a relatively low threshold for considering that CVD may be playing some role, even if just modifying the expression of another neurodegenerative process such as AD (Lopez *et al.*, 2000a). The reason for this point is that reduction of vascular risk factors could be of benefit to such patients despite our inability to effectively alter the course of the neurodegenerative condition.

In general, cases with clear multiple clinical strokes and step-wise course are the easiest to detect and diagnose. These cases may be considered classic VaD. A straightforward scenario is when a patient presents with a clinical stroke followed by an abrupt change in cognition. Because subjects with strokes can improve over time, the determination of the cognitive deficits must be done after the acute phase of the vascular episode. Again, it is generally accepted that the cognitive deficits must occur within 3 months of the stroke to establish the causal nature of the vascular event. To qualify for dementia, these cognitive deficits would have to be severe enough to disrupt the patient's social and occupational functioning (APA, 1994). The diagnosis of dementia can be done at the bedside using global cognitive measures (e.g. Mini-Mental State Examination: Folstein *et al.*, 1975), but sometimes it will require detailed neuropsychological testing.

Conditions that make diagnosis of VaD difficult

Subcortical vascular cognitive impairment

Cases which are primarily due to subcortical disease without discrete clinical events are more difficult to clearly diagnose. These patients tend to have a more gradual course, making their differentiation from neurodegenerative processes difficult. Nonetheless, consideration of the above cognitive profile and neuroimaging establishing significant white matter disease can lead to appropriate classification. Given the role of the neuropsychological profile for diagnosis in such patients, more extensive testing is often helpful.

VaD and other disease processes

The most difficult aspect in the diagnosis of VaD is to separate the presence of an ongoing neurodegenerative disease (e.g. AD, Parkinsons's disease (PD)) from true VaD. The presence of VaD superimposed on a neurodegenerative process is not unusual. This is particularly important in the early stages of the neurodegenerative process when subjects with mild dementia can progress abruptly to a more severe stage. The family members have a tendency to report the onset of the symptoms at the time of the vascular event, although the dementia symptoms have already started. Table 3.1 shows the most salient cognitive differences among AD, VaD and PD.

Patients with PD or other neurodegenerative disorders that present with extrapyramidal signs (e.g. progressive supranuclear palsy, dementia with Lewy bodies, frontotemporal dementia, corticobasal degeneration) can have superimposed VaD. In addition, mild parkinsonism can be secondary to multiple subcortical infarcts and/or diffuse subcortical white matter disease (Binswanger's disease, or subcortical ischemic vascular dementia;

De Reuck *et al.*, 1980). A subcortical dementia and gait disturbance, characterized by apraxia and lower-body parkinsonism can occur in association with Binswanger's disease.

Normal pressure hydrocephalus (NPH) can be quite difficult to differentiate from subcortical VaD, as both involve pathology to similar deep white matter structures (Friedland, 1989). A similar cognitive profile and the presence of gait abnormalities and incontinence is common to both etiologies. Imaging may not clearly differentiate these conditions and a low threshold for an NPH work-up should be pursued for this potentially reversible cause of dementia. Other non-degenerative conditions include HIV dementia, multiple sclerosis with dementia, progressive multifocal leukoencephalopathy, and head trauma encephalopathy. History usually allows for differentiation of these conditions. An additional diagnostic consideration are less common etiologic conditions producing cerebrovascular disease, such as genetic conditions (e.g. CADASIL) and inflammatory causes (e.g. vasculitis).

VaD and aphasia

Subjects with aphasia are difficult to evaluate, since they usually have problems understanding how to complete simple neuropsychological tests that assess impairments in other cognitive areas (e.g. memory). Patients with transcortical sensory aphasia without other focal neurological signs can mimic the language deficits often seen in neurodegenerative disorders. This is a non-fluent aphasia that may develop from infarcts in the vascular border zone between the middle cerebral artery and posterior cerebral artery. These subjects can present with naming, reading, and writing deficits, with intact repetition, echolalia, and good comprehension.

Patients with aphasia can also present with behavioral and psychiatric problems that in and of themselves can disrupt the subjects' activities of daily living. Subjects with Wernicke's aphasia (apparent effortless speech, chaotic grammatical construction, paraphasias, unintelligible jargon) have difficulty understanding social and emotional

Table 3.1 Cognitive functions and behavioral abnormalities among subjects with Alzheimer's disease, vascular dementia, and Parkinson's disease.

	Alzheimer's disease	Vascular dementia	Parkinson's disease
Abstract thinking and reasoning	Could be normal in early stages. Always abnormal in moderate/severe stages. Unawareness of cognitive deficits	Could be normal	Could be normal
Executive functions	Abnormal, even in early stages. Slow cognitive flexibility	Generally abnormal. Reduced psychomotor speed. Poor initiative and cognitive flexibility	Poor planning and cognitive flexibility
Memory	Abnormal episodic and semantic memory. Encoding and retention deficits (free recall and recognition). Significant false positives and intrusions	Memory could be normal. Poor organizational retrieval strategies. Immediate and delayed recall can be equally impaired. Recognition > recall	Inconsistent recall. Recognition > recall. Poor spatial working memory, and spatial organization
Attention	May be normal in early stages. Always abnormal in moderate/severe stages	May be impaired, even in non-demented subjects	Generally impaired, even in non-demented subjects
Visuospatial and visuoconstructional functions	Copy better than spontaneous drawing (e.g. clock drawing). Borderline in early stages, and always impaired in moderate/severe stages	May be impaired, even in non-demented subjects	Generally impaired, even in non-demented subjects
Language	Impaired. Category fluency worse than letter, or supermarket items. Impaired confrontation naming	Could be normal. Different types of aphasia. Dysarthria, poor letter fluency, may have reduced naming skills	Poor comprehension with complex sentence structure. Borderline verbal fluency
Psychiatric symptoms	Apathy, depressed mood (major depression <15%), delusions and hallucinations, aggression, anxiety, agitation	Apathy, depressed mood (major depression: VaD> AD), mental and physical slowness. Psychotic symptoms and aggression are rare	Apathy, depressed mood (major depression: PD> VaD), mania, anxiety, vivid dreams, abnormal REM behavior, hallucinations, hypersexuality, agitation, aggression is rare

VaD: Vascular dementia; AD: Alzheimer's disease; PD: Parkinson's disease.

situations, and can develop agitation with delusional ideas. Furthermore, the presence of aphasia does not necessarily mean that the patient has VaD; although severe language can significantly disrupt the subject's functioning. These patients can have a relative preservation of the other cognitive abilities (e.g. memory) with minimal deterioration in their activities of daily living. The diagnosis of dementia in aphasic patients is usually done by reports from the informants, and not by formal cognitive testing.

VaD and depression

Patients with cerebrovascular accidents can develop post-stroke depression, especially if the infarcts are localized in the left frontal lobe (Starkstein *et al.*, 1988b). However, depression can be seen in subjects with supra- and infra-tentorial infarcts (Starkstein *et al.*, 1988a). These depressive symptoms can have significant motivational (apathy; Starkstein *et al.*, 1993) and mood-related components. These symptoms can worsen mild cognitive function associated with vascular disease, and lead the patients to frank dementia. The treatment of depression can ameliorate the cognitive symptoms. Strokes can also occur in subjects with depression, or with lifetime history of psychiatric illness (e.g. bipolar disorders), with the subsequent exacerbation of the psychiatric symptomatology, and new onset of cognitive deficits.

Focal neurological signs and symptoms

The presence of focal neurological signs and symptoms of abrupt onset are frequently associated with VaD and, obviously, support the diagnosis. The presence of hemiparesis, asymmetric deep tendon reflexes, Babinski sign, and gait abnormalities support the diagnosis of VaD. These signs and symptoms can have a parallel course to the cognitive deficits, either progressing in stepwise fashion or improving over time.

Ancillary studies

The work-up for VaD is somewhat different than that for AD. Usually, patients with VaD have suffered strokes, and they have had extensive blood, cardiovascular, and neuroimaging assessments. Nevertheless, neuroimaging is at the center of the diagnosis of VaD, and physicians should perform cognitive assessments and other laboratory tests to rule out the presence of other clinical disorders that may worsen the symptoms of VaD (e.g. hypothyroidism).

Neuroimaging

The MRI or CT scan of the brain are essential for the diagnosis of VaD (see also Chapter 5). The presence of a single or multiple infarcts that are thought to be etiologically related to the cognitive disturbance is critical for the diagnosis of VaD (APA, 1994). These neuroimaging findings usually correlate with a clinical event that marked the onset of VaD. However, multiple infarcts in cortical or subcortical areas, not related to a specific vascular event, or severe white matter disease, can also support the diagnosis of VaD.

These neuroimaging studies also serve to clarify the etiology of dementia in subjects whose symptoms appeared abruptly, according to the informants (sudden recognition vs. sudden onset). Positron emission tomography (PET) and single photon computerized tomography (SPECT) can be useful to identify a neurodegenerative pattern (e.g. temporoparietal hypoperfusion) in a context of vascular disease, where we expect patchy damage, or hypoperfusion circumscribed to a specific vascular territory (see also Chapter 6).

Laboratory studies

Other studies of value in the work-up include serological tests for so-called reversible causes of dementia, such as vitamin B-12 level and thyroid function testing. The utility of checking a homocysteine level and treatment if elevated remains controversial despite the relationship of this marker with stroke and white matter disease (Hogervorst *et al.*, 2002; McMahon *et al.*, 2006; Parnetti *et al.*, 1997). Tests for evidence of systemic vascular disease, such as electrocardiogram, or echocardiogram are useful to determine the possible sources of emboli. Carotid Doppler images should be obtained in patients with large-vessel events. Work-up for other causes of CVD, including coagulation and inflammatory markers, should be dictated by the history. Tests for the possibility of diabetes mellitus, such as a hemoglobin A1C, may be of value. Genetic testing and muscle or skin

Table 3.2 Frequently reported risk factors for vascular dementia in population studies.

Authors	Constitutional factors	Cardiovascular risk factors	CVD	APOE-4
Ross *et al.* (1997)	Age	Coronary artery disease Post-prandial glucose level		N/E
Luchsinger *et al.* (2001)		Diabetes mellitus		N/E
Posner *et al.* (2002)		Hypertension, hypertension + heart disease		N/E
Hebert *et al.* (2000)	Age	Diabetes mellitus, hypertension for women, heart disease for men,		S
Tatemichi *et al.* (1993)	Age, education, race	Diabetes mellitus		N/E
Desmond *et al.* (2000)	Age, education, race	Diabetes mellitus	Previous stroke	N/E
Kuller *et al.* (2003)*	Age		Prior stroke, cerebral ventricular size, white matter lesions	NS
Barba *et al.* (2000)	Age	Atrial fibrillation	Previous stroke	NS
Lindsay *et al.* (1997)		Hypertension, heart disease		N/E

N/E: not examined; S: significant association, NS: not associated.

* Clinical and radiological factors present 4–5 years before the diagnosis of VaD.

biopsy for CADASIL is reasonable in the appropriate context. Finally, a lumbar puncture may be of added value in at least two incidences. First, a lumbar puncture or lumbar drain may be critical in differentiating VaD from NPH. Second, the measurement of Aβ and tau may allow for assessment of the potential contribution of AD to the clinical picture (Galasko *et al.*, 1998).

Risk factors

Risk factors can be used to support the diagnosis of VaD. Constitutional (e.g. age, education level, race) and cerebrovascular risk factors and previous strokes have been associated with the presence of VaD. Table 3.2 shows the risk factors for VaD identified in population studies. Although the majority of the studies agreed that cerebrovascular factors were associated with the development of VaD, diabetes

mellitus appears to be the strongest risk factor. Neuroradiological factors associated with the presence of VaD were left hemisphere strokes, anterior and posterior cerebral arteries territories versus other vascular territories, and large-artery atherosclerosis (Desmond *et al.*, 2000). Studies that examined the radiological features that precede the diagnosis of VaD in approximately 4–5 years found that cerebral ventricular volume and white matter lesions were associated with VaD (Kuller *et al.*, 2003, 2005). Furthermore, VaD increases the risk of stroke recurrence (Moroney *et al.*, 1997), and death (Aguerro-Torres *et al.*, 1998; Freels *et al.*, 2002; Molsa *et al.*, 1995; Tatemichi et al., 1994). The APOE 4 allele has been found elevated in younger (i.e. <65) patients with VaD, and AD with CVD compared to non-demented individuals (Isoe *et al.*, 1996; Myers *et al.*, 1996; Slooter *et al.*, 1997). However, studies conducted in older individuals (>70 years) have not found an association between VaD and the APOE 4 allele (Stengard *et al.*, 1995). Furthermore, there have been no associations between angiotensin-converting enzyme genotypes and VaD (Barba *et al.*, 2000), and the association between the sortilin-related receptor SORL1 genotypes and VaD has not been explored yet (Rogaeva *et al.*, 2007). Inheritable variants in the SORL1 neuronal sorting receptor have been found to be associated with late-onset AD.

Comments

Although clinicians have been aware that CVD can lead to cognitive deficits for several centuries, the clinical diagnosis of VaD is still difficult. The critical factors about the diagnosis of VaD are centered on two issues: the presence of dementia, and determination of vascular disease. Whether the dementia syndrome is secondary to a "pure" vascular pathology or to an underlying neuro-degenerative process associated with vascular disease is difficult to determine. In addition, patients with strokes can develop a wide variety of abnormal behaviors and motor deficits, which can affect their normal functioning, although they can have a relative preservation of their cognitive functions. Therefore, detailed clinical, laboratory, neuro-imaging, and neuropsychological assessments are necessary for the accurate diagnosis of VaD.

ACKNOWLEDGMENTS

This work was funded, in part, by Grants AG20098, AG028018, and AG05133 from the National Institute on Aging.

REFERENCES

Aguerro-Torres H, Fratiglioni L, Guo A, Viitanen M, Winblad B. Prognostic factors in very old demented adults: a seven-year follow-up from a population-based survey in Stockholm. *J Am Geriatr Soc* 1998; **46**: 444–52.

American Psychiatric Association (APA). *DSM-IV: Diagnostic and Statistic Manual of Mental Disorders*, Fourth Edition. Washington, D.C.; American Psychiatric Association, 1994.

Attems J, Jellinger KA. Only cerebral capillary amyloid angiography correlates with Alzheimer pathology – a pilot study. *Acta Neuropathol* 2004; **107**: 83–90.

Barba R, Martinez-Espinosa S, Rodriguez-Garcia E, Pondal M, Vivancos J, Del Ser T. Poststroke dementia. Clinical features and risk factors. *Stroke* 2000; **31**: 1494–501.

Benson DF, Cummings JL, Tsai SY. Angular gyrus syndrome simulating Alzheimer's disease. *Arch Neurol* 1982; **39**: 616–20.

Bogousslavsky J, Bernasconi A, Kumral E. Acute multiple infarction involving the anterior circulation. *Arch Neurol* 1996; **53**: 50–7.

Boiten J, Lodder J. Large striatocapsular infarcts: clinical presentation and pathogenesis in comparison with lacunar and cortical infarcts. *Acta Neurol Scand* 1992; **86**: 298–303.

Buffon F, Porcher R, Hernandez K, *et al*. Cognitive profile in CADASIL. *J Neurol Neurosurg Psychiatry* 2006; **77**: 175–80.

Chui HC, Mack W, Jackson JE, *et al*. Clinical criteria for the diagnosis of vascular dementia. *Arch Neurol* 2000; **57**: 191–6.

Chui HC, Victoroff JI, Margolin D, Jagust W, Shankle R, Katzman R. Criteria for the diagnosis of ischemic vascular dementia proposed by the State of California Alzheimer's Disease Diagnostic and Treatment Centers. *Neurology* 1992; **42**: 473–80.

Chui HC, Zarow C, Mack WJ, *et al*. Cognitive impact of subcortical vascular and Alzheimer's disease pathology. *Ann Neurol* 2006; **60**: 677–87.

Cordoliani-Mackowiak M-A, Henon H, Pruvo J-P, Pasquier F, Leys D. Poststroke dementia: the influence of hippocampal atrophy. *Arch Neurol* 2003; **60**: 585–90.

Damasio AR, Damasio H. The anatomic basis of pure alexia. *Neurology* 1983; **33**: 1573–83.

Damasio AR, Eslinger PJ, Damasio H, Van Hoesen GW, Cornell S. Multimodal amnesic syndrome following bilateral temporal and basal forebrain damage. *Arch Neurol* 1985; **42**: 252–9.

de Groot JC, de Leeuw FE, Oudkerk M, *et al*. Cerebral white matter lesions and cognitive function: the Rotterdam Scan Study. *Ann Neurol* 2000; **47**: 145–51.

De Reuck J, Crevits L, De Coster W, Sieben G, and van der Ecken H. Pathogenesis of Binswanger chronic progressive subcortical encephalopathy. *Neurology* 1980; **30**: 920–8.

del Ser T, Bermejo F, Portera A, Arredondo JM, Bouras C, Constantinidis J. Vascular dementia. A clinicopathological study. *J Neurol Sci* 1990; **96**: 1–17.

Desmond DW, Moroney JT, Paik MC, *et al.* Frequency and clinical determinants of dementia after ischemic stroke. *Neurology* 2000; **54**: 1124–31.

Erkinjunnti T, Inzitari D, Pantoni L, *et al.* Research criteria for subcortical vascular dementia in clinical trials. *J Neural Transm (Suppl)* 2000; **59**: 23–30.

Esiri MM, Wilcock GK, Morris JH. Neuropathological assessment of the lesions of significance in vascular dementia. *J Neurol Neurosurg Psychiatry* 1997; **63**: 749–53.

Folstein MF, Folstein SE, McHugh PR. Mini-mental state: a practical method grading the cognitive state of patients for the clinician. *J Psychiatr Res* 1975; **12**: 189–98.

Freels S, Nyenhuis DL, Gorelick PE. Predictors of survival in African American patients with AD, VaD, or stroke without dementia. *Neurology* 2002; **59**: 1146–53.

Friedland RP. "Normal'-pressure hydrocephalus and the saga of the treatable dementias. *JAMA* 1989; **262**: 2577–93.

Galasko D, Chang L, Motter R, *et al.* High cerebrospinal fluid tau and low amyloid B42 levels in the clinical diagnosis of Alzheimer disease and relation to apolipoprotein E genotype. *Arch Neurol* 1998; **55**: 937–45.

Galasko D, Hansen LA, Katzman R. Clinical–neuropathological correlations in Alzheimer's disease and related dementias. *Arch Neurol* 1994; **51**: 888–95.

Gold G, Bouras C, Canuto A, *et al.* Clinicopathological validation study of four sets of clinical criteria for vascular dementia. *Am J Psychiatry* 2002; **159**: 82–7.

Graff-Radford NR, Eslinger PJ, Damasio AR, Yamada T. Nonhemorrhagic infarction of the thalamus: Behavioral, anatomic, and physiologic correlates. *Neurology* 1984; **34**: 14–23.

Graham NL, Emery T, Hodges JR. Distinctive cognitive profiles in Alzheimer's disease and subcortical vascular dementia. *J Neurol Neurosurg Psychiatry* 2004; **75**: 61–71.

Groves WC, Brandt J, Steinberg M, *et al.* Vascular dementia and Alzheimer's disease: is there a difference? A comparison of symptoms by disease duration. *J Neuropsychiatry Clin Neurosci* 2000; **12**: 305–15.

Hachinski VC, Lassen NA. Multi-infarct dementia. A cause of mental deterioration in the elderly. *Lancet* 1974; **2**: 207–10.

Hebert R, Lindsay J, Varreault R, Rockwood K, Hill G, Dubois M-F. Vascular dementia: Incidence and risk factor in the Canadian study of Health and Aging. *Stroke* 2000; **31**: 1487–93.

Henon H, Durieu I, Guerouaou D, Lebert FFP, Leys D. Poststroke dementia: incidence and relationship to prestroke cognitive decline. *Neurology* 2001; **57**: 1216–22.

Hogervorst E, Bandelow S, Combrinck M, Irani S, Smith AD. The validity and reliability of 6 sets of clinical criteria to classify Alzheimer's disease and vascular dementia in cases confirmed post-mortem: added value of a decision tree approach. *Dement Geriatr Cogn Disord* 2003; **16**: 170–80.

Hogervorst E, Ribeiro HM, Molyneux A, Budge M, Smith AD. Plasma homocysteine levels, cerebrovascular risk factors, and cerebral white matter changes (leukoaraiosis) in patients with Alzheimer's disease. *Arch Neurol* 2002; **59**: 787–93.

Holmes C, Cairns N, Lantos P, Mann A. Validity of current clinical criteria for Alzheimer's disease, vascular dementia, and dementia with Lewy bodies. *Br J Psychiatry* 1999; **174**: 45–50.

Hulette C, Nochlin D, McKeel DW, *et al.* Clinical–neuropathologic findings in multi-infarct dementia: a report of six autopsied cases. *Neurology* 1997; **48**: 668–72.

Isoe K, Urikami K, Sato K, Takahashi K. Apolipoprotein E in patients with dementia of the Alzheimer type and vascular dementia. *Acta Neurol Scand* 1996; **93**: 133–7.

Jokinen H, Kalska H, Mantyla R, *et al.* Cognitive profile of subcortical ischaemic vascular disease. *J Neurol Neurosurg Psychiatry* 2006; **77**: 28–33.

Katz DI, Alexander MP, Mandell AM. Dementia following strokes in the mesencephalon and diencephalon. *Arch Neurol* 1987; **44**: 1127–33.

Knopman DS, Parisi JF, Boeve BF, *et al.* Vascular dementia in a population-based autopsy study. *Arch Neurol* 2003; **60**: 569–75.

Knopman DS, Rocca WA, Cha RH, Edland SD, Kokmen E. Incidence of vascular dementia in Rochester, Minn, 1985–1989. *Arch Neurol* 2002; **59**: 1605–10.

Kuller LH, Lopez OL, Jagust WJ, *et al.* Determinants of vascular dementia in the Cardiovascular Health Cognition Study. *Neurology* 2005; **64**: 1548–52.

Kuller LH, Lopez OL, Newman A, *et al.* Risk factors for dementia in the cardiovascular health cognition study. *Neuroepidemiology* 2003; **22**: 13–22.

Kumral E, Evyapan D, Balkir D, Kutluhan S. Bilateral thalamic infarction: Clinical, etiological and MRI correlates. *Acta Neurol Scand* 2001; **103**: 35–42.

Kumral E, Evyapan D, Balkir K. Acute caudate vascular lesions. *Stroke* 1999; **30**: 100–08.

Libon DJ, Price CC, Davis GK, Giovannetti T. From Binswanger's disease to leukoaraiosis: what we have learned about subcortical vascular disease. *Clin Neuropsychol* 2004; **18**: 83–100.

Lindsay J, Hebert R, Rockwood K. The Canadian Study of Health and Aging: risk factors for vascular dementia. *Stroke* 1997; **28**: 526–30.

Liu CK, Miller BL, Cummings JL, *et al.* A quantitative MRI study of vascular dementia. *Neurology* 1992; **42**: 138–43.

Lopez OL, Becker JT, Klunk W, *et al.* Research evaluation and diagnosis of possible Alzheimer's disease over the last two decades: II. *Neurology* 2000a; **55**: 1863–9.

Lopez OL, Becker JT, Klunk W, *et al.* Research evaluation and diagnosis of probable Alzheimer's disease over the last two decades: I. *Neurology* 2000b; **55**: 1854–62.

Lopez OL, Claassen D. Cerebral amyloid angiopathy in Alzheimer's disease: clinicopathological correlations. *Dementia* 1991; **2**: 285–90.

Lopez OL, Kuller LH, Becker JT, *et al.* Classification of vascular dementia in the Cardiovascular Health Study cognition study. *Neurobiology* 2005; **64**: 1531–47.

Lopez OL, Kuller LH, Fitzpatrick A, Ives D, Becker JT, Beauchamp N. Evaluations of dementia in the cardiovascular health cognition study. *Neuroepidemiology* 2003; **22**: 1–12.

Lopez OL, Larumbe MR, Becker JT, *et al.* Reliability of NINDS-AIREN criteria for vascular dementia. *Neurology* 1994; **44**: 1240–45.

Luchsinger JA, Tang M-X, Stern Y, Shea S, Mayeux R. *Am J Epidemiol* 2001; **154**: 635–41.

McMahon JA, Green TJ, Skeaff CM, Knight RG, Mann JI, Williams SM. A controlled trial of homocysteine lowering and cognitive performance. *N Engl J Med* 2006; **354**: 2764–72.

Min WK, Park KK, and Kim YS. Atherothrombotic middle cerebral artery territory infarction: topography diversity with common occurrence of concomitant small cortical and subcortical infarcts. *Stroke* 2000; **31**: 2055–61.

Molsa PK, Marttila RJ, Rinne UK. Long-term survival and predictors of mortality in Alzheimer's disease and multi-infarct dementia. *Arch Neurol Scand* 1995; **91**: 159–64.

Moroney JT, Bagiella E, Tatemichi TK, Paik MC, Stern Y, Desmond DW. Dementia after stroke increases the risk of long-term stroke recurrence. *Neurology* 1997; **48**: 1317–25.

Myers RH, Schaefer EJ, Wilson PWF, *et al.* Apolipoprotein E e4 association with dementia in a population-based study: the Framingham Study. *Neurology* 1996; **46**: 673–7.

Nordahl CW, Ranganath C, Yonelinas AP, DeCarli C, Reed BR, Jagust WJ. Different mechanisms of episodic memory failure in mild cognitive impairment. *Neuropsychologia* 2005; **43**: 1688–97.

Ott BR, Saver JL. Unilateral amnesic stroke. Six new cases and a review of the literature. *Stroke* 1993; **24**: 1033–42.

Parnetti L, Bottiglieri T, Lowenthal D. Role of homocysteine in age-related vascular and non-vascular diseases. *Aging (Milano)* 1997; **9**: 241–57.

Peters N, Herzog J, Opherk C, Dichgans M. A two-year clinical follow-up study in 80 CADASIL subjects. *Stroke* 2004; **35**: 1603–08.

Petrovitch H, Ross GW, Steinborn SC, *et al.* AD lesions and infarcts in demented and non-demented Japanese-American men. *Ann Neurol* 2005; **57**: 98–103.

Pfeifer LA, White LR, Ross GW, Petrovitch H, Launer LJ. Cerebral amyloid angiopathy and cognitive function: The HAAS autopsy study. *Neurology* 2002; **58**: 1629–34.

Pohjasvaara T, Mantyla R, Salonen O, *et al.* How complex interactions of ischemic brain infarcts, white matter lesions, and atrophy relate to poststroke dementia. *Arch Neurol* 2000; **57**: 1295–300.

Pohjasvaara T, Ritta M, Ylikoski R, Markku K, Erkinjuntti T. Clinical features of MRI-defined subcortical vascular disease. *Alzheimer Dis Assoc Disord* 2003; **17**: 236–42.

Posner HB, Tang M-X, Luchsinger J, Lantigua R, Mayeux R. The relationship of hypertension in the elderly to AD, vascular dementia, and cognitive function. *Neurology* 2002; **58**: 1175–81.

Prins N, van Dijk E, den Heijer T, *et al.* Cerebral small-vessel disease and decline in information processing speed, executive function, and memory. *Brain* 2005; **128**: 2034–41.

Prins N, van Dijk E, den Heijer T, Vermeer S, Koudtsal P, Oudkerk M. Cerebral white matter lesions and the risk of dementia. *Arch Neurol* 2004; **61**: 1503–04.

Reed BR, Eberling JL, Mungas D, Weiner M, Jagust WJ. Effects of white matter lesions and lacunes on cortical function. *Arch Neurol* 2004a; **58**: 545–50.

Reed BR, Mungas DM, Kramer JH, *et al.* Clinical and neuropsychological features in autopsy-defined vascular dementia. *Clin Neuropsychol* 2004b; **18**: 63–74.

Rogaeva E, Meng Y, Lee JH, *et al.* The neuronal sortilin-related receptor SORLI is genetically associated with Alzheimer Disease. *Nature Genetics* 2007; **39**: 168–77.

Roman GC. From UBOs to Binswanger's disease: impact of magnetic resonance imaging on vascular dementia research. *Stroke* 1996; **27**: 1269–73.

Roman GC, Tatemichi TK, Erkinjuntti T, *et al.* Vascular dementia: diagnostic criteria for research studies: report of the NINDS-AIREN International Workshop. *Neurology* 1993; **43**: 250–60.

Ross GW, Petrovich H, White LR, *et al.* Characterization of risk factors for vascular dementia: the Honolulu-Asia Aging Study. *Neurology* 1993; **53**: 337–43.

Schneider JA, Wilson RS, Cochran EJ, *et al.* Relation of cerebral infarctions to dementia and cognitive function in older persons. *Neurology* 2003; **60**: 1082–88.

Selnes OA, Vinters HV. Vascular cognitive impairment. *Nat Clin Pract Neurol* 2006; **2**: 538–47.

Slooter AJC, Tang M, van Dujin CM, *et al.* Apolipoprotein E epsilon4 and the risk of dementia with stroke: a population based investigation. *JAMA* 1997; **277**: 818–21.

Snowdon DA, Grainer LH, Mortimer JA, Riley KP, Grainer PA, Markesbery WR. Brain infarction and the clinical expression of Alzheimer disease: the nun study. *JAMA* 1997; **277**: 813–17.

Starkstein SE, Robinson RG, Berthier ML, Price TR. Depressive disorders following posterior circulation as compared with middle cerebral artery infarcts. *Brain* 1988a; **111**: 375–87.

Starkstein SE, Robinson RG, Price TR. Comparison of patients with and without poststroke major depression matched for size and location of lesion. *Arch Gen Psychiat* 1988b; **45**: 247–52.

Starkstein SE, Federoff JP, Price TR, Leiguarda R, Robinson RG. Apathy following cerebrovascular lesions. *Stroke* 1993; **24**: 1625–30.

Stengard JH, Pekkanen J, Sulkava R, Ehnholm C, Erkinjuntti T. Apolipoprotein E polymorphism, Alzheimer's disease and vascular dementia among elderly Finnish men. *Acta Neurol Scand* 1995; **92**: 297–8.

Tatemichi TK, Desmond DW, Mayeux R, *et al.* Dementia after stroke: baseline frequency, risks, and clinical features in a hospitalized cohort. *Neurology* 1992a; **42**: 1185–93.

Tatemichi TK, Desmond DW, Stern Y, Paik M, Bagiella E. Cognitive impairment after stroke: frequency, patterns, and relationship to functional abilities. *J Neurol Neurosurg Psychiatry* 1994; **57**: 202–07.

Tatemichi TK, Steinke W, Duncan C, *et al.* Paramedian thalamopeduncular infarction: clinical syndromes and magnetic resonance imaging. *Ann Neurol* 1992b; **32**: 162–71.

Tierney MC, Black SE, Szalai JP, *et al.* Recognition memory and verbal fluency differentiate probable Alzheimer disease from subcortical ischemic vascular dementia. *Arch Neurol* 2001; **58**: 1654–9.

Tomlinson BE, Blessed G, Roth M. Observations on the brain of demented old people. *J Neurol Sci* 1970; **11**: 205–42.

van Straaten ECW, Schelters P, Knol DL, *et al.* Operational definitions for the NINDS-AIREN criteria for vascular dementia. *Stroke* 2003; **34**: 1907–16.

Verhey FR, Lodder J, Rozendaal N, Jolles L. Comparison of seven sets of criteria used for the diagnosis of vascular dementia. *Neuroepidemiology* 1996; **15**: 166–72.

Vermeer SE, Prins ND, den Heijer T, Hofman A, Koudstaal PJ, Breteler MMB. Silent brain infarcts and the risk of dementia and cognitive decline. *N Engl J Med* 2003; **348**: 1215–22.

World Health Organization. *The ICD-10 Classification of Mental and Behavioral Disorders: Diagnostic Criteria for Research.* Geneva WHO, 1993.

Willis T. *The London Practice of Physick.* London, Dring Harper & Leigh, 1984.

Zekry D, Duyckaerts C, Belmin J, *et al.* The vascular lesions in vascular and mixed dementia: the weight of functional neuroanatomy. *Neurobiol Aging* 2003; **24**: 213–19.

4

Cognitive functioning in vascular dementia before and after diagnosis

Erika J. Laukka, Sari Karlsson, Stuart W. S. MacDonald and Lars Bäckman

Introduction

Describing cognitive functioning in vascular dementia (VaD) is a non-trivial task, as VaD encompasses a range of brain changes that may affect cognition in various ways. The cognitive profile of VaD patients is not homogenous, but depends on the VaD subtype and regions of the brain affected. In addition, individuals identified as belonging to the VaD group may differ as a function of the diagnostic criteria employed.

The possible origins of cognitive impairment in VaD are numerous as cognitive deficits may reflect multiple infarcts, a single strategic infarction, white matter lesions (WML), and co-morbid illness (e.g. depression, physical illness). In addition, brain atrophy due to co-existing Alzheimer's disease (AD) pathology may influence the extent and type of cognitive impairment. This review will focus primarily on cognitive functioning in multi-infarct dementia (MID) and subcortical (small-vessel disease) VaD, the most extensively studied subtypes.

Cognition in clinical VaD

Multi-infarct dementia versus subcortical VaD

Multi-infarct dementia

For many years, MID (Hachinski *et al.*, 1974) was the predominant focus of research on VaD. The traditional view of MID is that multiple completed thromboembolic infarctions cause a stereotypically step-wise course of cognitive decline and dementia. Although infarctions can occur both in cortical and subcortical areas, most investigators consider MID to be primarily a result of cortical damage (Desmond, 2004). The cognitive profile in MID is characterized by a patchy pattern of cognitive deficits, thought to reflect the location, size, and number of brain infarcts. Unlike the cognitive impairment seen in AD, there is no common pathway; rather, the pattern and progression of cognitive deficits can be very different from one patient to another. MID patients also exhibit fluctuations in cognitive performance more frequently than AD patients.

The course of cognitive decline in patients with AD is characterized by an insidious onset and a gradual progressive worsening of cognitive functioning. By contrast, the clinical picture in MID is often described as an acute onset of cognitive impairment followed by a step-wise worsening of symptoms, as recurrent strokes cause changes in the patient's level of functioning. After each drop, the cognitive decline reaches a plateau, with the potential for partial recovery of function after each stroke. However, an insidious onset and a gradually progressive course of decline have been found to occur in patients with MID (Fischer *et al.*, 1990). Gradual progression in MID may be due to clinically silent recurrent strokes, cerebral hypoxia or ischemia, and concomitant AD (Desmond, 1999).

Vascular Cognitive Impairment in Clinical Practice, ed. Lars-Olof Wahlund, Timo Erkinjuntti and Serge Gauthier. Published by Cambridge University Press. © Cambridge University Press 2009.

Subcortical VaD

With more extensive use of neuroimaging in dementia diagnosis, attention has shifted from MID toward subcortical VaD. Subcortical VaD results from small-vessel disease, which produces complete infarctions (lacunes and microinfarcts) in subcortical areas or widespread incomplete infarctions in deep cerebral white matter. The patient is characterized by motor and cognitive slowing, forgetfulness, dysarthria, mood changes, urinary symptoms, and short-stepped gait (Roman *et al.*, 2002).

The onset of cognitive symptoms in subcortical VaD is insidious, mimicking the typical course in AD. In many cases, patients with subcortical VaD experience a series of lacunar infarcts resulting in increased cognitive deficits, with each event followed by a slight improvement. However, compared to MID, the temporal relationship between evidence of brain lesions and cognitive deficits is less clear.

An important difference in the manifestation of subcortical VaD compared to MID is the effect of a single infarct on cognition. Whereas the effect of a cortical infarct in MID is restricted to the region of infarction, a strategically located subcortical infarct can have clinical effects remote from and disproportionate to its location and size due to the metabolic abnormalities that may result from pathway disruption (Desmond, 2004).

CADASIL

Cerebral autosomal dominant arteriopathy with subcortical infarcts and leukoencephalopathy (CADASIL) is an inherited small-vessel disease caused by mutation of the NOTCH3 gene on chromosome 19. Clinical symptoms typically emerge in early or middle adulthood with migraine or an ischemic event (e.g. Chabriat *et al.*, 1995). Later, it manifests itself through recurrent subcortical ischemic strokes leading to step-wise or progressive decline and a dementia syndrome with frontal lobe features. Magnetic resonance imaging (MRI) reveals a combination of small lacunar lesions and diffuse white matter abnormalities.

CADASIL has been put forward as a model of pure subcortical ischemic VaD. A common problem when performing clinical trials on patients with VaD is the frequently coexisting AD pathology. As the onset of dementia in CADASIL occurs relatively early, such confounding is less likely. The cognitive profile of CADASIL has been found to be very similar to that presented by patients with subcortical ischemic VaD, at least when a stroke has occurred in the CADASIL patients (Charlton *et al.*, 2006). In particular, both subcortical VaD patients and CADASIL patients were impaired on tasks measuring executive function and speed (Trails Switching test, Trails Motor Speed test, and verbal fluency). Both groups also showed impairment on tasks assessing episodic memory function, although this impairment was less pronounced (Charlton *et al.*, 2006). Findings from a study using Diffusion Tensor Imaging (DTI), an MRI technique sensitive to small changes in the integrity of cerebral tissue, suggest that executive dysfunction in CADASIL is due to damage to executive networks in the white matter (O'Sullivan *et al.*, 2005).

Frontal-executive function and episodic memory are two cognitive domains frequently assessed when trying to discriminate between VaD and other dementia types, and between different VaD subtypes. The following two sections will describe these domains in more detail, as well as their manifestation in VaD.

Frontal-executive function

Frontal-executive function is a summary term for processes that are sensitive to frontal-lobe damage and involve the control and regulation of cognitive activities. The adjectives "frontal" and "executive" are often used interchangeably, although there is no conclusive definition of these terms. Factor-analytic work has demonstrated the existence of three correlated but clearly separable executive functions: shifting (the ability to shift between tasks and mental sets), updating (the ability to update and monitor information), and inhibition (the ability to inhibit dominant responses; Miyake *et al.*, 2000).

Impaired frontal-executive function is often described as the primary cognitive syndrome in VaD. Patients show difficulties on tasks that involve planning and sequencing, speed of processing, attention, as well as on tasks that lack an inherent structure (Desmond, 2004). However, this pattern may not apply to all patients with VaD. For patients with MID, the type of cognitive impairment is dependent on the location of the lesions. Unless a MID patient has a frontal-lobe lesion, executive dysfunction should not dominate the clinical picture. Frontal-executive dysfunction may, however, be the most prominent type of cognitive impairment in subcortical VaD, as the lacunar infarcts in this subtype often occur in structures and connecting pathways of frontal–subcortical circuits that mediate executive function (Cummings, 1993). Cognitive functions depending on a circuit of connections are vulnerable, as lesions at any point may influence the integrity of the entire circuit. A study investigating cognitive functioning in subcortical ischemic vascular disease found that, although this group showed some impairment on episodic recall tasks, the largest impairment was seen on tasks measuring executive functioning (Stroop interference, card sorting; Kramer *et al.*, 2002).

Episodic memory

Episodic memory involves the conscious retrieval of information acquired at a certain time in a certain place (e.g. to recall what you had for lunch two days ago; Tulving, 2002). In the laboratory, episodic memory is typically assessed by having the participant recall or recognize some information (e.g. a list of words) acquired in the experimental setting.

Episodic memory impairment is considered to be the cardinal feature of AD. However, episodic memory is frequently impaired in VaD too. The memory impairment in VaD may have several different origins, such as concomitant AD, medial–temporal lobe infarction, and WML. Studies have shown that WML affect most cognitive domains,

including memory (e.g. de Groot *et al.*, 2000). Which cognitive domain is affected depends on the location and distribution of the WML. For example, memory impairment has been associated with the volume of temporal WML (Burton *et al.*, 2004).

Memory impairment may also be secondary to an existing frontal-executive dysfunction. Most complex tasks require the involvement of several cognitive functions and impaired frontal-executive functioning is likely to affect performance on tasks assessing episodic memory functioning. In addition, the relationship between brain changes and behavioral outcome is complex, making it possible for the same underlying pathology to cause impairment in more than one domain. Analogously, different types of brain pathologies may cause the same type of cognitive impairment. Episodic remembering draws on a large distributed network, including both prefrontal and medial–temporal regions (Cabeza and Nyberg, 2000). Alterations at any location in this network may cause episodic memory impairment. To illustrate, a study comparing AD and subcortical stroke observed a double dissociation between memory dysfunction and regional glucose metabolic activity. Whereas performance on an episodic memory task correlated with left-hippocampal and middle-temporal gyrus metabolism in AD patients, it correlated with prefrontal lobe metabolism in patients with subcortical stroke (Reed *et al.*, 2000). Thus, the same cognitive deficit may have different neurological underpinnings depending on the etiology of the disorder.

VaD versus AD

One of the challenges in clinical practice is to separate between VaD and other dementia types, most often AD. Making a correct differential diagnosis may be critical for tailoring the most effective intervention and for informing patients about their prognosis. For example, different pharmaceutical strategies may differentially modify the course of these diseases. Many studies have compared cognitive functioning in clinical VaD and AD, with divergent results. In a comprehensive review (Sachdev and Looi, 2003), research regarding this issue published before December 2000 was summarized. It was found that, for similar levels of cognitive deficit, VaD patients were more likely to have relative preservation of verbal episodic memory and greater deficits in frontal-executive functioning compared to AD patients. The VaD patients were also inferior in motor function, although few studies had examined this domain. In the other cognitive domains examined, the majority of studies showed no significant differences between the groups (language, attention, conceptual function, arithmetic function, constructional abilities, working memory and concentration, and visual perception), or there was insufficient evidence to draw any conclusions (intelligence, non-verbal episodic memory, orientation, and tactile perception).

Of totally 21 studies on verbal episodic memory, 14 showed superior performance for the VaD patients and only one showed an advantage for the AD patients. Memory tests in which the VaD patients did better included story recall, the California Verbal Learning Test (lower rates of false positives and intrusions, better overall performance), the Rey Auditory Verbal Learning Test (better overall performance, slower forgetting rate), and the Fuld Retrieval Test. Of nine studies investigating differences in frontal-executive tasks, eight showed inferior performance for the VaD patients. Examples of tasks where VaD patients performed poorer included the Porteus maze, Graphical Sequence Test, and Wisconsin Card Sorting Test (Sachdev and Looi, 2003).

Verbal fluency taxes processes such as initiation of behavior in response to a novel request, cognitive speed, and generation of efficient search strategies. Therefore, it is often regarded as a frontal-executive task. However, in the Sachdev and Looi review (2003), verbal fluency was classified as a language task. No differences in verbal fluency were found between VaD and AD patients. Nor were there any group differences in working memory and attention, two cognitive processes

drawing heavily on frontal regions (Cabeza and Nyberg, 2000). This lack of difference might reflect a frontal involvement in AD as well. Previous studies have shown that brain changes in the earliest stages of AD are not limited to the medial–temporal lobe, and that frontal-executive deficits are prominent already during the prodromal period (Bäckman *et al.*, 2005).

The observed differences in cognitive performance between VaD and AD may be explained by the different etiologies of these two disorders. In AD, medial–temporal lobe structures, such as the entorhinal cortex and hippocampus, are the first to be affected. These structures are known to be vital to episodic memory functioning (Squire and Zola, 1996). Consequently, early memory impairment is regarded as the cardinal feature of AD, although most cognitive functions are affected later in the dementia process. In VaD, the pathology is more heterogeneous, involving angiopathy, hemorrhage, microscopic and macroscopic infarctions, and white matter disease. However, the cognitive manifestations of subcortical VaD is believed to be more homogeneous than that of MID and primarily associated with frontal-executive dysfunction. The entorhinal cortex and hippocampus may be affected in subcortical VaD, but to a lesser extent than in AD (Du *et al.*, 2002). Instead, there are often lesions in structures and connecting pathways that comprise the dorso-lateral prefrontal circuit. This circuit consists of neuronal connections from prefrontal cortex via basal ganglia to the thalamus, with feedback from the thalamus to the prefrontal cortex (Cummings, 1993). Frontal-executive dysfunction can occur due to damage to any part of the circuit. Evidence from neuroimaging studies suggests that both frontal and total WML volume is associated with poorer executive function (Tullberg *et al.*, 2004) as well as with poorer attention and speed (Burton *et al.*, 2004). In addition, VaD patients with frontal lesions have been found to perform worse on tasks of executive function (e.g. Porteus maze) compared to non-frontal VaD patients (Villardita, 1993).

Possible explanations for the conflicting results from studies comparing cognitive functioning in VaD and AD are that differently recruited samples have been used in these comparisons, as well as divergent diagnostic criteria for VaD. Variability in choice of cognitive tasks and matching procedures for severity of dementia might also have contributed to the mixed findings. For example, three recent studies yielded quite divergent results regarding differences in executive functioning between VaD and AD. All three studies included at least one task taxing frontal-lobe integrity (verbal fluency or Trail Making–B) but used different diagnostic criteria for VaD (Hachinski Ischemic Score [HIS], ICD-10, the National Institute of Neurological Disorders and Stroke [NINDS] and Association Internationale pour la Recherche et l'Enseignement en Neurosciences [AIREN]) as well as different recruiting techniques (population-based, memory clinic). One of the studies found no difference in executive functions (Fahlander et al., 2002); one yielded an advantage for the VaD patients (Baillon et al., 2003); and another suggested an advantage for the AD patients (Canning et al., 2004). These findings illustrate the need for comparable samples, diagnostic criteria, matching procedures, and cognitive tasks when performing studies in this area.

A meta-analysis summarized the results from 16 studies comparing VaD and AD on subtests from the Wechsler Adult Intelligence Scale. The authors found that the VaD group performed at a lower level compared to the AD group on subtests involving executive components (e.g. Digit Span-backward, Object Assembly). This difference was enhanced when they only included studies comparing subcortical VaD and AD (Oosterman and Scherder, 2006).

The review by Sachdev and Looi (2003) did not differentiate between different VaD subtypes. However, the reported differences in verbal episodic memory and frontal-executive functions between AD and VaD patients were observed both in studies targeting MID and studies targeting subcortical VaD. Several recent studies have explicitly studied differences between subcortical VaD and AD, employing standardized research criteria for subcortical VaD as proposed by the NINDS-AIREN workshop (Roman et al., 1993). A general finding is that patients with subcortical VaD perform relatively worse on tasks measuring frontal-executive function (Graham et al., 2004; Tierney et al., 2001; Traykov et al., 2005), although some studies found no significant differences (Schmidtke and Hüll, 2002; Yuspeh et al., 2002). Another robust finding is that subcortical VaD patients have relatively spared episodic recognition memory compared to AD patients (Schmidtke and Hüll, 2002; Tierney et al., 2001; Yuspeh et al., 2002). Recognition performance has been reported to be within normal limits although the subcortical VaD patients performed at a lower level compared to controls on episodic memory tasks involving less retrieval support, such as free recall (Traykov et al., 2005; Vanderploeg et al., 2001). This relatively spared recognition memory has also been reported in a study involving CADASIL patients (Buffon et al., 2006).

The results from these studies suggest that the memory impairment in subcortical VaD and AD has different mechanisms. For subcortical VaD, the encoding process may be relatively spared, whereas the main difficulty lies in conscious retrieval. By contrast, consolidation and storage are major problems in AD. The observed difference may reflect that the episodic memory deficit in AD is driven largely by hippocampal pathology, whereas the deficit in subcortical VaD is more related to frontal–subcortical damage. Interruption of the dorsolateral–prefrontal circuit would cause impairment in self-initiation and effortful search critical to free recall. Increased retrieval support and task structure (e.g. cued recall, recognition) would, thus, benefit the VaD patients (see also Chapter 2).

Proposed new research criteria

Given the large variation in etiology and clinical outcome both within and between different VaD subtypes, it has been suggested that more focus should be directed toward patients with a subcortical, small-vessel basis for their deficits. Subcortical VaD (incorporating the two overlapping clinical entities of Binswanger's disease and lacunar state) is a more homogeneous subgroup compared to, for example, MID, and may thus be more suitable for clinical trials (Erkinjuntti *et al.*, 2000).

A modification of the NINDS-AIREN criteria for probable VaD has been proposed as new research guidelines for subcortical VaD (Erkinjuntti *et al.*, 2000). One difference from the NINDS-AIREN criteria is that the requirement of a temporal relationship between time of stroke and dementia onset has been omitted, as this is often less obvious in subcortical VaD. In contrast to most other criteria for dementia, the memory deficit may be mild and dominated by impaired recall with relatively intact recognition. Instead, a dysexecutive syndrome may be the predominant cognitive deficit. A study employing these new criteria found that a subcortical VaD group performed at a lower level compared to a control group for all cognitive domains measured (speed, executive functions, short-term memory/working memory, immediate episodic recall, delayed episodic recall, verbal intellectual functions, and visuospatial functions), with prominent deficits observed in the frontal-executive domain. Although episodic memory impairment was present, it could partly be explained by medial–temporal lobe atrophy, suggesting that subcortical damage was not driving the memory deficit (Jokinen *et al.*, 2006).

Cognition in preclinical VaD

For AD, numerous studies have demonstrated the existence of a preclinical phase with cognitive deficits during the years prior to a dementia diagnosis (Bäckman *et al.*, 2005). However, few studies have investigated a potential preclinical period in VaD. One reason to focus on the preclinical phase in dementia is that early detection and intervention is vital for the possibility of modifying the course of

the disorder. This is especially important in VaD, as many vascular risk factors are amenable to treatment. Another reason to focus on the preclinical phase is that it may be easier to identify distinguishing characteristics for different dementia types early on in the dementia process. Not surprisingly, studies have shown that patients with VaD and AD become more cognitively similar as the diseases progress.

In two studies using data from the Kungsholmen Project, we compared cognitive functioning in preclinical VaD, preclinical AD, and normal controls three years before dementia diagnosis. The VaD diagnosis was mainly a diagnosis of post-stroke dementia (MID or strategic single infarct). A key finding was that cognitive deficits were present three years before diagnosis of VaD, both for a measure of global cognition (Jones *et al.*, 2004) and for measures of episodic memory functioning (Laukka *et al.*, 2004). Further, the pattern of cognitive deficits in preclinical VaD was similar to that observed for preclinical AD. Both preclinical dementia groups performed at a lower level in comparison to the controls on the Mini-Mental State Examination total score. Performance on the episodic memory item delayed recall was the best predictor of incident dementia three years later for both VaD and AD, and there were no significant differences in cognitive performance between the two dementia groups (Jones *et al.*, 2004). In Laukka *et al.* (2004), a comprehensive cognitive test battery was administered. The general pattern indicated poorer cognitive performance for both preclinical dementia groups compared to the controls (see Figure 4.1). However, whereas the preclinical AD group performed worse than the controls on all measures of episodic memory, verbal fluency, and visuospatial functioning (except clock reading), the preclinical VaD group only performed worse than the controls on three episodic memory measures (random recall, word recognition, and face recognition). Although the results suggested a somewhat more pronounced cognitive deficit in preclinical AD, there were no reliable differences between the two dementia groups. In addition, both VaD

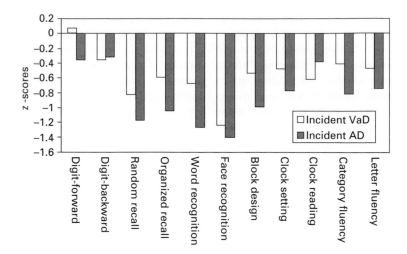

Figure 4.1 Cognitive performance 3 years before diagnosis (*z*-scores) for preclinical vascular dementia and Alzheimer's disease persons relative to a reference group (control means set at 0). (Adapted from Laukka et al., 2004 with permission).

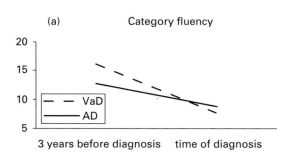

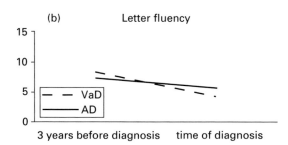

Figure 4.2(a) and (b) Performance on two verbal fluency tasks 3 years before diagnosis and at the time of diagnosis for vascular dementia and Alzheimer's disease persons. (Adapted from Jones *et al.*, 2006 with permission.)

and AD showed the largest impairment within the episodic memory domain three years before diagnosis (Laukka *et al.*, 2004).

An exception to the findings of similar levels of cognitive impairment was observed in a study comparing the effect of preclinical dementia on two verbal fluency tasks. Although both preclinical dementia groups showed poorer performance on letter fluency, the preclinical VaD persons outperformed the preclinical AD persons on category fluency three years before diagnosis (Jones *et al.*, 2006; Figure 4.2). The finding that the preclinical AD persons were disproportionally impaired in category fluency is in agreement with observations that the medial–temporal lobe is involved in this task (Pihlajamäki *et al.*, 2000). A possible reason thereof is that the search process in a category fluency task (in this case supermarket fluency) invokes personal experiences and thus involves episodic memory retrieval. Given that the medial–temporal lobe is relatively more affected in preclinical AD compared to VaD, this might explain the larger category fluency impairment for the preclinical AD persons.

The studies described above show that VaD is preceded by a preclinical phase with cognitive deficits. This is not an unexpected finding, given that persons with VaD are likely to be exposed to vascular risk factors many years before diagnosis. A number of vascular conditions, such as diabetes (Logroscino *et al.*, 2004), WML (de Groot *et al.*, 2000) and silent strokes (Vermeer *et al.*, 2003) have been shown to exert negative influences on cognitive performance in the absence of a dementia disorder. The prevalence of these conditions should be high in a sample of persons with impending VaD. However, it cannot be excluded that some VaD persons were also affected by degenerative processes characteristic of AD. Overlap in brain pathology might have obscured potential differences in cognitive functioning between preclinical VaD and preclinical AD.

Our finding that impairment on an episodic memory task predicted future VaD and AD alike (Jones *et al.*, 2004; Laukka *et al.*, 2004) has also been reported in other studies (e.g. Sacuiu *et al.*, 2005). A meta-analysis on cognitive functioning in preclinical AD demonstrates that most cognitive domains are already impaired at the preclinical stage, with the largest impairment seen for executive functioning, episodic memory, and speed (Bäckman *et al.*, 2005). Thus, separating between preclinical VaD and AD on the basis of neuropsychological test performance is a challenging task, even at a preclinical stage.

To our knowledge, there are no studies focusing on preclinical subcortical VaD. However, findings from CADASIL patients suggest that working memory and executive function are impaired in a very early phase of the disease, before a transient ischemic attack or stroke has occurred, whereas episodic memory functioning is relatively well preserved (Amberla *et al.*, 2004).

Diagnostic limitations

A major problem in VaD research has been the lack of harmonization of diagnostic procedures. The agreement between existing diagnostic criteria is low and the prevalence of VaD varies considerably depending on the specific criteria used. Divergent diagnostic criteria may identify different types of VaD patients. In addition, these patients may be at different stages of dementia development. Whereas some criteria are more general in nature (e.g. ICD-10), others target specific subtypes, such as MID (e.g. HIS), or subcortical VaD (e.g. Erkinjuntti *et al.*, 2000). The NINDS-AIREN criteria (Roman *et al.*, 1993) represent an attempt to resolve the heterogeneity in diagnostic procedures, but the debate is still ongoing. The use of standardized diagnostic criteria will facilitate comparison between studies. With more widespread access to neuroimaging in dementia diagnosis, the possibility of identifying different subtypes of VaD has much improved. However, population-based studies on the prevalence of different VaD subtypes are still lacking.

A problem in making differential diagnosis between VaD and other dementia types, particularly AD, is the overlap in dementia pathology. Autopsy evidence suggests that cerebrovascular pathology is common in patients with AD. Conversely, concomitant AD pathology is often present in clinically diagnosed VaD patients, with pure vascular pathology being very uncommon. Separating between the two dementia disorders is especially difficult in the oldest age groups (Agüero-Torres *et al.*, 2006). Because the prevalence of both AD and cerebrovascular disease (CVD) increases with advancing adult age, mixed dementia pathologies become increasingly common. In addition, the subtypes of VaD are not pure, and mixtures of vascular pathologies contribute to the heterogeneous clinical picture.

Besides the issue of overlapping pathology, one possible reason for the difficulty in detecting differences in cognitive performance between VaD and AD patients concerns the characteristics of the diagnostic criteria for dementia. The criteria for dementia are based on the concept of AD and require the presence of prominent memory impairment, which is not necessarily a prime symptom in VaD. This state of affairs results in a diagnostic bias, where patients with memory impairment are more likely to be recognized as demented compared to patients with executive dysfunction. This will lead to an over-representation of VaD patients with more AD-type symptomatology, which of course renders detection of differences more difficult. A possible way to avoid this problem is to employ diagnostic criteria for VaD that do not require a memory deficit (e.g. Erkinjuntti *et al.*, 2000). Another possibility is to focus on the relationship between vascular pathology and cognition regardless of dementia status. Such an approach would provide important information about the associations between different types of brain alterations and deficits on specific cognitive tasks.

The type of sample used for studying cognition in VaD is also relevant for the obtained results. For example, patients from memory clinics may more closely resemble AD patients compared to patients recruited from stroke clinics. Large population-based studies on VaD would provide more unbiased samples.

Practical implications and future research directions

The studies demonstrating cognitive deficits before a diagnosis of VaD illustrate that the cognitive deficits in VaD are the result of a lengthy process. Because many vascular causes of cognitive impairment are treatable, it should be most useful to focus on those individuals not yet fulfilling the diagnostic criteria for VaD. This might prevent the occurrence of VaD in some cases. Vascular cognitive impairment (VCI) is a relatively new concept that encompasses all cases where vascular factors could be assumed to contribute to the cognitive impairment observed. The concept includes the whole spectrum of cognitive impairment, from the brain-at-risk stage through full-blown dementia. However, common standards for the description and study of individuals with VCI have been lacking. Recently, such standards were proposed by a workshop organized by the NINDS and the Canadian Stroke Network (Hachinski *et al.*, 2006). They included recommendations regarding which cognitive tasks should be used in investigations of potential patients with VCI, both in clinical and research settings. It was suggested that neuropsychological protocols should cover a wide range of cognitive abilities, and be especially attuned to the assessment of executive functions. In particular, timed executive tasks may be sensitive to VCI-related impairment. Three protocols of different length were proposed. The 5-min protocol is devised as a quick screening and includes a 5-word memory task, a 6-item orientation task, and a letter fluency task. The longer test batteries comprise additional as well as more time-consuming tasks, including category fluency, a longer word list, the Digit–Symbol substitution test (30 min), and the Trail-Making Test, Boston Naming Test, and the Rey–Osterrieth Complex Figure (60 min). These protocols need to be validated and may later serve as a basis for provisional criteria for VCI (Hachinski *et al.*, 2006).

Including the same cognitive tasks in studies of VCI and VaD is important in order to obtain comparable results among studies when, for example, evaluating different kinds of interventions. Studies focusing on VaD also need to use standardized diagnostic criteria in order to facilitate between-study comparisons. Given the heterogeneity of VaD, it would be useful to study different subtypes of VaD separately. This would provide greater insight as to what type of cognitive impairment is associated with different kinds of brain damage. The patterns of cognitive deficits also need to be studied at different stages of VaD. In particular, it would be interesting to see more studies on cognitive functioning in preclinical VaD. Conceivably, the possibility to detect differences between VaD and AD and between different subtypes of VaD would be greatest in the prodromal phases.

Given that VaD is a preventable disorder, the study of the earliest stages becomes even more important. In an ongoing longitudinal study, we will investigate the earliest vascular changes in the brain, even prior to the appearance of WML, and onset of cognitive impairment. This will be

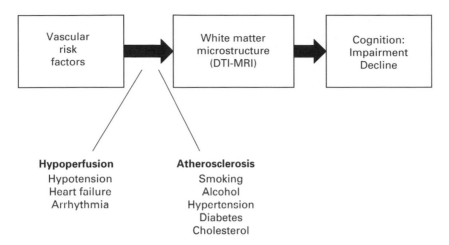

Figure 4.3 Schematic representation of the relationships among vascular risk factors, DTI (index of white-matter integrity), and cognition. The two clusters of risk factors represent two mechanisms through which vascular risk factors may influence cognitive functioning via white-matter alterations.

accomplished by using diffusion tensor imaging (DTI), which is a more sensitive neuroimaging technique for detecting subtle white matter alterations compared to conventional MRI. A reason for performing this study is that the mechanisms linking vascular risk factors, vascular brain injury, and cognitive impairment are not well understood. The aim is to study the onset of VCI and its relationship to vascular risk factors. An overarching goal is to determine whether the link between vascular risk factors and cognitive impairment and decline is mediated through measures of white matter integrity. Two major mechanisms linking vascular disorders to DTI alterations will be taken into account: atherosclerosis and hypoperfusion (see Figure 4.3). An additional goal is to understand how the relationship between vascular risk factors and cognitive functioning is modified by genetic, inflammatory, toxic, neurodegenerative and psychosocial factors. For example, specific genetic polymorphisms affecting the integrity of the vascular systems (e.g. APOE, cystatin C, a-fibrinogen) may attenuate or exacerbate the cognitive repercussions of vascular pathology. Neurodegenerative pathology may worsen the effect of vascular path-

ology in an additive or synergistic fashion. In contrast, psychosocial factors, such as physical and cognitive activity, might mitigate the negative impact of white-matter alterations on cognitive functioning.

Summary

The cognitive profile of VaD is heterogeneous and depends on the subtype and region of the brain affected. Studies comparing cognitive functioning in VaD and AD have found it difficult to distinguish between the two dementia types. However, in some studies, greater deficits in frontal-executive functioning and a relative advantage on verbal episodic memory tasks have been observed for patients with VaD. The pattern of cognitive impairment may be more distinct in subcortical VaD compared to MID. Recent studies suggest that frontal-executive dysfunction is the primary cognitive deficit in subcortical VaD and that the observed episodic memory deficit is largely due to retrieval problems. Separating VaD patients into subcortical and cortical types may facilitate comparisons between AD and VaD.

Cognitive deficits are present several years before a person can be classified with VaD. Future studies should seek to study the whole range of cognitive impairments associated with CVD, especially the earlier stages when the person still does not fulfill the criteria for dementia. This is where interventions would render the largest benefits.

ACKNOWLEDGMENTS

Writing of this chapter was supported by grants from the Swedish Council for Working Life and Social Research, and Swedish Brain Power to Lars Bäckman.

REFERENCES

Agüero-Torres H, Kivipelto M, von Strauss E. Rethinking the dementia diagnosis in a population-based study: what is Alzheimer's disease and what is vascular dementia? A study from the Kungsholmen Project. *Dementia Geriatr Cogn Disord* 2006; **22**: 244–9.

Amberla K, Wäljas M, Tuominen S, *et al*. Insidious cognitive decline in CADASIL. *Stroke* 2004; **35**: 1598–602.

Bäckman L, Jones S, Berger A-K, *et al*. Cognitive impairment in preclinical Alzheimer's disease: a meta-analysis. *Neuropsychology* 2005; **19**: 520–31.

Baillon S, Muhommad S, Marudkar M, *et al*. Neuropsychological performance in Alzheimer's disease and vascular dementia: comparisons in a memory clinic population. *Int J Geriatr Psychiatry* 2003; **18**: 602–8.

Buffon F, Porcher R, Hernandez K, *et al*. Cognitive profile in CADASIL. *J Neurol Neurosurg Psychiatry* 2006; **77**: 175–80.

Burton EJ, Kenny RA, O'Brien J, *et al*. White matter hyperintensities are associated with impairment of memory, attention, and global cognitive performance in older stroke patients. *Stroke* 2004; **35**: 1270–5.

Cabeza R, Nyberg L. Imaging cognition II: an empirical review of 275 PET and fMRI studies. *J Cogn Neurosci* 2000; **12**: 1–47.

Canning SJ, Leach L, Stuss D, *et al*. Diagnostic utility of abbreviated fluency measures in Alzheimer disease and vascular dementia. *Neurology* 2004; **62**: 556–62.

Chabriat H, Vahedi K, Iba-Zizen MT, *et al*. Clinical spectrum of CADASIL: a study of 7 families. *Lancet* 1995; **346**: 934–9.

Charlton RA, Morris RG, Nitkunan A, *et al*. The cognitive profiles of CADASIL and sporadic small vessel disease. *Neurology* 2006; **66**: 1523–6.

Cummings JL. Frontal–subcortical circuits and human behavior. *Neurol Rev* 1993; **50**: 873–80.

de Groot JC, de Leeuw F-E, Oudkerk M, *et al*. Cerebral white matter lesions and cognitive function: the Rotterdam Scan Study. *Ann Neurol* 2000; **47**: 145–51.

Desmond DW, The cognitive syndrome of vascular dementia: Implications for clinical trials. *Alzheimer Dis Assoc Disord* 1999; **13** (Suppl. 3): 21–9.

Desmond DW. The neuropsychology of vascular cognitive impairment: is there a specific cognitive deficit? *J Neurol Sci* 2004; **226**: 3–7.

Du AT, Schuff N, Laakso MP, *et al*. Effects of subcortical ischemic vascular dementia and AD on entorhinal cortex and hippocampus. *Neurology* 2002; **58**: 1635–41.

Erkinjuntti T, Inzitari D, Pantoni L, *et al*. Research criteria for subcortical vascular dementia in clinical trials. *J Neural Transm* 2000; **59** (Suppl.): 23–30.

Fahlander K, Wahlin Å, Almkvist O, *et al*. Cognitive functioning in Alzheimer's disease and vascular dementia: further evidence for similar patterns of deficits. *J Clin Exp Neuropsychol* 2002; **24**: 734–44.

Fischer P, Gatterer G, Marterer A, *et al*. Course characteristics in the differentiation of dementia of the Alzheimer type and multi-infarct dementia. *Acta Psychiatr Scand* 1990; **81**: 551–3.

Graham NL, Emery T, Hodges JR. Distinctive cognitive profiles in Alzheimer's disease and subcortical vascular dementia. *J Neurol Neurosurg Psychiatry* 2004; **75**: 61–71.

Hachinski V, Lassen NA, Marshall J. Multi-infarct dementia: a cause of mental deterioration in the elderly. *Lancet* 1974; **2**: 207–10.

Hachinski V, Iadecola C, Petersen RC, *et al*. National Institute of Neurological Disorders and Stroke–Canadian Stroke Network Vascular cognitive impairment harmonization standards. *Stroke* 2006; **37**: 2220–41.

Jokinen H, Kalska H, Mäntylä R, *et al*. Cognitive profile of subcortical ischaemic vascular disease. *J Neurol Neurosurg Psychiatry* 2006; **77**: 28–33.

Jones S, Laukka EJ, Small BJ, *et al*. A preclinical phase in vascular dementia: cognitive impairment three years before diagnosis. *Dementia Geriatr Cogn Disord* 2004; **18**: 233–9.

Jones S, Laukka EJ, Bäckman L. Differential verbal fluency deficits in the preclinical stages of Alzheimer's disease and vascular dementia. *Cortex* 2006; **42**: 347–55.

Kramer JH, Reed BR, Mungas D, *et al.* Executive dysfunction in subcortical ischaemic vascular disease. *J Neurol Neurosurg Psychiatry* 2002; **72**: 217–20.

Laukka EJ, Jones S, Small BJ, *et al.* Similar patterns of cognitive deficits in the preclinical phases of vascular dementia and Alzheimer's disease. *J Int Neuropsychol Soc* 2004; **10**: 382–91.

Logroscino G, Kang JH, & Grodstein F. Prospective study of type 2 diabetes and cognitive decline in women aged 70–81 years. *British Medical Journal* 2004; **328**: 548.

Miyake A, Friedman NP, Emerson MJ, *et al.* The unity and diversity of executive functions and their contributions to complex "frontal lobe" tasks: a latent variable analysis. *Cogn Psychol* 2000; **41**: 49–100.

Oosterman JM, Scherder EJA. Distinguishing between vascular dementia and Alzheimer's disease by means of the WAIS: a meta-analysis. *J Clin Exp Neuropsychol* 2006; **28**: 1158–75.

O'Sullivan M, Barrick TR, Morris RG, *et al.* Damage within a network of white matter regions underlies executive dysfunction in CADASIL. *Neurology* 2005; **65**: 1584–90.

Pihlajamäki M, Tanila H, Hänninen T, *et al.* Verbal fluency activates the left medial temporal lobe: a functional magnetic resonance imaging study. *Ann Neurol* 2000; **47**: 470–6.

Reed BR, Eberling JL, Mungas D, *et al.* Memory failure has different mechanisms in subcortical stroke and Alzheimer's disease. *Ann Neurol* 2000; **48**: 275–84.

Roman GC, Tatemichi TK, Erkinjuntti T, *et al.* Vascular dementia: diagnostic criteria for research studies. Report of the NINDS-AIREN international workshop. *Neurol* 1993; **43**: 250–60.

Roman GC, Erkinjuntti T, Wallin A, *et al.* Subcortical ischaemic vascular dementia. *Lancet Neurol* 2002; **1**: 426–36.

Sachdev PS & Looi JCL. Neuropsychological differentiation of Alzheimer's disease and vascular dementia. In Bowler JV, Hachinski V, eds. *Vascular Cognitive Impairment: Preventable Dementia*. New York: Oxford University Press, 2003.

Sacuiu S, Sjögren M, Johansson B, *et al.* Prodromal cognitive signs of dementia in 85-year-olds using four sources of information. *Neurol* 2005; **65**: 1894–900.

Schmidtke K, Hüll M. Neuropsychological differentiation of small vessel disease, Alzheimer's disease and mixed dementia. *J Neurol Sci* 2002; **203–4**: 17–22.

Squire LR, Zola SM. Structure and function of declarative and non-declarative memory systems. *Proc Nat Acad Sci USA* 1996; **93**: 1315–22.

Tierney MC, Black SE, Szalai JP, *et al.* Recognition memory and verbal fluency differentiate probable Alzheimer disease from subcortical ischemic vascular dementia. *Arch Neurol* 2001; **58**: 1654–59.

Traykov L, Baudic S, Raoux N, *et al.* Patterns of memory impairment and perseverative behavior discriminate early Alzheimer's disease from subcortical vascular dementia. *J Neurol Sci* 2005; **229–230**: 75–9.

Tullberg M, Fletcher E, DeCarli C, *et al.* White matter lesions impair frontal lobe function regardless of their location. *Neurol* 2004; **63**: 246–53.

Tulving E. Episodic memory: from mind to brain. *Annu Rev Psychol* 2002; **53**: 1–25.

Vanderploeg RD, Yuspeh RL, and Schinka JA. Differential episodic and semantic memory performance in Alzheimer's disease and vascular dementias. *J Int Neuropsychol Soc* 2001; **7**: 563–73.

Vermeer SE, Prins ND, den Heijer T, *et al.* Silent brain infarcts and the risk of dementia and cognitive decline. *N Engl J Med* 2003; **348**: 1215–22.

Villardita C. Alzheimer's disease compared with cerebrovascular dementia. Neuropsychological similarities and differences. *Acta Neurol Scand* 1993; **87**: 299–308.

Yuspeh RL, Vanderploeg RD, Crowell TA, *et al.* Differences in executive functioning between Alzheimer's disease and subcortical ischemic vascular dementia. *J Clin Exp Neuropsychol* 2002; **24**: 745–54.

5

Structural neuroimaging: CT and MRI

Wiesje M. van der Flier, Salka S. Staekenborg, Frederik Barkhof and
Philip Scheltens

Vascular dementia (VaD) is generally viewed as the second most common cause of dementia in elderly people, surpassed by Alzheimer's disease (AD) only. VaD can be caused by hypoxic–ischemic pathology or hemorrhagic brain lesions that may result in heterogeneous clinical syndromes. Traditionally, VaD has been recognized to develop after multiple strokes. The name "multi-infarct dementia" became synonymous with all dementias of vascular origin (Hachinski *et al.*, 1974). It is increasingly becoming acknowledged, however, that in addition to large-vessel infarcts, subcortical ischemic vascular disease may also cause dementia, and separate diagnostic criteria have been proposed (Erkinjuntti *et al.*, 2000; Roman *et al.*, 2002). In the diagnostic work-up of VaD, imaging – preferably MRI – plays an important role, as it is necessary to demonstrate the presence of cerebrovascular disease (CVD). Absence of CVD on MRI or CT is strong evidence against VaD, and is the most important brain imaging characteristic to distinguish VaD from AD. The criteria of the National Institute of Neurological Disorders and Stroke – Association Internationale pour la Recherche et l'Enseignement en Neurosciences (NINDS-AIREN) which are often used in VaD studies, define – in addition to clinical criteria – radiological criteria for VaD (Table 5.1) (Roman *et al.*, 1993). Topographic and severity criteria are defined, but it has been shown that, in practice, considerable inter-observer variability exists for their assessment. Operational definitions have been proposed, and their use improves agreement, especially for experienced observers (Van Straaten *et al.*, 2003). In this chapter, we describe brain abnormalities that can be observed on MRI in patients with VaD. VaD is a heterogeneous disorder, meaning that diverse cerebrovascular abnormalities can lead to a diagnosis of VaD. An overview of MRI abnormalities indicative of cerebrovascular disease is given.

Scan protocol

Computed tomography (CT) is usually sufficient to rule out causes of cognitive decline other than VaD or neurodegenerative types of dementia, such as a tumor, subdural hematoma, or hydrocephalus. In addition, infarcts can be observed on CT, and small-vessel disease and atrophy are appreciable to some extent. However, if available, MRI is the neuroimaging method of choice, as it provides far better spatial resolution, and (cerebrovascular) brain changes can be appreciated in more detail.

The MR protocol should include at least: axial T2-weighted images and axial fluid attenuated inversion recovery (FLAIR) images, or proton density-weighted images (Figure 5.1). Also, coronal 3D T1-weighted images, and finally, gradient-echo T2*-weighted

Vascular Cognitive Impairment in Clinical Practice, ed. Lars-Olof Wahlund, Timo Erkinjuntti and Serge Gauthier. Published by Cambridge University Press. © Cambridge University Press 2009.

Table 5.1 Radiological criteria of CVD sufficient for a diagnosis of probable VaD (Roman *et al.*, 1993; Van Straaten *et al.*, 2003).

Large-vessel disease

1. Topography–radiological lesions associated with dementia include any of the following or combinations thereof:

Anterior cerebral artery	Bilateral
Posterior cerebral artery, including	Paramedian thalamic infarctions
	Inferior medial temporal lobe lesions
Association areas	Parietotemporal
	Temporo-occipital
	Angular gyrus
Watershed carotid territories	Superior frontal
	Parietal region

2. Severity – in addition to the above, relevant radiological lesions associated with dementia
   Large-vessel lesions of the dominant hemisphere
   Bilateral large-vessel hemispheric strokes

Small-vessel disease

1. Topography
   Multiple basal ganglia and frontal white matter lacunes
   Extensive periventricular white matter lesions
   Bilateral thalamic lesions

2. Severity
   Leukoencephalopathy involving at least 1/4 of the total white matter

For the fulfillment of large-vessel disease, both a topography and a severity criterion for large-vessel disease have to be met. In the case of small-vessel disease, for white matter lesions both topography and severity criteria have to be met; for multiple lacunes and bilateral thalamic lesions only the topography criterion is sufficient.

images. To detect CVD, T2-weighted images and FLAIR or proton density-weighted images are used. Cortical infarcts can be appreciated on T2-weighted images and FLAIR. The scan sequence of choice to evaluate white matter hyperintensities (WMH) is FLAIR. FLAIR sequences suppress the signal of cerebrospinal fluid (CSF), allowing distinction of lacunes and perivascular spaces from WMH, all of which are bright on standard T2-weighted images, while only WMH appear bright on FLAIR. On the other hand, especially thalamic lesions may remain undetected on FLAIR, and are more easily discerned on T2 (Figure 5.2) (Bastos Leite *et al.*, 2004). For the detection of microbleeds and calcifications, gradient-echo T2*-weighted images are best suited. Finally, the coronal T1-weighted images, oriented perpendicular to the long axis of the hippocampal formation, can be used to evaluate atrophy of the medial temporal lobe. Global atrophy can be appreciated on axial FLAIR.

Large-vessel disease

Traditionally, VaD has almost exclusively been attributed to large-vessel disease, as the term "multi-infarct dementia" (MID) implies. The type of cognitive impairment observed in VaD due to large-vessel disease is variable, depending on the specific location of the infarcts. The NINDS-AIREN criteria recognize that VaD may be caused by multiple large-vessel infarcts, or by a single strategically placed infarct. Large-vessel infarcts include arterial territorial infarcts and watershed infarcts. Arterial territorial infarcts that may lead to a diagnosis of VaD include infarcts in the anterior cerebral artery

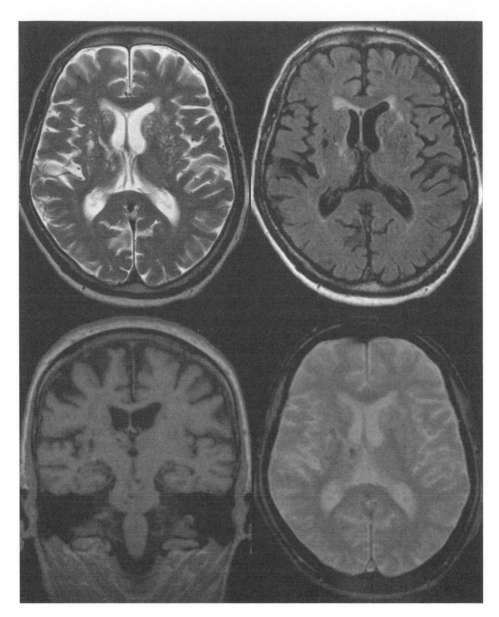

Figure 5.1 The MR scan protocol for the diagnosis of vascular dementia should include at least: axial T2-weighted images (upper left), axial fluid attenuated inversion recovery (FLAIR) images (upper right), coronal high-resolution T1-weighted images (lower left), and, finally, gradient-echo T2*-weighted images (lower right). In this example, mild white matter hyperintensities, lacunae and microbleeds can be observed. The basal ganglia area shows an example of état criblé.

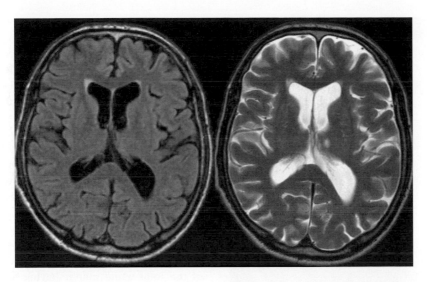

Figure 5.2 Thalamic lesions are best appreciated on T2-weighted (right), and may be easily missed on FLAIR (left).

territories, thalamic infarctions, inferior medial temporal lobe infarcts (Figure 5.3), and infarcts in the association areas (parietotemporal, temporo-occipital and angular gyrus).

Watershed infarcts are ischemic lesions that occur in the border zone regions between the main arterial territories (Figure 5.4). Posterior watershed infarcts (parietal region) are those located between the cortical supply of the middle cerebral artery and the posterior cerebral artery. Watershed infarcts in the superior frontal area are located between the cortical supply of the anterior cerebral artery and the middle cerebral artery. For large-vessel infarcts to be sufficient for a diagnosis of VaD, they are required to be located in the dominant hemisphere or – in the case of anterior cerebral artery territories – to be bilateral. Conversely, infarcts in the non-dominant hemisphere are not sufficient radiological support for a diagnosis of VaD.

Small-vessel disease

Apart from large-vessel disease, small-vessel disease may also account for VaD. Traditionally, this

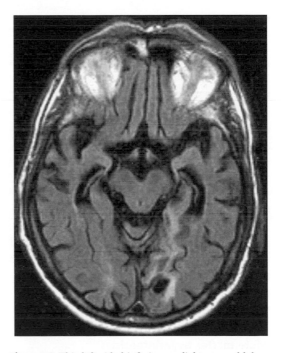

Figure 5.3 This left-sided inferior medial temporal lobe infarct is an example of an arterial territorial infarct that may lead to a diagnosis of VaD.

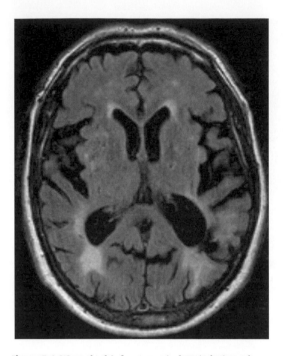

Figure 5.4 Watershed infarcts are ischemic lesions that occur in the borderzone regions between arterial territories. In this example, a left posterior watershed infarct (parietal region) can be observed, which is located between the cortical supply of the middle cerebral artery and the posterior cerebral artery.

type of dementia was referred to as *Binswanger's disease* in cases of severe leukoaraiosis, or *lacunar state* when multiple lacunes were present. The NINDS-AIREN criteria acknowledge multiple lacunes, extensive WMH and bilateral thalamic lesions as sufficient for a diagnosis of VaD. In fact, nowadays, it is recognized that small-vessel disease accounts for the largest proportion of VaD, and specific diagnostic criteria have been coined for subcortical ischemic vascular dementia (Erkinjuntti *et al.*, 2000) On MRI, several types of expression of small-vessel disease can be observed.

White matter hyperintensities

White matter hyperintensities (WMH) refer to areas in the white matter that appear hyperintense

(bright) on T2-weighted, proton density-weighted and FLAIR images. Frequently used synonyms are white matter lesions (WML) or white matter changes. On CT, changes in the white matter can also be observed when severe, but here they occur as *hypo*-densities, and are referred to as leukoaraiosis. The occurrence of WMH increases steadily with age, and they are frequently observed in the elderly. WMH have been shown to be related to subtle cognitive impairment, depressive symptoms and motor deficits. Patients with dementia have more WMH than healthy elderly subjects, and patients with VaD have more WMH than patients with other types of dementia (Barber *et al.*, 1999a). For WMH to be sufficient as a cause of VaD, an arbitrary cut-off has been set, with 25% of the total white matter having to be involved (Roman *et al.*, 1993).

WMH can be observed around the lateral ventricles (periventricular WMH) and in subcortical areas (subcortical or deep WMH). Periventricular WMH typically involve frontal and occipital caps, and bands along the lateral side of the ventricles. The pencil-thin lining or smooth halo along the ventricles that is often observed in healthy elderly subjects is probably innocent, and may not be of vascular origin. Subcortical WMH can occur as punctiform lesions, beginning confluent lesions or confluent areas (diffuse involvement of the entire region) (Figure 5.5). Periventricular and subcortical WMH are thought to have separate etiologies, and consequentially, also specific clinical sequelae.

WMH can be assessed using visual rating scales or using a volumetric method. Although some fully automated methods for the assessment of WMH volumes exist, most volumetric methods are semi-automatic at best, require high-quality scans, and involve quite some operator intervention. The advantage of these methods is that an exact volume of WMH is obtained, which is desirable when one is looking for subtle associations. Rating scales, on the other hand, offer a simple alternative to assess the severity (and location) of WMH. They have the advantage of being quite fast and reliable, when performed by an experienced rater. Furthermore,

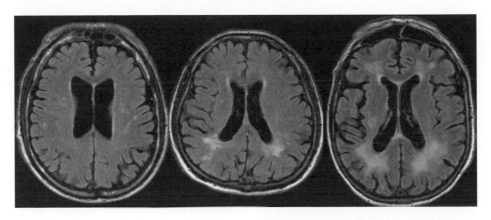

Figure 5.5 White matter hyperintensities appear as bright areas on FLAIR images. Examples of mild (punctiform), moderate (beginning confluent) or severe (confluent) subcortical white matter hyperintensities are shown. The panel on the right is from a patient who received a diagnosis of VaD based on involvement of 25% of the white matter.

they do not require sophisticated image post-processing facilities, and scans of moderate quality can often be used. Therefore, visual rating scales are widely applicable, also in clinical settings. Finally, it seems that clinico radiological associations are of comparable strength, regardless of the use of volumetrics or rating scales, favoring the use of a simpler rating scale (Gouw *et al.*, 2006). There are many different rating scales estimating the degree and distribution of WMH, and they differ in many aspects (Scheltens *et al.*, 1998). Among the most simple and straightforward rating scales is the scale developed by Fazekas *et al.* (1987). Subcortical WMH are rated as mild (punctiform), moderate (beginning confluent) or severe (confluent), and periventricular WMH can be rated on a separate four-point rating scale. Some years ago, an effort was made to construct a new rating scale combining the strengths of several existing rating scales. The age-related white matter changes (ARWMC) scale was developed to be used for both MRI and CT (Wahlund *et al.*, 2001). The simple four-point rating scale was adopted from the Fazekas scale as decribed above, but now, the presence of WMH is rated in five different areas (frontal, parieto-occipital, temporal, infratentorial and basal ganglia), for left and right hemisphere separately. In this way, the maximum total score is 30. As

an operationalization of the 25% criterion in the NINDS-AIREN criteria, it has been suggested to require as a minimum twice a score of 2 and twice a score of 3 in the left and right frontal and parieto-occipital areas.

Lacunes

Lacunes are small subcortical infarcts measuring 3–20 mm in diameter, occurring in territories supplied by the small perforating arteries (Longstreth *et al.*, 1998). On MRI, they can be defined as round or oval lesions with CSF-like intensity on all sequences, surrounded by white matter or subcortical gray matter, sometimes surrounded by a rim of high signal (gliosis) on T2 and FLAIR (Figure 5.6). Lacunes can be located in the basal ganglia, internal capsule, thalamus, paramedian and lateral regions of the brain stem, corona radiata, and centrum semi-ovale. They may be clinically silent, but sometimes are accompanied by a history of transient ischemic attack or stroke. Lacunes in the thalamic area deserve special attention, as the thalamus plays a crucial role in many cognitive functions, and even small lesions in this structure may result in cognitive deficits (Van der Werf *et al.*, 2003). For a diagnosis of VaD to be based on the presence of lacunes, there

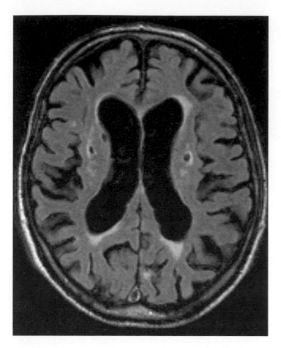

Figure 5.6 Lacunes are small subcortical infarcts measuring 3–20 mm in diameter, occurring in territories supplied by the small perforating arteries. On MRI, they appear as round or oval lesions with CSF-like intensity on all sequences, surrounded by white matter or subcortical gray matter.

should be evidence of multiple (at least two) basal ganglia and frontal white matter lacunes.

Lacunes should be distinguished from Virchow–Robin spaces (VRS), which typically occur at the vertex and around the anterior commissure near the substantia perforata. VRS are dilated perivascular spaces. An association between VRS and WMH has been described in healthy elderly subjects, but the number of VRS were not independently related to cognitive function (Maclullich *et al.*, 2004). Recently, it was shown that VRS are omnipresent, even in young healthy subjects, and are to be considered a normal finding (Groeschel *et al.*, 2006). When VRS appear in large numbers (*état criblé*, occurring especially in the basal ganglia), this probably reflects focal brain atrophy around blood vessels.

Microbleeds

Microbleeds are small, dot-like lesions of low signal intensity in the brain that can be observed on T2*-weighted images (Figure 5.7). Histologically, they represent focal leakage of hemosiderin from abnormal small blood vessels affected by lipohyalinosis or arising from arteries affected by amyloid deposition (Fazekas *et al.*, 1999). Microbleeds can be observed in cortical/subcortical, basal ganglia/thalamus and infratentorial areas, and should be distinguished from calcification or iron deposits that are often observed symmetrically in the globi pallidi, and flow void artefacts of the pial blood vessels. Microbleeds are associated with other expressions of small vessel disease such as WMH, and with future intracerebral hemorrhagic stroke (Cordonnier *et al.*, 2006; Fan *et al.*, 2003; Wardlaw *et al.*, 2006). In community-based populations, prevalence of microbleeds is relatively low, in the order of 5% (Koennecke, 2006). Prevalence of microbleeds in stroke populations and in VaD is far higher, around 50–70% (Cordonnier *et al.*, 2006; Koennecke, 2006). Microbleeds are the radiological key feature of cerebral amyloid angiopathy (CAA). Although highly prevalent among patients with VaD, microbleeds are not described in the radiological NINDS-AIREN criteria.

CADASIL

Cerebral autosomal dominant arteriopathy with subcortical infarcts and leukoaraiosis (CADASIL) is a hereditary form of VaD, presenting in young patients in the absence of vascular risk factors. Clinically, CADASIL presents with recurrent stroke, dementia, migraine with aura, and mood disturbances (Chabriat *et al.*, 1995). On imaging, diffuse white matter hyperintensities involving the U-fibers are characteristically observed, mainly in the temporal, temporopolar, and frontal regions (Figure 5.8) (Skehan *et al.*, 1995; Yousry *et al.*, 1999). In addition, lacunes are present in the semiovale center, the thalamus, the basal ganglia, and the pons (van Den *et al.*, 2002). Finally, microbleeds are observed in a

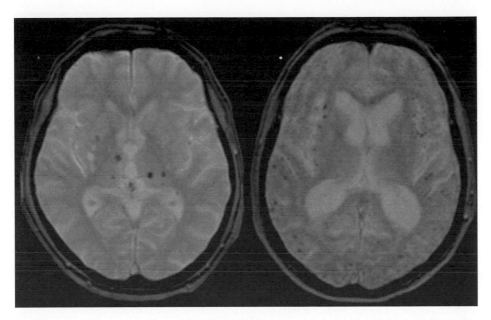

Figure 5.7 Microbleeds are small, dot-like lesions of low signal intensity in the brain that can be observed on T2*-weighted images. Microbleeds can be observed in basal ganglia/thalamus (left panel), cortical/subcortical (right panel), and infratentorial areas.

considerable proportion of these patients (Lesnick Oberstein *et al.*, 2001).

Neurodegeneration

Atrophy of the brain is usually regarded as evidence of neurodegenerative disease. More specifically, atrophy of the medial temporal lobe, including the hippocampus, is regarded as indicative of Alzheimer-type pathology. The volume of the hippocampus has been shown to be associated with the burden of Alzheimer-type pathology (Gosche *et al.*, 2002). However, evidence is mounting that hippocampal atrophy may not be specific for AD. In fact, hippocampal atrophy has been observed in other types of dementia including VaD, and a similar neuronal loss has been shown in both patients with AD and VaD (Barber *et al.*, 1999b; Du *et al.*, 2002; Kril *et al.*, 2002). It is unclear whether hippocampal atrophy in VaD is due to concomitant Alzheimer-type pathology, or if

another type of neuropathology has the same result of neuronal loss, and eventually atrophy. The hippocampus is highly vulnerable to ischemia, which may contribute to hippocampal atrophy in VaD. In support of this hypothesis, it has been shown that vascular risk factors are related to hippocampal atrophy (den Heijer *et al.*, 2003; Korf *et al.*, 2004).

In addition to focal atrophy in the medial temporal lobe, general cerebral atrophy can also be observed in VaD, although only a few, small studies actually address global atrophy in VaD. Cerebral atrophy is observed in VaD to a similar extent as in AD (Barber *et al.*, 2000; Pantel *et al.*, 1998). Progression in brain atrophy over time has also been shown to be similar among patients with VaD and AD (O'Brien *et al.*, 2001). Although atrophy is not one of the hallmarks of VaD and is not described in the radiological criteria according to NINDS-AIREN, it seems to be an important aspect none the less. Atrophy is frequently observed in VaD, and studies assessing cognitive decline in subjects with

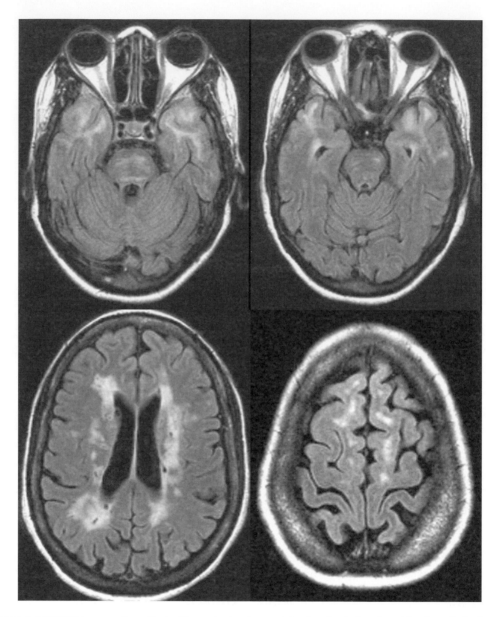

Figure 5.8 Axial FLAIR images of a patient with cerebral autosomal dominant arteriopathy with subcortical infarcts and leukoencephalopathy (CADASIL). Diffuse white matter hyperintensities are observed, mainly in the temporal, temporopolar, and frontal regions.

subcortical ischemic vascular disease and stroke have repeatedly suggested that atrophy (both medial temporal lobe atrophy and general cortical atrophy) is a stronger predictor of subsequent cognitive decline than baseline indicators of cerebrovascular disease (Gainotti *et al.*, 2004; Mungas *et al.*, 2007). Among the explanations is the possibility that atrophy is secondary to cerebrovascular disease, e.g. via

Wallerian degeneration or hypoperfusion. Alternatively, it is conceivable that although subcortical ischemic disease by itself is not able to cause dementia, the presence of vascular disease increases the expression of concomitant Alzheimer pathology.

New methods

The usefulness of conventional MRI (e.g. FLAIR, T2) in assessing and monitoring disease severity in patients with small-vessel disease is limited, as only modest associations between small-vessel disease and clinical symptoms exist. Two aspects may contribute to this so-called clinico-radiological dissociation. First, the high signal intensity observed in areas of WMH probably reflects a wide spectrum of pathological changes. In other words, WMH that appear similar on conventional MRI, are probably heterogeneous in their etiology and histopathology, with some WMH representing severe disease, whereas others are relatively benign. On the other end of the spectrum, white matter that appears normal on conventional MRI (i.e. normal appearing white matter or NAWM) may not be entirely normal. Subtle changes, invisible to the human eye, may already have occurred. Although currently not used in the diagnostic work-up of (vascular) dementia, quantitative methods such as diffusion tensor imaging (DTI) and magnetization transfer imaging provide valuable new ways to assess the integrity of white matter in more detail.

Magnetization transfer imaging (MTI) is based on the exchange of magnetization between a pool of free water protons and a pool of bound macromolecular (e.g. myelin) protons in biological tissues (Grossman et al., 1994). The amount of magnetization transfer depends on the concentration as well as on the surface chemistry and biophysical dynamics of macromolecules, and may be quantified by calculating the magnetization transfer ratio (MTR). The MTR is low in areas with no bound protons, such as CSF, and high in myelinated areas, e.g. the white matter. Reduced MTR indicates disruption of brain tissue. The MTR of WMH is lower than that of NAWM and decreases with increasing WMH severity (Fazekas et al., 2005). In addition, using MTI, heterogeneity in WMH that appeared similar on conventional MRI could be demonstrated (Spilt et al., 2006). Finally, even in the normal appearing white matter, subtle abnormalities have been shown.

DTI is another technique that provides quantitative information on the integrity and/or disruption of white matter tracts (Basser and Pierpaoli, 1996). It is based on measurement of the diffusivity of water. In tracts of parallel fibers, such as the white matter, diffusion occurs preferentially along the direction of the fibers. This directionality can be quantified as fractional anisotropy, which varies from zero, where diffusion is equal in all directions (e.g. CSF), to one, where diffusion occurs along a single axis. In the brain, white matter has relatively high anisotropy, as diffusion is preferential along the white matter tracts. Damage to axons or myelin will lead to increased diffusion, and thus reduction in fractional anisotropy. Reduced fractional anisotropy has been shown in patients with subcortical ischemic vascular disease and in patients with CADASIL (Chabriat et al., 1999; O'Sullivan et al., 2001). In addition, correlations with cognitive decline have been shown (Holtmann Spotter et al., 2005; O'Sullivan et al., 2004).

Summary

- A number of different types of cerebrovascular abnormalities can be observed on MRI, reflecting the heterogeneity in neuropathology underlying VaD.
- The diagnostic MR scan protocol should include at least axial FLAIR, T2-weighted and T2*-weighted imaging to appreciate the different types of vascular abnormalities. Coronal T1-weighted imaging is recommended to evaluate atrophy of the medial temporal lobe.
- Typical MR characteristics of VaD include large-vessel infarcts (arterial territorial and watershed infarcts) and expressions of small-vessel disease: white matter hyperintensities, lacunes and microbleeds.

- In addition, evidence of neurodegeneration (i.e. general atrophy, medial temporal lobe atrophy) is frequently observed.

REFERENCES

Barber R, Scheltens P, Gholkar A, *et al*. White matter lesions on magnetic resonance imaging in dementia with Lewy bodies, Alzheimer's disease, vascular dementia, and normal aging. *J Neurol Neurosurg Psychiatry* 1999a; **67**(1): 66–72.

Barber R, Gholkar A, Scheltens P, Ballard C, McKeith IG, O'Brien JT. Medial temporal lobe atrophy on MRI in dementia with Lewy bodies. *Neurology* 1999b; **52**(6): 1153–58.

Barber R, Ballard C, McKeith IG, Gholkar A, O'Brien JT. MRI volumetric study of dementia with Lewy bodies: a comparison with AD and vascular dementia. *Neurology* 2000; **54**(6): 1304–09.

Basser PJ, Pierpaoli C. Microstructural and physiological features of tissues elucidated by quantitative-diffusion-tensor MRI. *J Magn Reson B* 1996; **111**(3): 209–19.

Bastos Leite AJ, Van Straaten EC, Scheltens P, Lycklama G, Barkhof F. Thalamic lesions in vascular dementia: low sensitivity of fluid-attenuated inversion recovery (FLAIR) imaging. *Stroke* 2004; **35**(2): 415–19.

Chabriat H, Vahedi K, Iba-Zizen MT, *et al*. Clinical spectrum of CADASIL: a study of 7 families. Cerebral autosomal dominant arteriopathy with subcortical infarcts and leukoencephalopathy. *Lancet* 1995; **346**(8980): 934–9.

Chabriat H, Pappata S, Poupon C, *et al*. Clinical severity in CADASIL related to ultrastructural damage in white matter: in vivo study with diffusion tensor MRI. *Stroke* 1999; **30**(12): 2637–43.

Cordonnier C, van der Flier WM, Sluimer JD, Leys D, Barkhof F, Scheltens P. Prevalence and severity of microbleeds in a memory clinic setting. *Neurology* 2006; **66**(9): 1356–60.

den Heijer T, Vermeer SE, van Dijk EJ, *et al*. Type 2 diabetes and atrophy of medial temporal lobe structures on brain MRI. *Diabetologia* 2003; **46**(12): 1604–10.

Du AT, Schuff N, Laakso MP, *et al*. Effects of subcortical ischemic vascular dementia and AD on entorhinal cortex and hippocampus. *Neurology* 2002; **58**(11): 1635–41.

Erkinjuntti T, Inzitari D, Pantoni L, *et al*. Research criteria for subcortical vascular dementia in clinical trials. *J Neural Transm Suppl* 2000; **59**: 23–30.

Fan YH, Zhang L, Lam WW, Mok VC, Wong KS. Cerebral microbleeds as a risk factor for subsequent intracerebral hemorrhages among patients with acute ischemic stroke. *Stroke* 2003; **34**(10): 2459–62.

Fazekas F, Chawluk JB, Alavi A, Hurtig HI, Zimmerman RA. MR signal abnormalities at 1.5 T in Alzheimer's dementia and normal aging. *Am J Roentgenol* 1987; **149**(2): 351–6.

Fazekas F, Kleinert R, Roob G, *et al*. Histopathologic analysis of foci of signal loss on gradient-echo T2*-weighted MR images in patients with spontaneous intracerebral hemorrhage: evidence of microangiopathy-related microbleeds. *Am J Neuroradiol* 1999; **20**(4): 637–42.

Fazekas F, Ropele S, Enzinger C, *et al*. MTI of white matter hyperintensities. *Brain* 2005; **128**(Pt 12): 2926–32.

Gainotti G, Acciarri A, Bizzarro A, *et al*. The role of brain infarcts and hippocampal atrophy in subcortical ischaemic vascular dementia. *Neurol Sci* 2004; **25**(4): 192–7.

Gosche KM, Mortimer JA, Smith CD, Markesbery WR, Snowdon DA. Hippocampal volume as an index of Alzheimer neuropathology: findings from the Nun Study. *Neurology* 2002; **58**(10): 1476–82.

Gouw AA, van der Flier WM, Van Straaten EC, *et al*. Simple versus complex assessment of white matter hyperintensities in relation to physical performance and cognition: the LADIS study. *J Neurol* 2006; **253**(9): 1189–96.

Groeschel S, Chong WK, Surtees R, Hanefeld F. Virchow–Robin spaces on magnetic resonance images: normative data, their dilatation, and a review of the literature. *Neuroradiology* 2006; **48**(10): 745–54.

Grossman RI, Gomori JM, Ramer KN, Lexa FJ, Schnall MD. Magnetization transfer: theory and clinical applications in neuroradiology. *Radiographics* 1994; **14**(2): 279–90.

Hachinski VC, Lassen NA, Marshall J. Multi-infarct dementia. A cause of mental deterioration in the elderly. *Lancet* 1974; **2**(7874): 207–10.

Holtmannspotter M, Peters N, Opherk C, *et al*. Diffusion magnetic resonance histograms as a surrogate marker and predictor of disease progression in CADASIL: a two-year follow-up study. *Stroke* 2005; **36**(12): 2559–65.

Koennecke HC. Cerebral microbleeds on MRI: prevalence, associations, and potential clinical implications. *Neurology* 2006; **66**(2): 165–71.

Korf ES, White LR, Scheltens P, Launer LJ. Midlife blood pressure and the risk of hippocampal atrophy: the Honolulu Asia Aging Study. *Hypertension* 2004; **44**(1): 29–34.

Kril JJ, Patel S, Harding AJ, Halliday GM. Patients with vascular dementia due to microvascular pathology have significant hippocampal neuronal loss. *J Neurol Neurosurg Psychiatry* 2002; **72**(6): 747–51.

Lesnik Oberstein SA, van Den BR, van Buchem MA, *et al.* Cerebral microbleeds in CADASIL. *Neurology* 2001; **57** (6): 1066–70.

Longstreth WT, Jr., Bernick C, Manolio TA, Bryan N, Jungreis CA, Price TR. Lacunar infarcts defined by magnetic resonance imaging of 3660 elderly people: the Cardiovascular Health Study. *Arch Neurol* 1998; **55**(9): 1217–25.

Maclullich AM, Wardlaw JM, Ferguson KJ, Starr JM, Seckl JR, Deary IJ. Enlarged perivascular spaces are associated with cognitive function in healthy elderly men. *J Neurol Neurosurg Psychiatry* 2004; **75**(11): 1519–23.

Mungas D, Jagust WJ, Reed BR, *et al.* MRI predictors of cognition in subcortical ischemic vascular disease and Alzheimer's disease. *Neurology* 2001; **57** (12): 2229–35.

O'Brien JT, Paling S, Barber R, *et al.* Progressive brain atrophy on serial MRI in dementia with Lewy bodies, AD, and vascular dementia. *Neurology* 2001; **56**(10): 1386–88.

O'Sullivan M, Summers PE, Jones DK, Jarosz JM, Williams SC, Markus HS. Normal-appearing white matter in ischemic leukoaraiosis: a diffusion tensor MRI study. *Neurology* 2001; **57**(12): 2307–10.

O'Sullivan M, Morris RG, Huckstep B, Jones DK, Williams SC, Markus HS. Diffusion tensor MRI correlates with executive dysfunction in patients with ischaemic leukoaraiosis. *J Neurol Neurosurg Psychiatry* 2004; **75** (3): 441–47.

Pantel J, Schroder J, Essig M, *et al.* In vivo quantification of brain volumes in subcortical vascular dementia and Alzheimer's disease. An MRI-based study. *Dement Geriatr Cogn Disord* 1998; **9**(6): 309–16.

Roman GC, Tatemichi TK, Erkinjuntti T, *et al.* Vascular dementia: diagnostic criteria for research studies. Report of the NINDS-AIREN International Workshop. *Neurology* 1993; **43**(2): 250–60.

Roman GC, Erkinjuntti T, Wallin A, Pantoni L, Chui HC. Subcortical ischaemic vascular dementia. *Lancet Neurol* 2002; **1**(7): 426–36.

Skehan SJ, Hutchinson M, MacErlaine DP. Cerebral autosomal dominant arteriopathy with subcortical infarcts and leukoencephalopathy: MR findings. *Am J Neuroradiol* 1995; **16**(10): 2115–19.

Spilt A, Goekoop R, Westendorp RG, Blauw GJ, de Craen AJ, van Buchem MA. Not all age-related white matter hyperintensities are the same: a magnetization transfer imaging study. *Am J Neuroradiol* 2006; **27**(9): 1964–8.

Scheltens P, Erkinjunti T, Leys D, *et al.* White matter changes on CT and MRI: an overview of visual rating scales. European Task Force on Age-Related White Matter Changes. *Eur Neurol* 1998; **39**(2): 80–9.

van Den Boom, Lesnik Oberstein SA, van Duinen SG, *et al.* Subcortical lacunar lesions: an MR imaging finding in patients with cerebral autosomal dominant arteriopathy with subcortical infarcts and leukoencephalopathy. *Radiology* 2002; **224**(3): 791–6.

Van der Werf YD, Scheltens P, Lindeboom J, Witter MP, Uylings HB, Jolles J. Deficits of memory, executive functioning and attention following infarction in the thalamus; a study of 22 cases with localised lesions. *Neuropsychologia* 2003; **41**(10): 1330–44.

Van Straaten EC, Scheltens P, Knol DL, *et al.* Operational definitions for the NINDS-AIREN criteria for vascular dementia. An interobserver study. *Stroke* 2003; **34**(8): 1907–12.

Wahlund LO, Barkhof F, Fazekas F, *et al.* A new rating scale for age-related white matter changes applicable to MRI and CT. *Stroke* 2001; **32**(6): 1318–22.

Wardlaw JM, Lewis SC, Keir SL, Dennis MS, Shenkin S. Cerebral microbleeds are associated with lacunar stroke defined clinically and radiologically, independently of white matter lesions. *Stroke* 2006; **37** (10): 2633–6.

Yousry TA, Seelos K, Mayer M, *et al.* Characteristic MR lesion pattern and correlation of T1 and T2 lesion volume with neurologic and neuropsychological findings in cerebral autosomal dominant arteriopathy with subcortical infarcts and leukoencephalopathy (CADASIL). *Am J Neuroradiol* 1999; **20**(1): 91–100.

6

Functional imaging in vascular dementia: clinical practice

Lars-Olof Wahlund and Rimma Axelsson

Introduction

Functional imaging is sometimes used in dementia work-ups. The technique has been mostly used in tertiary dementia units such as university clinics. The majority of studies in this area have been performed on Alzheimer's disease (AD), far fewer papers have focused on vascular dementia (VaD). Functional imaging is used to investigate regional cerebral blood flow and glucose metabolism changes. It reflects vascular and neuronal metabolic functions which should provide a sound basis for the method/diagnostic analysis.

Background

The purpose of functional imaging in clinical practice is to increase diagnostic accuracy when differentiating between dementia disorders. The techniques most often used are imaging of regional cerebral blood flow (rCBF), using single photon emission computed tomography (SPECT), and imaging of glucose metabolism using positron emission tomography (PET). There are also other modalities able to image brain function: functional magnetic resonance imaging (fMRI), diffusion-weighted imaging based on MRI, and perfusion imaging based on MRI (see also Chapter 5).

The present chapter focuses on regional cerebral blood flow (rCBF) with SPECT and glucose metabolism with PET.

The SPECT technique is based on the fact that a radioactively labeled compound will be trapped in brain tissue during its first passage through the vessels. The most common radionuclide used for labeling is 99m-Tc (Technetium). The concentration of the labeled compound is proportional to the blood flow in the area. Patients are examined in a device (gamma camera) which detects the gamma rays emitted from the radioactively labeled compound. Registration of radioactivity is performed by a two- or three- headed gamma camera, after which images are reconstructed and displayed on a computer screen. Different dementias are characterized by specific blood flow patterns. Alzheimer's disease typically has reduced blood flow in the temporal and parietal areas, while frontotemporal lobe degeneration is characterized by a reduced blood flow in the frontal and anterior temporal parts of the brain.

Glucose metabolism is imaged by a glucose analog labeled with a positron emitting nuclide, preferably Fluor-18. Radioactivity is detected with a positron emission tomography (PET) camera. The pathological changes in Alzheimer's disease and frontotemporal lobe degeneration are similar to those seen with SPECT.

Vascular Cognitive Impairment in Clinical Practice, ed. Lars-Olof Wahlund, Timo Erkinjuntti and Serge Gauthier. Published by Cambridge University Press. © Cambridge University Press 2009.

Regional cerebral bloodflow (rCBF) detected with SPECT

Technetium-labeled agents – hexametyl-propylen-aminoxin =HMPAO (Tc-99m-HMPAO, commercial name Ceretec®) or N,N'-1,2-ethylenediylbis-ı-cysteine diethyl ester dihydrochloride (commercial name Neurolite®) – are usually used to investigate cerebral blood flow. The amount of these compounds trapped in the tissue is in direct relation to the rCBF in the area. The images can be evaluated in several ways. The most common evaluation technique has been to visually judge the reduction of blood flow using specific rating scales. Lately, other techniques have been introduced; e.g. a quotient calculated between the signal intensity in the affected area and that found in a reference area (usually the cerebellum). In recent years, more sophisticated evaluation methods have been introduced, statistical parametric mapping (SPM) (Yoshikawa *et al.*, 2003b). Another alternative SPECT technique utilizes a Xenon isotope. This method has been used in clinical practice, usually either with visual ratings or with quotient calculations (Komataui *et al.*, 1998).

It is difficult to categorize a specific perfusion pattern in vascular dementia with the aim of differentiating it from Alzheimer's disease, other dementias, or healthy controls. In an early review by Jagust *et al.* from 1995, it was reported that it was difficult to differentiate multiple infarct dementias (MID) from Alzheimer's disease using SPECT, due to a variety of different findings in VaD patients (Jagust *et al.*, 1995). These findings included temporal/parietal and multiple focal hypoperfusion as well as patchy and global rCBF reductions. Reductions in the basal ganglia and frontal lobes were also reported.

Lojkowska *et al.* reported that vascular dementia patients had "patchy" blood flow changes in different regions compared to Alzheimer's patients. In this study, it was also reported that vascular dementia patients had a pronounced reduction of blood flow in the motor cortex, something that has not been reported elsewhere.

A reduction in the cerebral blood flow in the frontal lobes seems to be the most consistent finding in vascular dementia (Talbot *et al.*, 1998; Yoshikawa *et al.*, 2003a, 2003b). Another common feature is what is described as "scattered diffuse" or patchy rCBF pattern. Examples of vascular dementia and a normal healthy subject imaged with HMPAO-SPECT are presented in Figures 6.1 and 6.2, respectively.

As mentioned earlier, visual rating or simple activity quotients were the evaluation techniques most utilized in the past. During the last decade several other more sophisticated methods have been introduced. In one study, SPM has been used to analyze the rCBF pattern in VaD patients. In this study a relationship between the reduction of cerebral blood flow in the anterior and posterior associating areas (Yang *et al.*, 2002) and the severity of dementia was reported. The same authors report in a publication from 2006 that when subcortical ischemic vascular dementias were compared with controls, a significant reduction of blood flow in the thalamus, the anterior cingulate gyrus, the head of caudate nucleus and the left para-hippocampus was found in VaD subjects (Shim *et al.*, 2006).

Some researchers have used computerized image analysis to increase the ability of rCBF to differentiate between vascular dementia and other dementias (Hanyu *et al.*, 2004). These authors described a technique in which a "stereotactic surface projection" method was used. The method evaluates images by carrying out a pixel-by-pixel analysis of the severity, extent and localization of abnormal rCBF. In this study the authors were able to divide the perfusion pattern into three groups:
- anterior cerebral hypoperfusion,
- posterior cerebral hypoperfusion,
- diffuse cerebral hypoperfusion.

It was also reported that patients with Binswanger's disease (as VaD was earlier designated) showed decreased blood flow in the frontal lobes and in the anterior cingulate cortex, while Alzheimer patients showed a decrease in the temporo-parietal and the posterior cingulate cortices.

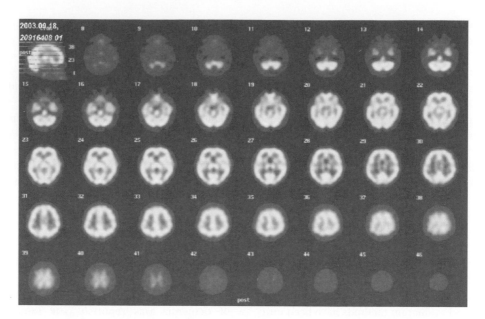

Figure 6.1 99m-Tc-HMPAO Transaxial SPECT slices in a patient with non-altered cerebral blood flow. See Figure 6.1 in the color plate section.

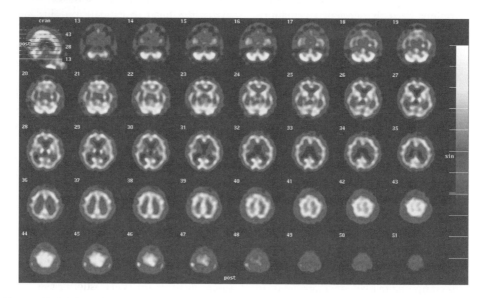

Figure 6.2 99m-Tc-HMPAO Transaxial SPECT slices in a patient with VaD. The patchy distribution pattern is seen in the whole brain, with small areas of mild hypoperfusion in several cortical and subcortical regions: right posterior frontal, left lateral temporal, parietal bilateral, occipital bilateral. See Figure 6.2 in the color plate section.

Table 6.1 Parameters of importance for evaluation of diagnostic tests.

Sensitivity: The probability to find an abnormal result in individuals with the disease. The test finds all those who are sick
Specificity: The probability to find a normal result in those who are without the disease. The test finds all those who are healthy (or without a specific disease)
Positive and negative likelihood ratios, LR+/− : LR for a test combines information from sensitivity and specificity and is expressed as quotients:

LR+ = sensitivity/(1–specificity)
LR− = 1–sensitivity/specificity

LR+ is commonly stratified as follows:
1–5 low, 5–9 medium, and high >10

Low values indicate the method does not generally contribute to the diagnostics. High values indicate that the method is good at separating given diagnostic groups

Another computerized image method, known as "Fractal dimension analysis" (FD) has been reported by Yoshikawa *et al.* (2003c). In this study, Alzheimer's disease was compared with vascular dementia patients. Fractal dimension is an index of the heterogeneity of rCBF; a higher FD indicates uneven rCBF in SPECT images. It was reported that higher FD values were found in VaD and AD subjects compared to controls. Moreover, the heterogeneity of rCBF SPECT images was larger in the anterior parts of the brain in VaD compared to AD.

These analysis methods confirm earlier findings that in patients with VaD a reduction in rCBF appears in the anterior parts of the brain and that the rCBF reductions are more heterogeneously distributed.

Diagnostic value of SPECT

In a systematic review by Dougall *et al.* (2004), the regional cerebral blood flow in vascular dementia patients was compared to Alzheimer's disease to assess its diagnostic usefulness. After a thorough and systematic search of the literature, the authors reported the results of 13 studies. The overall pooled weighted sensitivity for VaD compared to AD was 71% and the pooled weighted specificity 76%, resulting in positive and negative likelihood ratios

(LR+ and LR−) of 3.0 and 0.4 respectively. For an explanation of likelihood ratios, see Table 6.1.

According to the authors, these likelihood ratios are small but sometimes important in shifting the pre-test to post-test probabilities. However, it is important to note that meta reviews are conservative in their conclusions since the most recent publications are usually not included. Another aspect of the studies included is that severely demented patients were sometimes investigated, resulting in one thing. The pathological changes are often more evident, as is the clinical picture. In other words, the usefulness of a test in such cases is less than when the patients are investigated earlier in the disease process. However, it is in the early cases that the need for an efficient diagnostic tool is more important.

The results from Dougall *et al.* (2004) were, to some extent, supported by a study from Talbot *et al.* (1998) in which the authors compared rCBF as a diagnostic tool in VaD and other dementias including Alzheimer's disease, Lewy body disease, frontotemporal dementia and progressive aphasia. They reported the diagnostic usefulness in likelihood ratios and found that a reduction in bilateral anterior rCBF differentiated vascular dementia from Alzheimer's disease with a positive likelihood ratio (LR) of 7.3. When comparing Lewy body disease with VaD, bilateral posterior and unilateral anterior reductions in rCBF differentiated the two diseases with an LR+ of 9.8. When comparing FTD and VaD, the bilateral anterior blood flow was similar, resulting in an LR+ of 2.2, indicating that VaD and frontotemporal dementia showed similar rCBF pathology in the anterior parts of the brain.

SPECT and vascular reactivity

Regional cerebral blood flow assessed with SPECT has also been used to study vascular reactivity. Vascular reactivity is dependent on pathological changes in the vessels (usually due to arteriosclerosis), resulting in their losing the ability to change diameter in response to metabolic demands.

Vascular reactivity can be studied by ascertaining the effect of acetazolamide on rCBF. Acetazolamide normally induces the vessels to dilatate, resulting in an increase in rCBF. In areas with vascular lesions, acetazolamide is unable to increase blood flow.

In one study, the basal rCBF of vascular dementia patients' was compared to acetazolamid rCBF (Pavics *et al.*, 1998). A quantitative evaluation of VaD and AD dementia subjects showed that approximately 70% of the VaD patients had decreased reactivity while the corresponding figure for AD was 22%.

The use of SPECT in following treatment

rCBF-SPECT has also been used to evaluate the effect of dementia treatment. In one study, published by Lojkowska *et al.* (2003), the effect of treatment in eight patients with Alzheimer's disease was evaluated by assessing the change in regional cerebral blood flow in the temporal, frontal and motor cortex. The patients were imaged before and after 12 months of treatment with cholinesterase inhibitors (AchEI). Only in AD subjects was a significant ($p < 0.03$) increase in rCBF found in temporal areas. In the frontal cortex and in the motor cortex, a non-significant increase was noted in both VaD and AD subjects. It was

suggested that the reported increase in rCBF was a result of improved functionality in the cholinergic innervation of the vessels, which in turn was caused by the AchEI.

SPECT and CADASIL

rCBF has also been studied in CADASIL, a hereditary form of VaD (Scheid *et al.*, 2006). In a study of three CADASIL subjects, it was found that they all had reduced rCBF in the cingulate cortex. In one patient, decreased blood flow was also seen in the temporal cortex bilaterally, and in another additional deficits were found in thalamic and fronto-parietal areas. The authors concluded that functional imaging might be important in the diagnosis of CADASIL, but that it was not related to the disease-associated cognitive decline.

PET imaging in VaD

Generally, PET shows the same disease pattern as SPECT when ligands are used for investigating regional cerebral blood flow (see Figure 6.3). PET is also used to study regional glucose metabolism using Fluoro-Deoxy-D-Glucose (FDG), oxygen

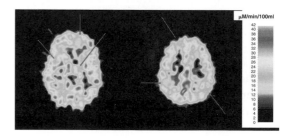

Figure 6.3 Two transaxial slices of 18F-FDG-PET in a patient with VaD. Multiple small uptake defects can be seen in different regions: frontal bilateral, right medial temporal, parietal cortex and left basal ganglia (arrows). The picture was taken at Uppsala University PET-Center, Sweden, by Henry Engler. See Figure 6.3 in the color plate section.

metabolic extraction rate and cerebral oxygen metabolic rate. A study by De Reuck *et al.* (1999) showed that rCBF, regional oxygen extraction rate and regional cerebral oxygen metabolic rate are decreased in VaD (actually multi-infarct dementia). There was a reduction in rCBF and regional cerebral oxygen metabolic rate, and a generalized increase of regional oxygen extraction rate in dementia caused by lacunar infarcts. The authors concluded that there are two different pathophysiological mechanisms in vascular dementia. PET was also used to study vascular reactivity. This was accomplished by evaluating the effect on rCBF of the inhalation of $^{13}NH_3$. A reduction in vascular reactivity was found in both MID patients and patients with lacunar infarctions. The latter group was more severely impaired.

In a small but interesting study, the diagnostic usefulness of FDG-PET and HMPAO SPECT was compared. Alzheimer patients, VaD patients and controls were compared and PET was found to be superior to SPECT in differentiating AD from VaD. The most significant areas were the temporoparietal and occipital association cortices where a reduction was detected in the AD group compared to the VaD subjects (Mielke *et al.*, 1994).

Summary

Despite the fact that functional imaging reflects brain perfusion and vascular dementia is the result of pathological changes in brain vessels, there is little consensus regarding a specific brain perfusion pattern in vascular dementia. This is in contrast to primary degenerative disorders such as Alzheimer's disease and frontotemporal lobe degeneration which usually show a clear pattern of brain perfusion.

In clinical practice rCBF-SPECT of vascular dementia shows a reduction in the anterior lobes and a patchy reduction of blood perfusion. According to the meta review by Dougall *et al.* (2004) it is clear that the clinical usefulness of SPECT in differentiating vascular dementia from Alzheimer's disease is limited. Despite this fact, SPECT might be considered a complement to dementia work-ups, when differentiating between different primary degenerative disorders and vascular dementia. It sometimes yields relevant and useful information.

PET scanning of glucose metabolism shows the same pattern of reduction in glucose metabolism as is seen with rCBF-SPECT.

Other aspects of the comparison between PET and SPECT are cost and availability. SPECT is much more available and less costly than PET imaging and, therefore, more applicable to the dementia work-up in primary and secondary settings. The efficacy of modern PET imaging with new ligands, such as Pittsburgh Compound B (PIB) imaging of amyloid, in the evaluation of VaD needs to be further investigated.

REFERENCES

De Reuck J, Decoo D, Hasenbroekx MC, *et al.* Acetazolamide vasoreactivity in vascular dementia: a positron emission tomographic study. *Eur Neurol* 1999; **41**(1): 31–6.

Dougall NJ, Bruggink S, Ebmeier KP. Systematic review of the diagnostic accuracy of 99mTc-HMPAO-SPECT in dementia. *Am J Geriatr Psychiatry* 2004; **12**(6): 554–70.

Hanyu H, Shimizu S, Tanaka Y, Takasaki M, Koizumi K, Abe K. Cerebral blood flow patterns in Binswanger's disease: a SPECT study using three-dimensional stereotactic surface projections. *J Neurol Sci* 2004; **220**(1–2): 79–84.

Jagust WJ, Johnson KA, Holman BL. SPECT perfusion imaging in the diagnosis of dementia. *J Neuroimaging* 1995; **5** Suppl 1: S45–52.

Komatani A, Yamaguchi K, Sugai Y, *et al.* Assessment of demented patients by dynamic SPECT of inhaled xenon-133. *J Nucl Med* 1988; **29**(10): 1621–6.

Lojkowska W, Ryglewicz D, Jedrzejczak T, *et al.* The effect of cholinesterase inhibitors on the regional blood flow in patients with Alzheimer's disease and vascular dementia. *J Neurol Sci* 2003; **216**(1): 119–26.

Mielke R, Pietrzyk U, Jacobs A, *et al.* HMPAO SPECT and FDG PET in Alzheimer's disease and vascular dementia: comparison of perfusion and metabolic pattern. *Eur J Nucl Med* 1994; **21**(**10**): 1052–60.

Pavics L, Grunwald F, Reichmann K, *et al*. rCBF SPECT and the acetazolamide test in the evaluation of dementia. *Nucl Med Rev Cent East Eur* 1998; **1**(1): 13–19.

Scheid R, Preul C, Lincke T, *et al*. Correlation of cognitive status, MRI- and SPECT-imaging in CADASIL patients. *Eur J Neurol* 2006; **13**(4): 363–70.

Shim YS, Yang DW, Kim BS, Shon YM, Chung YA. Comparison of regional cerebral blood flow in two subsets of subcortical ischemic vascular dementia: statistical parametric mapping analysis of SPECT. *J Neurol Sci* 2006; **250** (1–2): 85–91.

Talbot PR, Lloyd JJ, Snowden JS, Neary D, Testa HJ. A clinical role for 99m Tc-HMPAO SPECT in the investigation of dementia? *J Neurol Neurosurg Psychiatry* 1998; **64**(3): 306–13.

Yang DW, Kim BS, Park JK, Kim SY, Kim EN, Sohn HS. Analysis of cerebral blood flow of subcortical vascular dementia with single photon emission computed tomography: adaptation of statistical parametric mapping. *J Neurol Sci* 2002; **203–204**: 199–205.

Yoshikawa T, Murase K, Oku N, *et al*. Quantification of the heterogeneity of cerebral blood flow in vascular dementia. *J Neurol* 2003a; **250**(2): 194–200.

Yoshikawa T, Murase K, Oku N, *et al*. Statistical image analysis of cerebral blood flow in vascular dementia with small-vessel disease. *J Nucl Med* 2003b; **44**(4): 505–11.

Yoshikawa T, Murase K, Oku N, *et al*. Heterogeneity of cerebral blood flow in Alzheimer disease and vascular dementia. *AJNR* 2003c; **24**(7): 1341–7.

7

Biomarkers in vascular dementia

Anders Wallin and Tuula Pirttilä

Introduction

A biomarker can be defined as an indicator of health or pathology. Biomarkers primarily identify the existence or the absence of a given disease, but in a broader sense a biomarker may also reflect a pathophysiological process associated with the disease, or confirm the risk of developing the disease. Biomarkers can be classified, e.g. according to their relation to the illness: they can be primary and linked to the essential pathological processes, secondary (reflecting non-specific disease-associated pathological processes), or they can simply be epiphenomenal in nature.

The vast majority of biomarker research has focused on the development of markers for Alzheimer's disease (AD). Table 7.1 gives examples of possible markers for different types of brain pathologies. Many pathological processes – for example, oxidative stress, inflammation, or excitotoxic damage – are shared by different dementing disorders. Also, many patients with clinical dementia syndrome have mixed pathology consisting of, for example, AD pathology and cerebrovascular disease (CVD). The markers can be used for prognostic assessment of cognitive decline, early identification of specific diseases, differential diagnosis, detection of different pathological processes, and monitoring progression of the disease or therapeutic responses. However, it is unlikely that a single marker can be found that could be used for all purposes in any dementing disease. This review summarizes the data of some biomarkers that are associated with the presence of vascular disease, and potential markers of different brain pathologies relevant to vascular dementia (VaD) and for differential diagnosis.

Major types and pathogenesis of vascular dementia

Impaired blood flow resulting from partial blockage of the vessels supplying the brain dominated our concepts about the cause of VaD for decades. During the 1970s, as a result of thorough neuropathological studies, the concept of chronic brain ischemia as an explanation for VaD was abandoned. It was claimed that vascular disease could lead to cognitive disorders, not via blood-flow-related energy deficiency, but through repeated stroke episodes resulting in cerebral tissue damage. However, the demonstration of symptoms producing white matter changes not directly associated with stroke episodes, the increased number of elderly in the population, and changes in the cerebrovascular disease panorama has led to questioning about whether multiple infarctions are the essential cause of VaD. Instead of simplified disease categories, it is now asserted that vascular

Vascular Cognitive Impairment in Clinical Practice, ed. Lars-Olof Wahlund, Timo Erkinjuntti and Serge Gauthier. Published by Cambridge University Press. © Cambridge University Press 2009.

Table 7.1 Examples of possible biomarkers for brain pathology.

Pathology	Possible markers	Comments
Neurofibrillary pathology	tau, p-tau	Highest CSF levels reported in AD, exception CJD (extremely high CSF tau levels)
Amyloid pathology	βAPP, soluble Aβ-peptides	Measurable in plasma and CSF Decreased CSF levels in brain amyloid diseases
Axonal and neuronal pathology	tau, ASAT, neuron-specific enolase, (NSE), ubiquitin, 14-3-3 protein, neuromodulin (GAP-43), neurofilament, transglutaminase	CSF levels increase in various neurodegenerative diseases
Myelin damage	sulfatide, myelin basic protein	
Synaptic changes	synaptotagmin, rab3, SNAP25, synaptophysin, chromogranin A, neuromodulin (GAP-43), neurogranin	
Neurotransmitters	Cholinergic markers Monoamine metabolites 5-hydroxyindoleacetic acid (5-HIAA), homovanillic acid (HVA), and vanillylmandelic acid (VMA)	
Glial cell activation	GFAP, S-100β, glutamine synthetase	Measurable in plasma and CSF, sources in plasma unclear
Inflammation	acute-phase reactants, cytokines, complement factors, adhesion molecules, beta-2-microglobulin, matrix metalloproteinases, nitrioc oxide metabolites	Mainly produced by glial cells in the CNS and thus CSF levels may increase with glial activation
Oxidative damage	8-hydroxyguanoside, 4-hydroxynonenal, SOD, isoprostanes, nitrotyrosine	
Miscellaneous	neuronal thread protein, creatine kinase prostaglandins, 24S-hydroxycholesterol, heme-oxygenase 1, kallikrein, somatostatin, transthyretin, cystatin C, angiotensin converting enzyme, glutamic oxaloacetic transaminase (GOT), lactic dehydrogenase (LDH)	

Table 7.2 Vascular mechanisms for brain damage.

Thromboembolism
Vessel wall damage
• Atherosclerosis
• Hyalinosis
• Amyloid angiopathy
Cerebrovascular insufficiency
• Disturbance of systemic circulation
• Vascular anatomy of the brain
• Disturbed regulation of cerebral blood flow
Hyperviscosity
Bleeding

mechanisms leading to cognitive impairment are the basis for disease classification. Since several such mechanisms exist (Wallin and Blennow, 1993; Table 7.2), consequently, there are several types of VaD (Roman *et al.*, 2002; Table 7.3). In the past decade, particular attention has been given to post-stroke dementia with cognitive impairment following an identified stroke and subcortical vascular dementia with a more insidious disease course. In that respect, post-stroke dementia was considered to be a model for large-vessel (thromboembolic) and subcortical vascular dementia for small-vessel

Table 7.3 Clinicopathological classification of vascular dementia. Reprinted from *The Lancet Neurology*, Vol 1, Issue 7, Roman GC, Erkinjuntti T, Wallin A, Pantoni L, Chui HC. Subcortical ischemic vascular dementia. 426–36, 2002, with permission from Elsevier.

Large-vessel vascular dementia

Multi-infarct dementia – multiple large complete infarcts, cortical or subcortical in location, usually with perifocal incomplete infarction involving the white matter

Strategic infarct dementia – single infarct in functionally critical areas of the brain (angular gyrus, thalamus, basal forebrain, or territory of the posterior cerebral artery or anterior cerebral artery)

Small-vessel vascular dementia

SIVD

Binswanger's disease

Lacunar dementia or lacunar state (état lacunaire)

Multiple lacunes with extensive perifocal incomplete infarctions

Cerebral autosomal dominant arteriopathy with subcortical infarcts and leucoencephalopathy (CADASIL)

Cortical–subcortical

Hypertensive and arteriosclerotic angiopathy

Cerebral amyloid angiopathies (including familial British dementia)

Other hereditary forms

Collagen-vascular disease with dementia

Venous occlusions

Ischemic–hypoperfusive vascular dementia

Diffuse anoxic–ischemic encephalopathy

Restricted injury due to selective vulnerability

Incomplete white matter infarction

Border-zone infarction

Hemorrhagic vascular dementia

Traumatic subdural hematoma

Subarachnoid hemorrhage

Cerebral hemorrhage

(hypoperfusive) VaD. There are also less common types, such as, cerebral autosomal dominant arteriopathy with subcortical infarcts and leukoencephalopathy (CADASIL). In addition to that, several recent epidemiological and neuropathological studies have found that vascular factors and Alzheimer-type degenerative changes are common, simultaneous manifestations in patients with dementia. The term mixed-type dementia (or AD plus VaD, or AD with CVD) has been introduced for these patients. It is rather about a supertype than a subtype of VaD.

Post-stroke dementia

Several studies have shown an increased prevalence of dementia among stroke survivors. Three months after an episode of stroke, the prevalence of dementia (post-stroke dementia) has been found to range between 18% and 30%. At 3-year follow up in a group of stroke patients, dementia was reported in 29%. Insufficient stroke type, lesion location, total volume of infarcted tissue, incomplete impairment of tissue function are presumably essential factors underlying the development of post-stroke dementia.

In a study by Barba *et al.* (2000), progressive cognitive dysfunction following stroke episodes was found in only 1 of 10 patients, suggesting that cognitive disorders are a residual syndrome, i.e. not a sign of dementia in a strict sense. In the three-year follow-up study mentioned above, most of the patients developed dementia syndrome within the first half year, which also suggests that dementia syndrome is a residual syndrome. Approximately 10% of stroke patients followed up for cognitive ability showed signs of dementia even prior to the stroke episode. In investigating patients during the acute phase, Hénon *et al.* (1997) found signs of pre-stroke dementia in 15% of the patients.

Although several questions have yet to be answered, under certain conditions it is more or less apparent that a causal association exists between stroke and dementia:

- in young patients where there is small probability for concurrent Alzheimer's disease;
- when cognitive ability, which was normal prior to the stroke episode, was impaired immediately after stroke and cognitive dysfunction became worse with time;
- when a well-defined vasculopathy leading to dementia is demonstrated.

Strategic infarction dementia is sometimes explained as a special variety of post-stroke dementia. Isolated bilateral infarctions in the hippocampus can lead to dementia, but milder cognitive disturbances are more common. Bilateral thalamic infarctions, unilateral thalamic infarctions, basal frontal infarctions, infarctions in the angular gyrus, infarctions in the non-dominant parieto-temporal region, and infarctions in the dominant hemisphere are other examples of strategically localized infarctions that are reported to cause dementia. Strategic infarction dementia as a disease entity has been called into question since one generally ignores the influence from other lesions, e.g. white matter damage, that are not always investigated in studies (often case descriptions) addressing strategic infarction dementia (Pantoni *et al.*, 2001).

Subcortical vascular dementia

Subcortical vascular dementia is the most homogeneous subtype and probably also the most common (Roman *et al.*, 2002). Changes found in magnetic resonance imaging (MRI) within the subcortical area in patients with VaD have been found to be associated with impairment of executive-psychomotor capacity, but not with impairment of global cognitive capacity. Patients with subcortical vascular dementia have been found to show more pronounced impairment in their capacity to deal with complex information, formulate strategies, and exercise self-control in comparison to Alzheimer's patients whose executive dysfunction was mainly associated with attention deficit disorder and impaired working memory. Patients with subcortical vascular dementia have shown less pronounced episodic memory impairment, but more depressive symptomatology and more variability in progress speed than have patients with AD. It has been suggested that patients with subcortical microvascular disease are the ones that later develop dementia which, in the early phases of the disease, show signs of mild cognitive impairment (MCI). The findings speak in favor of disturbance of the executive control function in patients with subcortical vascular dementia, i.e. the control function for goal-oriented behavior, which coordinates cognitive functions such as planning, attention, working memory, abstraction capacity, flexibility, and the ability to take action.

The crucial mechanism of subcortical vascular dementia presumably involves damage to the arterioles as a result of aging, hypertension, and other factors such as diabetes, and genetic vulnerability leading to lumen constriction, impaired ability to change lumen diameter according to metabolic needs, and possible ischemic-hypoxic tissue damage within the vulnerable vascular architecture of the terminal areas of the long penetrating arteries (border-zone areas). The structural and physiological changes in the branches of the penetrating arteries, the arterioles, can also lead to degradation of the blood–brain barrier.

Mixed-type dementia

Not long ago, the occurrence of vascular risk factors/diseases was considered to be exclusion criteria for the diagnosis of AD. Longitudinal epidemiological studies have, however, shown that hypertension, diabetes, arterial fibrillation, and smoking are risk factors not only for vascular dementia but also for AD. It has been suggested that ischemic processes not only co-exist with AD, but also contribute to its development by decreasing the threshold for cognitive decline and possibly also by precipitating neurodegenerative changes. The "Nun Study" (Snowdon *et al.*, 1997) found that among deceased elderly nuns diagnosed with AD, based on neuropathological examination, only 57% had dementia. Among those who had been diagnosed with AD plus cortical infarctions, 75% had dementia, and of those who had AD plus lacunes in subcortical brain regions, 93% had dementia. Other studies have also shown that vascular lesions influence the effect of AD, or vice versa (Esiri *et al.*, 1999; MRC-CFAS, 2001).

Ischemia, via the vasoactive effects of amyloid, impaired blood flow, and reduced metabolism, inflammatory mechanisms, and changes in the blood–brain barrier are different factors that have been considered as the genesis of vascular tissue damage in AD. Some authors have even suggested that AD is primarily microvascular, where degeneration of the capillaries in the hippocampus and other brain regions with secondary neuronal hypometabolism comprise the central pathophysiological chain of events (de la Torre, 2002).

Identifying patients with AD and concurrent CVD is not easy when the patient lacks markers for AD. This can be a reason why the rate of mixed dementia has been underestimated. According to a relatively current review of clinical neuropathological studies, mixed dementia comprises between 20% and 40% of dementia cases (Zekry *et al.*, 2002), and may be the most common form of dementia in the very old population.

Markers for the presence of vascular disease

Markers of hypercoagulative state

Abnormalities of coagulation and the fibrinolytic system leading to a hypercoagulable state are associated with vascular disease. Serum or plasma markers of a hypercoagulable state include markers of activated coagulation, platelet activation, hypofibrinolysis and endothelial dysfunction.

Among the serum markers of hypercoagulability, serum fibrinogen has been most commonly studied. Fibrinogen, a precursor of fibrin and an acute-phase reactant, is a final step in the coagulation response to vascular and tissue injury. The Rotterdam Study showed that subjects with higher levels of fibrinogen had an increased risk of dementia, the hazard ratio for dementia per standard deviation increase of fibrinogen being 1.30 (95% CI, 1.13–1.50) after adjustment for age, gender, cardiovascular factors and stroke (Bots *et al.*, 1998). The risk was increased for VaD and AD. Other studies have shown that plasma fibrinogen levels are increased in patients with VaD (Smith *et al.*, 1997; Stott *et al.*, 2001). Plasma fibrinogen levels may correlate with the amount of white matter changes and some studies suggest that high fibrinogen levels are associated with the progressive phase of Binswanger's disease (Tomimoto *et al.*, 1999).

Other markers of hypercoagulable state include thrombin–antithrombin complex (TAT), fibrinogen degradation product (FDP), a breakdown product that is formed from fibrinogen cleavage by thrombin, and D-dimer, a marker of fibrin turnover. High FDP levels correlate with stroke and asymptomatic atherosclerosis (Lip *et al.*, 2001), and a recent study found almost 10-times higher levels in patients with VaD compared to controls, whereas the levels were only slightly increased in AD (Gupta *et al.*, 2005). The Rotterdam study showed that increased plasma levels of D-dimer were associated with increased risk of VaD and AD (Bots *et al.*, 1998). Increased levels were also found in patients with VaD in case control studies (Stott *et al.*, 2001). Another study (Barber *et al.*, 2004) showed that levels were higher in atrial fibrillation (AF) patients with dementia than those without dementia, but the assessment of cognition was performed by telephone screening and no classification of dementia was done. Increased levels of prothrombin factor I + II have been reported in patients with lacunar stroke, VaD and AD, and in AF patients with dementia (Barber *et al.*, 2004; Gupta *et al.*, 2005). Patients with Binswanger's disease who are at deteriorating stages may have increased TAT, prothrombin fragment I + II and D-dimer levels, whereas no changes were found in subjects without dementia and white matter changes and stable phase of Binswanger's disease (Tomimoto *et al.*, 1999). It has been hypothesized that coagulation activation may result in the formation of microthrombi and microcirculatory disturbances in the brains of these patients, and thus promote further tissue destruction.

Other abnormalities of hemostasis have also been described in association with VaD. Levels of a clotting factor VII were increased in VaD and AD in one study (Gupta *et al.*, 2005). Lipoprotein-a (Lp-a), an LDL-like particle and acute-phase reactant, has thrombogenic properties. It has structural homology to plasminogen and may compete with it for binding to plasminogen receptors, fibrinogen and fibrin. A recent meta-analysis of 27 prospective studies showed a risk ratio of 1.6 (95% CI, 1.4–1.8) for coronary heart disease for those with the top third concentrations of Lp-a as compared to those with the bottom third (Danesh *et al.*, 2000). Increased levels have been found also in VaD (Urakami *et al.*, 2000). Endothelial dysfunction may contribute to the development of vascular disease. Plasminogen-activator-inhibitor-1 (PAI-1) is the main inhibitor of the fibrinolytic pathway that is expressed by endothelial cells. Elevated plasma PAI-1 levels have been found in VaD but not in AD (Mari *et al.*, 1996). Von Willebrand factor is a marker of endothelial cell damage and promotes aggregation of platelets and coagulation. High serum levels have been found in VaD and AD (Gupta *et al.*, 2005; Mari *et al.*, 1996).

However, atherothrombosis is a systemic disease, and hence hemostasis abnormality may not be specific for any single vascular phenotype although some studies suggest that plasma fibrinogen levels may correlate with the presence of small vessel disease. Many patients with vascular cognitive impairment have co-existent ischemic heart disease, and this may contribute to the levels of these markers. Moreover, hemostatic abnormalities can also be found in patients with AD. None of the described markers has proven to be useful for diagnosing a significant cerebrovascular disease or planning therapeutic interventions in patients with or irrespective of cognitive impairment.

Homocysteine

Homocysteine is a sulfur-containing amino acid that occurs in a number of forms in plasma. It is formed from methionine and then metabolized via the B6-dependent trans-sulfuration pathway. Under negative methionine balance homocysteine is metabolized via remethylation pathways, one of which involves B12-dependent enzyme methionine synthase and the substrate 5-methyltetrahydrofolate. The intracellular concentration of homocysteine is under tight metabolic control and depends entirely upon methionine metabolism and the methylation cycle. Excess homocysteine is actively excreted into the extracellular compartment and the plasma concentration reflects the intracellular concentration. Hyperhomocysteinemia is used to refer to elevated levels in plasma, generally greater than 14–15 μmol l^{-1}. The levels are influenced by nutritional, genetic and drug-related factors, and various diseases. Plasma concentration is inversely correlated to dietary intake of folate and vitamins B6 and B12. The levels are higher in men than in women and increase with age.

Recent meta-analysis that included 13 prospective and retrospective studies with stroke outcomes published before January 1999 reported that lower plasma homocysteine levels were associated with a 19% lower stroke risk (OR 0.81; 95%

CI, 0.69–0.95, adjusted for known cardiovascular risk factors) (The Homocysteine Studies Collaboration, 2002). The meta-analysis also showed that the risks associated with homocysteine were significantly weaker in the prospective studies than the retrospective studies. Another meta-analysis included 12 of 21 studies with cerebrovascular outcomes published before July 1999 (Moller et al., 2000). The overall weighted odds-ratio with a concentration above the 95-percentile was 4.12 (2.94–5.77) for cross-sectional studies and 3.74 (2.53–5.54) for the longitudinal studies.

Case-control hospital cohort studies have suggested that elevated plasma homocysteine is associated particularly with subcortical vascular disease and white matter disease (WMD). The relationship between WMD and homocysteine has also been found in AD patients and community-based dwelling non-demented subjects (Hogerworst et al., 2002; Wright et al., 2005). However, in the Cardiovascular Health Study, homocysteine levels were not significantly associated with MRI findings after controlling for age and sex (Longstreth et al., 2004). There was a linear trend between homocysteine level and a pattern of MRI findings combining infarcts and high white matter grade. The influence of homocysteine may be mediated via endothelial dysfunction since, in one study, the inclusion of the endothelial markers intercellular adhesion molecule (ICAM 1) and thrombomodulin in a logistic regression model resulted in loss of significance for the association between homocysteine and subcortical vascular disease (Hassan et al., 2004).

It is still unclear whether homocysteine is causative in the pathogenesis of atherosclerosis and thus a risk factor, or a marker of existing vascular disease. One study showed that plasma homocysteine levels were not elevated within 24 h of acute stroke, but increased 3 months later (Meiklejohn et al., 2001). The other studies reported elevated levels in subjects with acute stroke, and higher levels of homocysteine within 24 h of acute stroke were associated with higher recurrence within 15 months of follow-up (Boysen et al., 2003). The Rotterdam Scan Study found a significant association between plasma homocysteine levels and new silent brain infarcts after a mean follow-up of 3.4 years (Vermeer et al., 2003). However, the Vitamin Intervention for Stroke Prevention (VISP) trial did not show efficacy of combined vitamin therapy consisting of high doses of folic acid, pyridoxine (vitamin B6), and cobalamin (vitamin B12), for recurrent vascular events in patients with non-disabling stroke despite a moderate reduction of total homocysteine after 2 years of treatment (Toole et al., 2004).

Homocysteine has also been related to cognitive decline, but the factors behind the association remain unclear. In prospective hospital cohorts, plasma homocysteine levels were not independently associated with post-stroke cognitive decline (Sachdev et al., 2006). One study found elevated homocysteine levels in patients with VaD, but also in stroke patients without dementia and AD patients (McIlroy et al., 2002). Many other studies have suggested hyperhomocysteinemia to be an independent risk factor for AD (Morris, 2003). Moreover, high homocysteine levels have been associated with low performance in cognitive tests independently of structural changes on MRI (Nurk et al., 2005).

In conclusion, elevated homocysteine levels appear to be strongly associated with existing vascular disease and may be a risk factor for cognitive decline. However, it is not a specific marker for vascular cognitive decline and the value of lowering homocysteine levels remains unclear.

Inflammatory and glial activation markers

Many prospective population-based studies have reported an association between increased plasma levels of inflammation markers and an increased risk of atherosclerotic vascular diseases and dementia. An association between increased C-reactive protein (CRP) and risk of all dementias, but particularly VaD, was found in The Rotterdam Study (Engelhart et al., 2004) and the Honolulu–Asia

Aging Study (Schmidt *et al.*, 2002). Other studies suggest that there is an interaction between inflammatory response and cardiovascular morbidity on the effect on cognition, and that vascular risk factors contribute to cognitive impairment in subjects that have evidence of inflammatory response (Yaffe *et al.*, 2004).

High plasma levels of interleukin *1β* (IL-*1β*), tumor necrosis factor *a* (TNF*a*) and IL-6 have been found to be associated with an increased likelihood of having VaD or AD (Gupta *et al.*, 2005; Zuliani *et al.*, 2006). Some studies have found increased plasma IL-6 levels to be more common in VaD than in AD (Zuliani *et al.*, 2007). However, it has also been found that there is an absence of changes in plasma IL levels in patients with these diagnoses (Tarkowski *et al.*, 1999). Other studies suggest that severity of the disease may influence plasma IL levels. In one of them, AD patients with moderate cognitive decline showed changes in IL-1β levels and IL-6 and TNF*a* release, but no changes were found in patients with mild cognitive decline (De Luigi *et al.*, 2002).

It is reasonable to assume that cerebrospinal fluid (CSF) may reflect inflammatory response in the brain better than plasma. In one study, increased intrathecal levels of TNF*a* and soluble TNF-receptor II (TNFR-II) were found in patients with AD or VaD, whereas there were no changes in plasma TNF*a*, IL-6 or IL-1β levels (Tarkowski *et al.*, 1999). Another study (Wada-Isoe *et al.*, 2004) found elevated CSF concentrations of IL-6 in patients with VaD, but no changes in patients with AD or non-demented patients with CVD. It has also been found that CSF levels of TNF*a* are inversely correlated with levels of Fas/APO-I, suggesting a neuroprotective role of TNF*a* (Tarkowski *et al.*, 1999). On the other hand, a significant correlation between CSF TNF*a* and sulfatide levels has been reported in patients with subcortical vascular dementia (Tarkowski *et al.*, 2003). Since TNF*a* may induce the death of oligodendrocytes, it may contribute to white matter degeneration. Other cytokines and inflammatory mediators that have shown increased CSF levels in AD and VaD include vascular endothelial growth factor (VEGF), transforming growth factor beta (TGF-beta), granulocyte macrophage colony-stimulating factor (GM-CSF) and matrix metalloproteinase 9 (MMP-9, gelatinase B) (Adair *et al.*, 2004; Tarkowski *et al.*, 2001, 2002). Interestingly, in one study, CSF MMP-9 levels were profoundly increased in VaD patients but not in AD patients, whereas the levels of MMP-2 were similar to those in controls (Adair *et al.*, 2004).

Glial fibrillary acidic protein (GFAP) is the structural protein of the astroglial intermediate filament and its levels increase in the brains that show astrogliosis. CSF levels of GFAP may be increased in patients with VaD and AD.

In conclusion, different dementias are associated with a complex inflammatory response but the inflammatory markers are not of help for diagnosis. Their role in monitoring progression of the disease or therapeutic response remains unclear.

Beta amyloid markers

Beta amyloid in cerebrospinal fluid

Accumulation of extracellular neuritic plaques with a core of fibrillar *β*-amyloid protein (A*β*) is a characteristic feature of AD. Soluble CSF A*β* is considered to reflect brain A*β* and may help in the differential diagnosis. Several studies have shown that CSF levels of A*β*42 are decreased in patients with clinical diagnosis of AD (Blennow and Hampel, 2003). The specificity for CSF A*β*42 to distinguish patients with AD from cognitively intact controls has varied from 42% to 88%, and the sensitivity from 72% to 100% in clinic-based studies (Blennow and Hampel, 2003). CSF A*β*42 levels are decreased already in asymptomatic subjects and patients with MCI who developed dementia, particularly AD, during the follow-up (Hansson *et al.*, 2006; Herukka *et al.*, 2005). Recent studies confirmed the rapid clearance of A*β* into CSF in vivo in the human central nervous system (Bateman *et al.*, 2006) and decreased levels may thus indicate dysregulation of production or clearance of A*β* in AD.

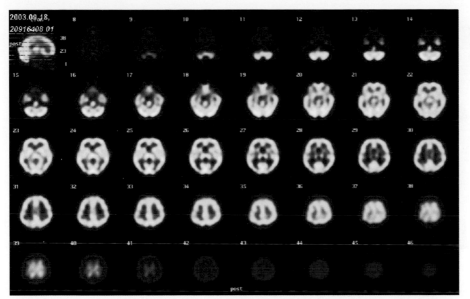

Figure 6.1 99m-Tc-HMPAO Transaxial SPECT slices in a patient with non-altered cerebral blood flow.

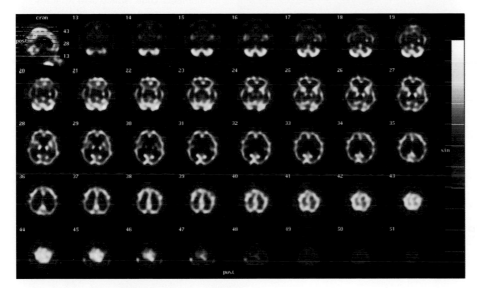

Figure 6.2 99m-Tc-HMPAO Transaxial SPECT slices in a patient with VaD. The patchy distribution pattern is seen in the whole brain, with small areas of mild hypoperfusion in several cortical and subcortical regions: right posterior frontal, left lateral temporal, parietal bilateral, occipital bilateral.

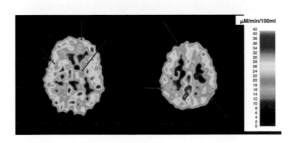

Figure 6.3 Two transaxial slices of 18F-FDG-PET in a patient with VaD. Multiple small uptake defects can be seen in different regions: frontal bilateral, right medial temporal, parietal cortex and left basal ganglia (arrows). The picture was taken at Uppsala University PET-Center, Sweden, by Henry Engler.

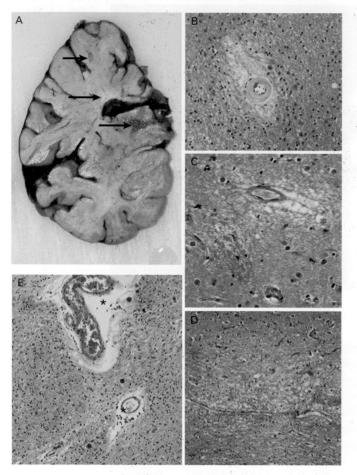

Figure 9.1 Pathological lesions associated with SVD. *A*, recent infarct (arrow) in the thalamus and lacunes (short arrows) in the white matter of a 78-year-old man with cognitive impairment. *B*, hyalinized vessel with severe demyelination in white matter. Moderate gliosis in the perivascular region is also evident. *C* and *D*, microinfarcts and perivascular rarefaction in the basal ganglia. *E*, dilated perivascular spaces (*) in small vessels in the subcortical white matter. Magnification Bar: A=2 cm; B=50 μm; C–D=100 μm; E=200 μm.

Figure 11.1 (below) Schematic representation of the APP molecule and location of known mutations in exons 16 and 17. The APP sequence 665–728 is indicated in one-letter code. Amino acid residues highlighted in red are found in the wild-type molecule, whereas the corresponding mutation(s) for each position are indicated in black letters. Aβ genetic variants primarily associated with CAA are shown in yellow squares. Whenever available, the given name of the mutation is specified. Location of the transmembrane domain (residues 700–723) is indicated by a green box.

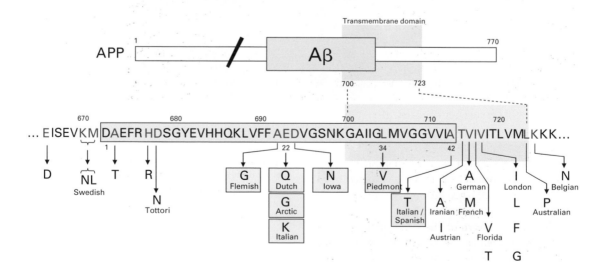

However, decreased Aβ42 levels in CSF have been reported in patients with clinical diagnosis of other dementias, including patients with subcortical vascular dementia. One problem in the studies relates to the fact that clinically examined control and patient populations are always contaminated with AD pathology given its frequency in asymptomatic individuals and patients with clinical phenotype of non-AD dementia. On the other hand, vascular changes are common in AD. Clinicopathological marker studies are sparse. Low postmortem Aβ42 in ventricular CSF correlated with amyloid load in the brain and cerebral vessels in one study (Strozyk et al., 2003). More recent studies found an inverse relation between CSF Aβ42 and in vivo amyloid load using positron emission tomography (PET) imaging of the amyloid-binding agent, Pittsburgh Compound-B (Fagan et al., 2006). We have recently examined the relationship between antemortem CSF Aβ42 and brain pathology in a series that included five patients with VaD. Two of them had low Aβ42 levels, but their brains were not completely free of amyloid pathology. Thus it seems that CSF Aβ42 is a reliable marker of brain amyloid pathology and may help to detect concomitant AD pathology in patients with cerebrovascular disease.

Beta amyloid in plasma

The main pool of plasma Aβ seems to originate from platelets although a proportion of it originates from CSF and brain. Many factors seem to influence plasma Aβ levels. The levels of Aβ40 and Aβ42 increase with age, although a recent longitudinal population based study suggested that the levels decreased during the 7 and 12 years follow-up in men aged 70 years of age at baseline. Plasma Aβ levels correlate with body mass index, creatinine and homocysteine levels in blood. The levels of Aβ42 may be increased in the users of insulin and biguanides and decreased in the users of statin and Gingko biloba.

The studies concerning the relationship between plasma Aβ, dementia and AD have yielded controversial results. The plasma Aβ levels are increased in

some patients with AD and in carriers of APP or presenilin gene mutations, but most AD subjects have similar levels as healthy controls (Scheuner et al., 1996; Sobow et al., 2005). One large population-based study reported increased plasma Aβ42 levels at baseline in cognitively healthy individuals who developed dementia after 3 years of follow-up as compared to those who remained cognitively intact (Mayeux et al., 1999). The levels decreased after the onset of AD. The other studies have shown that plasma Aβ42 or Aβ40 at baseline did not predict cognitive decline, but the increase of plasma Aβ42 in serial measurements may be associated with worsening cognition (Blasko et al., 2006). Thus it seems that the pattern of change of individual biomarkers over time may more accurately predict clinical course than single cross-sectional measurements.

In contrast, the Rotterdam study suggested that high concentrations of Aβ40 but not Aβ42 at baseline were associated with an increased risk of dementia, both AD and VaD (van Oijen et al., 2006). Compared with the first quartile of Aβ40, age- and sex-adjusted hazard ratios for dementia for the second, third, and fourth quartiles were 1.07 (95% CI 0.72–1.58), 1.16 (0.78–1.70), and 1.46 (1.01–2.12), respectively. The possible role for circulating Aβ in microvascular dysfunction and WMD is supported by other studies that showed an association between WMD and plasma Aβ40 concentrations in AD or AD/MCI and subjects with CAA after adjustment for potential confounders. The presence of lacunar infarcts has been associated with increased Aβ40.

Owing to controversial findings, the role of plasma Aβ in the assessment of risk or early detection of dementia remains unclear.

Markers of structural damage

Markers of axonal and neuronal damage

Tau and phospho-tau (p-tau)

Tau is a phosphoprotein that promotes assembly and stability of microtubules by binding to tubulin. Abnormally phosphorylated tau-protein is a core protein of neurofibrillary tangles (NFTs) in AD. CSF tau levels increase with age. Several studies have shown that CSF total tau levels are elevated in AD (Blennow and Hampel, 2003). However, an increase of CSF total tau is not specific for AD and the levels are increased in patients with many other neurodegenerative diseases. Sensitivities of CSF total tau in the diagnosis of AD have varied from 40% to 93%, specificities for non-demented controls from 70% to 98%, and specificities for other dementias from 57% to 85% (Blennow and Hampel, 2003). The levels are elevated in patients with MCI who developed dementia during the follow up (Hansson *et al.*, 2006; Herukka *et al.*, 2005).

Many studies have found elevated CSF tau levels in some patients with a clinical diagnosis of VaD although the levels are lower than in patients with AD (Blennow *et al.*, 1995; Hulstaert *et al.*, 1999; Tapiola *et al.*, 1998). However, several studies have reported normal values in patients with different types of VaD (Sjögren *et al.*, 2000; Wallin and Sjögren, 2001). One reason for the inconsistent results may be the contamination of VaD groups with patients with comorbid AD pathology or the heterogeneity of VaD. Yet, CSF total tau levels increase in diseases associated with extensive neuronal death, such as in Creutzfeld–Jakob's disease (CJD) (Otto *et al.*, 1997), and in patients with acute head trauma and stroke (Hesse *et al.*, 2000; Zemlan *et al.*, 1999). These findings suggest that CSF tau may be a marker of neuronal cell death and axonal degeneration rather than a disease-specific marker. One recent clinicopathological study found the highest tau levels in AD and slightly elevated levels in frontotemporal dementia and dementia with Lewy bodies in comparison with controls (Clark *et al.*, 2003). In our own clinicopathological study, one patient with severe vascular pathology had elevated CSF tau whereas the levels were normal in four other patients with VaD.

Hyperphosphorylation of tau is a characteristic feature for AD and measurement of soluble phosphorylated tau (p-tau) may thus offer better discrimination between AD and other neurodegenerative diseases including VaD. Recently, four different independent bioassays have been developed which reliably detect p-tau in CSF. These assays detect CSF tau phosphorylated at threonine 181, serine 199, threonine 231, and serine 396/404. The studies suggest that CSF p-tau increases specificity and provides added value in discrimination between AD and other dementias including VaD (Hu *et al.*, 2002; Nägga *et al.*, 2002).

Other markers for axonal and neuronal degeneration

Ubiquitin is a small, intracellular protein that has been found in all eukaryotic cells. Ubiquitin is required for ATP-dependent, non-lysosomal intracellular protein degradation, which eliminates most intracellular defective problems as well as normal proteins with a rapid turnover. Ubiquitin is involved in the pathogenesis of many neurodegenerative diseases that are characterized by abnormal protein aggregation. CSF levels of ubiquitin have been found to be increased in patients with VaD and AD.

Neuron-specific enolase (NSE) is a glycolytic enzyme that is localized in neurons and neuroendocrine cells. The serum levels are increased in acute stroke patients, and the levels correlate with volume of infarcted tissue (Anand and Stead, 2005). CSF NSE originates mainly from brain. One study found elevated levels in AD and subcortical VD (Blennow *et al.*, 1994), whereas other studies reported low levels in patients with VaD (Parnetti *et al.*, 1995).

The enzyme tissue transglutaminase (tTG) is a calcium-dependent enzyme that crosslinks substrate proteins into insoluble aggregates resistant to proteases. *N*(epsilon)(gamma-glutamyl)lysine isodipeptide is released from the breakdown of proteins cross-linked by transglutaminase. Transglutaminase is thought to be an indicator of acute cell death and a marker for apoptosis. One study found elevated levels of isodipeptide concentrations in patients with VD and AD, and significantly higher levels in AD than in VaD (Nemes *et al.*, 2001). Another study measured transglutaminase levels and found no difference between controls and VaD (Bonelli *et al.*, 2002).

Neurofilaments (NF) are a major cytoskeletal constituent of neuronal cells. NFs can be released into CSF during neuronal damage, and are therefore markers of neuronal degeneration. CSF levels of NFs may be increased in AD and subcortical vascular dementia as well as in other neurodegenerative diseases. The light subtype of NF (NFL) is found mainly in large myelinated axons, and it has been found that CSF NFL levels are associated with WMD (Sjögren *et al.*, 2001).

Markers of synaptic loss and dysfunction

The markers of synaptic integrity include the vesicle proteins (rab3a, synaptotagmin, synaptophysin and chromogranin A), the presynaptic membrane protein GAP-43 (located in presynaptic terminals and axons) and the postsynaptic protein neurogranin. Chromogranin A and GAP-43 are found in CSF but their levels have not been found to be changed in patients with VaD (Blennow *et al.*, 1995; Sjögren *et al.*, 2000).

The cholinergic system consists of neurons capable of synthesizing acetylcholine (ACh) for neurotransmission. These neurons contain acetylcholinesterase (AChE), an enzyme that degrades ACh and in nearly all cases also nicotinic and/or muscarinic receptors. There is growing evidence for a compromised cholinergic system in patients with VaD (Grantham and Geerts, 2002). Post-mortem studies have shown that patients with subcortical vascular dementia have decreased levels of choline acetyltransferase (ChAT) activity in the cortex, hippocampus and striatum compared to controls. In one clinical study, patients with subcortical vascular dementia have been found to have significantly lower levels of ACh in the CSF compared to controls (Tohgi *et al.*, 1996). In another study, the CSF-AChE activity was significantly decreased compared to controls in patients

with subcortical vascular dementia, but not in AD or frontotemporal dementia (Wallin *et al.*, 2003). In a third CSF study in patients with VaD and AD, a positive correlation between ACh deficit and cognitive impairment was found in both groups. The studies suggest that cholinesterase inhibitors may be a fruitful treatment strategy not only for AD, but also for VaD patients.

Markers of myelin loss

Sulfatide is the major acidic glycosphingolipid in the oligodendrocytes that constitute the myelin sheath, but it forms only a minor proportion of the membrane lipids in other brain cells. Post-mortem findings have indicated significantly reduced levels of the glycolipids in the white matter from the centrum semiovale of patients with VaD. This reduction is interpreted as a sign of demyelination in the subcortical white matter. White matter changes visualized by MRI indicated demyelination, but do not indicate whether this demyelination is ongoing. A possible marker of ongoing demyelination, i.e. an increased shedding of membrane fragments from myelin, is the CSF sulfatide. One study reported CSF concentrations of sulfatide of more than 200% of control values in patients with subcortical vascular dementia and normal concentrations in patients with pure AD (Fredman *et al.*, 1992). In patients with subcortical arteriosclerotic encephalopathy, the CSF levels of sulfatide were significantly higher than in patients with normal pressure hydrocephalus (Tullberg *et al.*, 2000).

Blood–brain barrier breakdown in VaD

The endothelial cells of the brain capillaries are sealed together by continuous tight junctions and there are few channels running through the cells. These restrictive characteristics constitute the basis of the blood–brain barrier (BBB). Pericytes and astrocytes maintain vascular integrity and release many biological-response modifiers that participate in vascular remodeling and regulation of blood flow in brain microcirculation. The BBB is a highly metabolic organ with two principal functions: a carrier and a barrier function. At its luminal (blood-facing) side, there are several transporters for specific classes of nutrients (e.g. for glucose, amino acids, vitamins and nucleosides) and receptors (e.g. for lipoproteins, regulatory peptides and proteins, hormones and metals such as iron) mediating transcellular influx of circulation substances into the brain. At the abluminal side of the BBB there are transport systems eliminating potentially toxic molecules (e.g. excitatory transmitters, Aβ and metabolic waste products) from brain interstitial fluid to blood. The numerous mitochondria in the endothelial cells of the brain allow energy supply for the various transport systems. Metabolic exchange has been found not only in capillaries, but also in arterioles, which implies that the latter have BBB features.

Integrity of the BBB can be measured by determining the CSF/serum ratio for albumin. An increased CSF/serum albumin ratio indicates impaired BBB function. Post-mortem studies have found a relation between VaD and arteriolosclerosis, lipohyalinosis, and hypertensive angiopathy of the intracerebral capillaries and arterioles of the brain (Olsson *et al.*, 1996). These changes may lead to dysfunction of the endothelial cells, with increased permeability and extravasation of serum proteins, i.e., BBB damage. An increased CSF/serum albumin ratio has been found in patients with VaD and in patients with white matter changes. Alzheimer patients with concomitant vascular disorders, e.g. arterial hypertension or white matter changes, have been found to have disturbed BBB function, whereas this function has been found to be normal in patients with pure AD.

Summary

- Homocysteine may be of value for risk assessment, since people with high levels of homocysteine in blood are more likely to have atherosclerosis and worse outcomes from arterial disease (Hansrani and Stansby, 2002).

Table 7.4 Usefulness of current biomarkers in dementia patients.

Classification of VaD	Detection of co-existent AD pathology	Monitoring disease progression and therapeutic response
NFL and sulfatide for subcortical vascular dementia	CSF Aβ42, tau, phospho-tau	Markers reflecting progression of brain pathology – not yet identified

- CSF tau, p-tau and Aβ42 may be used as an aid to reveal co-existing AD (or AD changes) in patients with VaD (Table 7.4).
- The presence of BBB damage supports the diagnosis of VaD.
- Subcortical vascular dementia is characterized by increased levels of NFL in CSF, and CSF sulfatide levels are also increased but relatively late in the disease process, when the white matter damage is more pronounced.
- The profile of tau and amyloid markers in CSF differ between subcortical vascular dementia and AD. Subcortical vascular disease is characterized by normal or slightly increased levels of tau, normal p-tau and decreased levels of Aβ42, whereas levels of tau and p-tau are increased in association with low Aβ42 in AD.
- Longitudinal biomarker studies are missing. Therefore it is not known what markers could reflect progression of the brain pathology and thus could be suitable as surrogate markers in therapeutic trials.

REFERENCES

Adair JC, Charlie J, Dencoff JE, *et al.* Measurement of gelatinase B (MMP-9) in the cerebrospinal fluid of patients with vascular dementia and Alzheimer disease. *Stroke* 2004; **35**: e159–62.

Anand N, Stead LG. Neuron-specific enolase as a marker for acute ischemic stroke: a systematic review. *Cerebrovasc Dis* 2005; **20**: 213–19.

Barba R, Martinez-Espinosa S, Rodriguez-Garcia E, Pondal M, Vivancos J, Del Ser T. Poststroke dementia: clinical features and risk factors. *Stroke* 2000; **31**: 1494–501.

Barber M, Tait RC, Scott J, *et al.* Dementia in subjects with atrial fibrillation: hemostatic function and the role of anticoagulation. *J Thromb Haemost* 2004; **2**: 1873–8.

Bateman EJ, Munsell LY, Morris JC, *et al.* Human amyloid-β synthesis and clearance rates as measured in cerebrospinal fluid in vivo. *Nature Med* 2006; **12**: 856–61.

Blasko I, Jellinger K, Kemmler G, *et al.* Conversion from cognitive health to mild cognitive impairment and Alzheimer's disease: Prediction by plasma amyloid beta 42, medial temporal lobe atrophy and homocysteine. DOI:10.1016/j.neurobiolaging/2006.09.002

Blennow K, Wallin A, Ekman R. Neuron specific enolase in cerebrospinal fluid: a biochemical marker for neuronal degeneration in dementia disorders? *J Neural Transm Park Dis Dement Sect* 1994; **8**: 183–91.

Blennow K, Wallin A, Ågren H, *et al.* Tau protein in cerebrospinal fluid. A biochemical marker for axonal degeneration in Alzheimer disease? Mol Chem Neuropathol 1995; **26**: 231–44.

Blennow K, Hampel H. CSF markers for incipient Alzheimer's disease. *Lancet Neurol* 2003; **2**: 605–13.

Bonelli RM, Aschoff A, Niederwieser G, Heuberger C, Jirikowski G. Cerebrospinal fluid tissue transglutaminase as a biochemical marker for Alzheimer's disease. *Neurobiol Dis* 2002; **11**: 106–10.

Bots ML, Breteler MM, van Kooten FR, *et al.* Coagulation and fibrinolysis markers and risk of dementia. *Haemostasis* 1998; **28**: 216–22.

Boysen G, Brander T, Christensen H, Gideon R, Truelsen T. Homocysteine and risk of recurrent stroke. *Stroke* 2003; **34**: 1258–61.

Clark CM, Xie S, Chittams J, *et al.* Cerebrospinal fluid tau and beta-amyloid: how well do these biomarkers reflect autopsy-confirmed dementia diagnoses? *Arch Neurol* 2003 Dec; **60**(12): 1696–702.

Danesh J, Collins R, Peto R. Lipoprotein(a) and coronary heart disease: meta-analysis of prospective studies. *Circulation* 2000; **102**: 1082–5.

De Luigi A, Pizzimenti S, Quadri P, *et al.* Peripheral inflammatory response in Alzheimer's disease and multiinfarct dementia. *Neurobiol Dis* 2002; **11**: 308–14.

Engelhart MJ, Geerlings MI, Meijer J, *et al.* Inflammatory proteins in plasma and the risk of dementia. The Rotterdam Study. *Arch Neurol* 2004; **61**: 668–72.

Esiri MM, Nagy Z, Smith MZ, Barnetson L, Smith AD. Cerebrovascular disease and threshold for dementia in the early stages of Alzheimer's disease. *Lancet* 1999; **354**: 919–20.

Fagan AM, Mintun MA, Mach RH, *et al.* Inverse relation between in vivo amyloid imaging load and cerebrospinal fluid Aβ42 in humans. *Ann Neurol* 2006; **59**: 512–9.

Fredman P, Wallin A, Blennow K, *et al.* Sulfatide as a biochemical marker in cerebrospinal fluid of patients with vascular dementia. *Acta Neurol Scand* 1992; **85**: 103–6.

Grantham C, Geerts H. The rationale behind cholinergic drug treatment for dementia related to cerebrovascular disease. *Neurol Sci* 2002; **202–204(C)**: 131–6.

Gupta A, Watkins A, Thomas P, *et al.* Coagulation and inflammation in Alzheimer's and vascular dementia. *Int J Clin Pract* 2005; **59**: 52–7.

Hansrani M, Stansby G. Homocysteine lowering interventions for peripheral arterial disease and bypass grafts. *Cochrane Database of Systematic Reviews* 2002; Issue 3: CD003285.

Hansson O, Zetterberg H, Buchhave P, *et al.* Association between CSF biomarkers and incipient Alzheimer's disease in patients with mild cognitive impairment: a follow-up study. *Lancet Neurol* 2006; **5**: 228–34.

Hassan A, Hunt BJ, O'Sullivan M, *et al.* Homocysteine is a risk factor for cerebral small vessel disease, acting via endothelial dysfunction. *Brain* 2004; **127**: 212–9.

Henon H, Pasquier F, Durieu I, *et al.* Preexisting dementia in stroke patients. Baseline frequency, associated factors, and outcome. *Stroke* 1997; **28**: 2429–36.

Herukka SK, Hallikainen M, Soininen H, Pirttilä T. The combination of CSF Ab42 and tau or phosphorylated tau helps to predict progressive mild cognitive impairment. *Neurology* 2005; **65**: 1294–7.

Hesse C, Rosengren L, Vanmechelen E, *et al.* Cerebrospinal fluid markers for Alzheimer's disease evaluated after acute ischemic stroke. *J Alzheimer Dis* 2000; **2**: 199–206.

Hogervorst E, Mendes Ribeiro H, Molyneux A, Budge M, Smith D. Plasma homocysteine levels, cerebrovascular risk factors, and cerebral white matter changes (leukoaraiosis) in patients with Alzheimer's disease. *Arch Neurol* 2002; **59**: 787–93.

Hu YY, He SS, Wang X, *et al.* Levels of nonphosphorylated and phosphorylated tau in cerebrospinal fluid of Alzheimer's disease patients: an ultrasensitive bienzyme–substrate recycle enzyme-linked immunosorbent assay. *Am J Pathol* 2002; **160**: 1269–78.

Hulstaert F, Blennow K, Ivanoiu A, *et al.* Improved discrimination of AD patients using β-amyloid1-42 and tau levels in CSF. *Neurology* 1999; **52**: 1555–62.

Lip GYH, Blann AD, Farooqi IS, *et al.* Abnormal haemorheology, endothelial function and thrombogenesis in relation to hypertension in acute stroke patients: the West Birmingham Stroke Project. *Blood Coagul Fibrinol* 2001; **12**: 307–15.

Longstreth WT Jr., Katz R, Olson J, *et al.* Plasma total homocysteine levels and cranial magnetic resonance imaging findings in elderly persons: the Cardiovascular Health Study. *Arch Neurol* 2004; **61**: 67–72.

Mari P, Parnetti L, Coppola R, *et al.* Haemostatic abnormalities in patients with vascular dementia and Alzheimer's disease. *Thromb Haemost* 1996; **75**: 216–8.

Mayeux R, Tang MX, Jacobs DM, *et al.* Plasma amyloid beta-peptide 1–42 and incipient Alzheimer's disease. *Ann Neurol* 1999; **46**(3): 412–16.

Mcllroy SP, Dynan KB, Lawson JT, *et al.* Moderately elevated plasma homocysteine, methylenetetrahydrofolate reductase genotype, and risk of stroke, vascular dementia, and Alzheimer disease in Northern Ireland. *Stroke* 2002; **33**: 2351–6.

Meiklejohn DJ, Vickers MA, Dijkhuisen R, Greaves M. Plasma homocysteine concentrations in the acute and convalescent periods of atherothrombotic stroke. *Stroke* 2001; **32**: 57–62.

Moller J, Nielsen GM, Tvedegaard KC, Andersen NT, Jorgensen PE. A meta-analysis of cerebrovascular disease and hyperhomocysteinaemia. *Scand J Clin Lab Invest* 2000; **60**: 491–500.

Morris MS. Homocysteine and Alzheimer's disease. *Lancet Neurol* 2003; **2**: 425–8.

Nemes Z, Fesus L, Egerhazi A, Keszthelyi A, Degrell IM. *N* (epsilon)(gamma-glutamyl)lysine in cerebrospinal fluid marks Alzheimer type and vascular dementia. *Neurobiol Aging* 2001 May–Jun; **22**(3): 403–06.

Neuropathology Group. Medical Research Council Cognitive Function and Aging Study. Pathological correlates of late-onset dementia in a multicentre, community-based population in England and Wales. Neuropathology Group of the Medical Research Council Cognitive Function and Ageing Study (MRC CFAS). *Lancet* 2001; **357**: 169–75.

Nurk E, Refsum H, Tell GS, *et al.* Plasma homocysteine and memory in the elderly: the Horhaland homocysteine study. *Ann Neurol* 2005; **58**: 847–57.

Nägga K, Gottfries J, Blennow K, Marcusson J. Cerebrospinal fluid phospho-tau, total tau and β-amyloid1–42 in the differentiation between Alzheimer's disease and vascular dementia. *Dementia Geriatr Cogn Disord* 2002; **14**: 183–90.

Olsson Y, Brun A, Englund E. Fundamental pathological lesions in vascular dementia. *Acta Neurol Scand Suppl* 1996; **168**: 31–8.

Otto M, Wiltfang J, Tumani H, *et al.* Elevated levels of tau-protein in cerebrospinal fluid of patients with Creutzfeldt–Jakob disease. *Neurosci Lett* 1997; **225**: 210–12.

Pantoni L, Basile AM, Romanelli M, *et al.* Abulia and cognitive impairment in two patients with capsular genu infarct. *Acta Neurol Scand* 2001; **104**: 185–90.

Parnetti L, Palumbo B, Cardinali L, *et al.* Cerebrospinal fluid neuron-specific enolase in Alzheimer's disease and vascular dementia. *Neurosci Lett* 1995; **183**: 43–5.

Roman GC, Erkinjuntti T, Wallin A, Pantoni L, Chui HC. Subcortical ischemic vascular dementia. *Lancet Neurol* 2002; **1**: 426–36.

Sachdev PS, Brodaty H, Valenzuela MJ, *et al.* Clinical determinants of dementia and mild cognitive impairment following ischemic stroke: the Sydney Stroke Study. *Dement Geriatr Cogn Disord* 2006; **21** (5–6): 275–83.

Sachdev PS, Valenzuela MJ, Brodaty H, *et al.* Homocysteine as a risk factor for cognitive impairment in stroke patients. *Dement Geriatr Cogn Disord* 2003; **15**: 155–62.

Scheuner D, Eckman C, Jensen M, *et al.* Secreted amyloid beta-protein similar to that in the senile plaques of Alzheimer's disease is increased in vivo by the presenilin 1 and 2 and APP mutations linked to familial Alzheimer's disease. *Nat Med* 1996; **2**(8): 864–70.

Schmidt R, Schmidt H, Curb JD, *et al.* Early inflammation and dementia: a 25-year follow-up of the Honolulu–Asia Aging Study. *Ann Neurol* 2002; **52**: 168–74.

Sjögren M, Minthon L, Davidsson P, *et al.* CSF levels of tau, β-amyloid 1–42 and GAP-43 in frontotemporal dementia, other types of dementia and normal aging. *J Neural Transm* 2000; **107**: 563–79.

Sjögren M, Blomberg M, Jonsson M, *et al.* Neurofilament protein in cerebrospinal fluid: a marker of white matter changes. *J Neurosci Res* 2001; **66**: 510–16.

Smith FB, Lee AJ, Fowkes FG, *et al.* Haemostatic factors as predictors of ischemic heart disease and stroke in the Edinburgh Artery Study. *Arterioscler Thromb Vasc Biol* 1997; **17**: 3321–5.

Snowdon DA, Greiner LH, Mortimer JA, Riley KP, Greiner PA, Markesbery WR. Brain infarction and the clinical expression of Alzheimer disease. The Nun Study. *JAMA* 1997; **277**: 813–17.

Sobow T, Flirski M, Kloszewska I, Liberski PP. Plasma levels of alpha beta peptides are altered in amnestic mild cognitive impairment but not in sporadic Alzheimer's disease. *Acta Neurobiol Exp (Wars)* 2005; **65**: 117–24.

Stott DJ, Spilg E, Campbell AM, *et al.* Haemostasis in ischemic stroke and vascular disease. *Blood Coagul Fibrinol* 2001; **12**: 651–7.

Strozyk D, Blennow K, White LR, Launer LJ. CSF Aβ 42 levels correlate with amyloid-neuropathology in a population-based autopsy study. *Neurology* 2003; **60**: 652–6.

Tapiola T, Lehtovirta M, Ramberg J, *et al.* CSF tau is related to apolipoprotein E genotype in early Alzheimer's disease. *Neurology* 1998; **50**: 169–74.

Tarkowski E, Blennow K, Wallin A, Tarkowski A. Intrathecal production of tumor necrosis factor-α, a local neuroprotective agent, in Alzheimer disease and vascular dementia. *J Clin Immunol* 1999; **19**: 223–30.

Tarkowski E, Wallin A, Regland B, Blennow K, Tarkowski A. Local and systemic GM-CSF increase in Alzheimer's disease and vascular dementia. *Acta Neurol Scand* 2001; **103**: 166–74.

Tarkowski E, Issa R, Sjogren M, *et al.* Increased intrathecal levels of the angiogenic factors VEGF and TGF-beta in Alzheimer's disease and vascular dementia. *Neurobiol Aging* 2002; **23**: 237–43.

Tarkowski E, Tullberg M, Fredman P, Wikkelso C. Correlation between intrathecal sulfatide and TNF-alpha levels in patients with vascular dementia. *Dement Geriatr Cogn Disord* 2003; **15**: 207–11.

The Homocysteine Studies Collaboration. Homocysteine and risk of ischemic heart disease and stroke. *JAMA* 2002; **288**: 2015–22.

Tohgi H, Abe T, Kimura M, Saheki M, Takahashi S. Cerebrospinal fluid acetylcholine and choline in vascular dementia of Binswanger and multiple small infarct types as compared with Alzheimer type dementia. *J Neural Transm* 1996; **103**: 1211–20.

Tomimoto H, Akiguchi I, Ohtani R, *et al.* Coagulation activation in patients with Binswanger disease. *Arch Neurol* 1999; **56**: 1104–08.

Toole JF, Malinow MR, Chambless LE, *et al.* Lowering homocysteine in patients with ischemic stroke to prevent recurrent stroke, myocardial infarction, and death: the Vitamin Intervention for Stroke Prevention (VISP) randomized controlled trial. *JAMA* 2004; **291**: 565–75.

de la Torre JC. Alzheimer disease as a vascular disorder: nosological evidence. *Stroke* 2002; **33**: 1152–62.

Tullberg M, Mansson JE, Fredman P, *et al.* CSF sulfatide distinguishes between normal pressure hydrocephalus and subcortical arteriosclerotic encephalopathy. *J Neurol Neurosurg Psychiatry* 2000; **69**: 74–81.

Urakami K, Wada Isoe K, Wakutani Y, *et al.* Lipoprotein (a) phenotype in patients with vascular dementia. *Dement Geriatr Cogn Disord* 2000; **11**: 135–8.

van Oijen M, Hofman A, Soares HD, Koudstaal PJ, Breteler MM. Plasma Abeta(1–40) and Abeta(1–42) and the risk of dementia: a prospective case-cohort study. *Lancet Neurol* 2006; **5**: 655–60.

Vermeer SE, Den Heijer T, Koudstaal PJ, *et al.* Incidence and risk factors of silent brain infarcts in the population based Rotterdam Scan Study. *Stroke* 2003; 34: 392–6.

Wada-Isoe K, Wakutani Y, Urakami K, Nakashima K. Elevated interleukin-6 levels in cerebrospinal fluid of vascular dementia patients. *Acta Neurol Scand* 2004 Aug; **110**(2): 124–7.

Wallin A, Blennow K. Heterogeneity of vascular dementia – mechanisms and subgroups. *Int J Geriatr Psychiatry Neurol* 1993; **6**: 177–88.

Wallin A, Sjögren M. Cerebrospinal fluid cytoskeleton proteins in patients with subcortical white matter dementia. *Mech Ageing Develop* 2001; **122**: 1937–49.

Wallin A, Sjögren M, Blennow K, Davidsson P. Decreased cerebrospinal fluid acetylcholinesterase In patients with subcortical ischemic vascular dementia. *Dement Geriatr Cogn Disord* 2003; **16**: 200–07.

Wright CB, Paik MC, Brown TR, *et al.* Total homocysteine is associated with white matter hyperintensity volume: the Northern Manhattan Study. *Stroke* 2005; **36**: 1207–11.

Yaffe K, Kanaya A, Lindquist K, *et al.* The metabolic syndrome, inflammation, and risk of cognitive decline. *JAMA* 2004; **292**: 2237–42.

Zekry D, Hauw JJ, Gold G. Mixed dementia: epidemiology, diagnosis, and treatment. *J Am Geriatr Soc* 2002; **50**: 1431–8.

Zemlan FP, Rosenberg WS, Luebbe PA, *et al.* Quantification of axonal damage in traumatic brain injury: affinity purification and characterization of cerebrospinal fluid tau proteins. *J Neurochem* 1999; **72**: 741–50.

Zuliani G, Ranzini M, Guerra G, *et al.* Plasma cytokines profile in older subjects with late onset Alzheimer's disease or vascular dementia. *J Psychiatr Res* 2007; **41**: 686–93.

Pathophysiology

Pathophysiology

8

Physiopathology of large-vessel vascular dementia

Leonardo Pantoni, Francesca Pescini and Anna Poggesi

Introduction

Definition of the topic of the chapter

Cerebrovascular diseases (CVDs) can cause cognitive impairment through a quite large number of mechanisms and underlying pathological processes. Diseases affecting the large arteries are one of the possible causes of vascular cognitive impairment and vascular dementia (VaD). Since this chapter is focused on large-vessel dementia, we will first give a definition of large vessels and an overview of their pathological processes, and then of what can be meant with the term large-vessel VaD.

In the description of the afferent circulation to the brain, the term *large vessels* is arbitrarily used with the principal aim of differentiating these vessels from those defined as small. One of the main reasons for making this distinction is that the pathological processes affecting the large vessels are different from those affecting the small ones. However, the anatomical differentiation between the two types of vessels is not straightforward. For the purpose of this review, the term *large vessels* will be used to include the large arteries of the neck and the intracranial arteries that form the circle of Willis and that depart from it to provide the blood supply to various regions of the brain (i.e. the anterior, middle, and posterior cerebral arteries). Therefore, we will not include the smaller arteries located at the surface of the brain and those penetrating the brain parenchyma.

The definition of *large vessel VaD* may apply to different pathological conditions. For example, this term can be used in a broad sense to also include conditions linked with vasculopathies other than those affecting the large arteries, such as those resulting from pathology of the veins (i.e. cerebral venous thrombosis) or from abnormal arterial–vein connections (e.g. fistulae). Moreover, occlusions of the large arteries not primarily depending on diseases of the occluded vessel also occur. This is the case of occlusion of a major cerebral artery from emboli originating in the heart or in the aortic arch; this might be difficult to differentiate from occlusion originating on the site of an underlying pathological process of the vessel wall. Finally, large-artery diseases may also contribute to, or be the cause of, a form of VaD linked with hypoperfusion. Cardio-embolic and hypoperfusive causes of VaD will be dealt with in another chapter of this book. In this chapter, we will touch upon hypoperfusion mechanisms of VaD only as they relate to the occurrence of border zone infarcts.

In summary, our chapter will be mainly focused on the description of large-artery VaD rather than

Vascular Cognitive Impairment in Clinical Practice, ed. Lars-Olof Wahlund, Timo Erkinjuntti and Serge Gauthier. Published by Cambridge University Press. © Cambridge University Press 2009.

on large-infarct VaD, even if this distinction is not always easy to carry out.

Clinical aspects of large-vessel vascular dementia

Having discussed some issues related to the definition of large-vessel VaD, other relevant concepts are to be examined hereafter.

In fact, large-vessel VaD is not a clinical concept, and is based on the pathophysiological assumption that the cognitive syndrome depends on a disease of the large vessels. This has to be put in the perspective of other, more commonly used, terms in this field, such as multi-infarct dementia (MID) and post-stroke dementia. The term multi-infarct dementia is a widely used term that is based on another physiopathological aspect, i.e. the multiplicity of brain infarcts and their putative additional effect on cognition (see below). The term and the concept were introduced in the early 1970s when researchers and clinicians began to differentiate between degenerative and vascular forms of dementia (Hachinski *et al.*, 1974). The concept that lies under the term multi-infarct dementia is that of the load of lost brain tissue caused by infarction, greater volumes being more likely to be associated with cognitive loss than smaller volumes. In most instances, MID refers to cases where multiple large cerebral infarcts are present. However, MID also includes, at least from the terminology point of view, cases where multiple small infarcts (or lacunes) are present, the so-called *multi-lacunar state* that is not related to large-vessel pathology.

Post-stroke dementia is instead a clinical term in which all the forms of dementia that follow a stroke in close time relationship are assembled. Therefore, the term encompasses all causes of VaD, from hemorrhagic to hypoperfusive to multi-infarct, and does not distinguish among causes of stroke. Because large-vessel pathology is a leading cause of stroke, many cases of large-vessel VaD may present as post-stroke dementia.

Still on clinical grounds, one single large cortico-subcortical brain ischemic lesion may present with

Table 8.1 The Hachinski ischemic score.

Hachinski ischemic score	Score
Abrupt onset	2
Step-wise deterioration	1
Fluctuating course	2
Nocturnal confusion	1
Relative preservation of personality	1
Depression	1
Somatic complaints	1
Emotional incontinence	1
History of hypertension	1
History of strokes	2
Evidence of associated atherosclerosis	1
Focal neurological symptoms	2
Focal neurological signs	2

an acute cognitive deterioration if located in an area that is functionally critical for cognition (so-called strategic infarct dementia). The location can be subcortical or involving the cortex and, in this instance, the lesion may be associated with large-vessel pathology. Locations of large infarcts associated with strategic infarct dementia are the angular gyrus, the medial frontal lobe, and the inferomedial portion of the temporal lobe (Roman *et al.*, 1993).

From a clinical point of view, large-vessel VaD is characterized by a step-wise cognitive deterioration, focal signs and symptoms which are the result of repeated ischemic strokes. As opposed to subcortical VaD, where the natural course can be progressive and characterized by the presence of pseudobulbar signs, dysexecutive syndrome, depression, emotional lability, and behavioral symptoms, large-vessel VaD is mostly characterized by the presence of cortical signs such as aphasia, apraxia, agnosia, abulia, amnesia, more or less associated with motor-sensory loss. The clinical distinction between VaD and Alzheimer's disease (AD) is important, but may be difficult. Differences considered as typical are the absence of focal neurological signs and symptoms in AD and its more progressive course which is in contrast with the usual stepwise deterioration of VaD. The ischemic score, Table 8.1 (Hachinski *et al.*, 1975) has been proposed as an instrument capable of differentiating VaD caused by multiple ischemic strokes (score >7) and AD (score <4).

Pathological processes of the parenchyma underlying large-vessel vascular dementia

In this part of the chapter we will give some descriptions of the pathological aspects of large cerebral infarcts and large-vessel pathology as they potentially relate to large-vessel VaD.

Large cerebral infarcts

A cerebral infarction can be defined as an area of brain parenchyma pathologically characterized by the presence of tissue necrosis consequent to ischemia. Thorough histological description of a brain infarct depends heavily on the time that has elapsed between the onset of the clinical manifestation (i.e. the stroke) and the time of the lesion assessment. In the first few weeks, large cerebral infarcts undergo a series of histological processes and changes, usually from early ischemic changes with preservation of the general architecture of the tissue to late complete necrosis with cavitation of the area. In this sense, a brain infarct has to be considered a lesion with a temporal evolution (Garcia *et al.*, 1993, 1995). A complete description of the temporal changes of a brain infarct is beyond the scope of this chapter. Moreover, the evolution of a brain infarct from the pathological viewpoint is difficult to study in a human specimen, and available data are scarce (Chuaqui and Tapia, 1993). More data are available from the neuroimaging viewpoint. CT is the technique routinely used, although new methods such as diffusion-weighted MRI may demonstrate ischemic brain tissue within a few minutes from the onset of the symptoms (Chalela *et al.*, 2007; Warach *et al.*, 1992). Within the first 6 h of stroke onset, early CT findings can be

found: loss of the gray–white differentiation in the cortical ribbon or the lentiform nucleus, effacement of sulci or slight ventricular compression as a result of localized brain swelling (Eckert and Zeumer, 1998; Masdeu *et al.*, 2006; von Kummer *et al.*, 1994). Moreover, in the case of a middle cerebral artery or basilar artery occlusion, hyperdense formation within the vessel lumen corresponding to the occluding thrombus or embolus can be seen (von Kummer *et al.*, 1994). After 24 h the full impact of the infarction is seen as a hypodense area mostly due to intra- and extracellular edema. From the histological viewpoint, in the first four days after the beginning of ischemia, phagocytosis of the necrotic area starts and newly formed vessels appear in the tissue. Dead cells, astrocyte proliferation, and enlarged macrophages are described at this time in the brain infarct area (Chuaqui and Tapia, 1993). Two to three weeks after the stroke, a "fogging effect" on CT scans can arise. This is a decrease of the density of the area consequent to the above-described tissue evolution, in particular to hyperemia and reduction of local edema (Becker *et al.*, 1979). After 3–4 weeks, cavitation of the tissue becomes prominent and the area appears on CT with a density similar to that of the cerebrospinal fluid.

From the histological viewpoint, brain infarcts produced by arterial occlusion can be classified as pale or hemorrhagic (red). The pale infarct consists of soft and swollen tissue with poorly demarcated anatomical structures. Occasional hemorrhages may be seen at the margin of the infarct. The hemorrhagic infarct consists of softening of the brain tissue, the majority of which is scattered by congested blood vessels and numerous petecchiae. Hemorrhages originate from the damaged small blood vessels in the ischemic area (del Zoppo, 1994) and may become confluent (Adams and Vander Eecken, 1953). Today, we know that reperfusion (spontaneous or therapeutic) may contribute or exacerbate hemorrhagic transformation of brain infarcts (Khatri *et al.*, 2007). In terms of cognition, there are no data showing that one type of infarct (ischemic or hemorrhagic) is more associated than the other with cognitive impairment, and it may be assumed that the extension of the damaged area remains the principal factor involved.

Cerebral infarction can also be divided on an anatomic basis into territorial and border zone infarctions. This distinction bears also a physiopathological significance. A territorial infarct is produced by the occlusion of a major artery or of branches of this artery. The extent of the brain infarct is determined by the site of the arterial occlusion and by the functional efficacy of collateral circulation through the leptomeningeal arteries, the circle of Willis, or the external carotid artery system, for example through the ophthalmic artery (Eckert and Zeumer, 1998). Typically, territorial infarcts are cortical–subcortical lesions more or less extending into the white matter. In large artery occlusion such as middle cerebral artery occlusion, the result is a massive infarct involving the entire territory supplied by the artery when poor collateral circulation is present, while in the case of adequate collateral circulation an infarct in the central territory (wedge-shaped on coronal sections) supplied by the artery develops. Border zone infarcts appear in the areas between the territories of the major intracranial cerebral arteries (external border zone), and in the area between the superficial and deep branches of the middle cerebral artery (internal border zone). Internal border zone infarcts also affect the areas between the branches of the vertebral artery and basilar artery in the cerebellum, and the areas between the deep branches supplying the subcortical gray matter (Ogata and Pantoni, in press).

Pathological processes affecting cerebro-afferent arteries

The parenchyma lesions described in the previous paragraph may be caused by different pathological diseases of the large vessels (Table 8.2), the most common of which by far is atherosclerosis. In the following paragraph we will briefly review some of these large-vessel diseases.

Atherosclerosis

Atherosclerosis is the commonest type of arteriosclerosis. It affects large and medium size arteries causing a progressive hardening of vessel walls. The pathologic lesion at the basis of atherosclerosis is the atheromatous plaque. The term atheroma comes from the Greek meaning "gruel", which describes the soft lipid core of the lesion. The atherosclerotic process starts in very young children with the fatty streaks. At more advanced ages, atherosclerosis of some degree is invariably found. Fatty streaks are focal areas of intracellular lipid collection (macrophages and smooth muscle cells). They gradually grow in number from childhood to the second and third decades of life. Subsequently, they decline in number and are replaced at some locations by the atherosclerotic plaques (Rajamani *et al.*, 1998). Macroscopically, the plaques appear white or yellowish white and protrude into the lumen of the vessel. The luminal surface is formed by the fibrous cap which covers the deep lipid core. Microscopically, three major constituents form the plaque: cells (macrophages, smooth muscle cells, leukocytes), connective tissue (collagen, elastic tissue, and proteoglycans), and lipid deposits both within and outside the cells. The fibrous cap is formed of smooth muscle cells, connective tissue, and leukocytes. The deeper lipid core is composed of extracellular lipid, cellular debris, lipid laden "foam cells", fibrin, and plasma proteins. The complicated lesions are more advanced and clinically relevant. These are lesions with added thrombosis, ulceration, calcification within the fibrous cap and the atheroma, and hemorrhage in the lesion. Plaques can enlarge and become confluent, thicken, and eventually cause stenosis and occlusion of the vessel. Because the media is involved progressively, the vessel wall may become weakened and lead to aneurysm formation (Garcia and Anderson, 1997; Rajamani *et al.*, 1998).

Table 8.2 Diseases and pathological processes affecting the cerebral large vessels that may cause ischemic strokes.

Disease	Subtypes	Age of stroke	Stroke pathogenesis
Atherosclerosis		Old age	Stenosis/occlusion Thromboembolism
Arterial dissection	Traumatic Spontaneous Associated conditions: Fibromuscular dysplasia Cystic medial degeneration Moyamoya syndrome Ehlers–Danlos syndrome Atherosclerosis Polyarteritis nodosa Arterial kinks, coils or tortuosity Myxoid degeneration Fibroelastic thickening Osteogenesis imperfecta Autosomal dominant polycystic kidney disease Systemic lupus erythematosus Gaps in the internal elastic lamina Marfan syndrome Luetic arteritis Tuberculous aneurysm Mycotic aneurysm Saccular aneurysm Pseudoxanthoma elasticum	Usually young age	Stenosis/occlusion Thromboembolism
Angiitis	See Table 8.3	Usually young age (except for giant cell arteritis)	See text
Moyamoya disease		Young age	Stenosis/occlusion
Moyamoya syndrome		All ages	Thrombosis
Fibromuscular dysplasia		Young age	Dissection Stenosis/occlusion
Migraine		Young age	Vasospasm
Neurofibromatosis		Young age	
Metabolic disorders	MELAS[a]	Young age	Stenosis/occlusion Stenosis/occlusion
	Homocystinuria	Young age	Thromboembolism
	Fabry disease	Young age	Thrombosis
Intracranial arterial dolichoectasia	Often associated with Fabry disease	All ages	Thrombosis

Table 8.2 (cont.)

Disease	Subtypes	Age of stroke	Stroke pathogenesis
Large-vessel stroke secondary to hematological alterations	Sickle-cell anemia, paroxysmal nocturnal hemoglobinuria, polycythemia vera, secondary polycythemia, essential thrombocytemia, secondary thrombocytosis, multiple myeloma, disseminated intravascular coagulation, protein S deficiency, protein C deficiency, antithrombin III deficiency, protein C activated resistance	Usually young age	Thrombosis Stenosis/occlusion (moyamoya syndrome)
Vascular malignant angioendothe-liomatosis		Usually old age	Stenosis/occlusion
Radiation		All ages	Angiitis Stenosis/occlusion
Drugs	Cocaine	Usually young age	Vasospasm, stenosis/occlusion
	Heroin		Arteritis, stenosis/occlusion
	Amphetamine		Arteritis, stenosis/occlusion Stenosis/occlusion
CADASIL[b]	LSD (lysergic acid diethylamide)	Young age	Stenosis

[a] MELAS: mitochondrial encephalopathy with lactic acidosis and stroke-like episodes syndrome.
[b] CADASIL: cerebral autosomal dominant arteriopathy with subcortical infarcts and leukoencephalopathy.

The initiation of atherosclerosis may result from blood flow oscillatory shear stress. Geometric aspects of the bifurcation of the carotid artery, including the ratio of the cross-section of the internal carotid artery to that of the common carotid artery and the angle of the carotid artery bifurcation, may be important factors in determining the sites of atherosclerosis (Fisher and Fierman, 1990; Strong, 1992). In the intracranial circulation, the occlusive disease is more frequent at the carotid siphon, and the proximal part of the middle, anterior, and basilar arteries (Adams and Vander Eecken, 1953).

Atherothrombotic strokes occur because the atherosclerotic plaques enlarge to produce significant stenosis of the lumen, and occlusion is often induced by superimposed thrombus. On the other side, atherosclerotic plaques may release embolic materials from the site of plaque rupture or superimposed thrombus (artery-to-artery embolism associated with atherosclerosis of the extracranial and intracranial large arteries). Aortic arch atheroma is also an important embolic source for ischemic stroke (Amarenco *et al.*, 1994; Jones *et al.*, 1995).

Arterial dissection

Arterial dissection is a frequent cause of stroke particularly in young people (Schievink, 2001). It is caused by a tear in the layers of the arteries with intramural bleeding within a tissue plane of the arterial wall or extravasation of blood through the endothelial surface (Adams *et al.*, 1998). The most likely type of dissection is the subintimal one that derives from the extension of the hematoma to the intima and eventually its connection with the original lumen (double lumen); less frequently, the dissection may have a subadventitial pattern (especially in intracranial vessels) when the hematoma extends to the adventitia. In the last case, a progression toward arterial dilatation may occur (dissecting aneurysm) (Ogata and Pantoni, in press). Both intra- and extracranial arteries may be involved, the latter being much more common in adults (Chaves *et al.*, 2002; Farrell *et al.*, 1985; Schievink *et al.*, 1994). Ischemic strokes derive from artery stenosis or occlusion due to the intramural hematoma or from thromboembolism, since intraluminal thrombosis can develop (Caplan, 2005; Lucas *et al.*, 1998). Artery dissection may occur spontaneously or in association with blunt trauma to the head or neck (including neck hyperextension) (Schievink, 2001; Ogata and Pantoni, in press).

From the histological viewpoint, artery dissection may be associated with a large number of conditions such as fibromuscular dysplasia, cystic medial necrosis, atherosclerosis or connective tissue abnormalities (see also Table 8.2), although often no specific underlying pathology is found (Berger and Wilson, 1984; Brandt *et al.*, 2001; Schievink, 2001).

Artery dissection can be diagnosed in vivo through MRI and MR angiography, even though angiography is still considered the gold standard (Adams *et al.*, 1998) and can also reveal the associated underlying arteriopathy (e.g. fibromuscular dysplasia).

Angiitis

Angiitis of the central nervous system are a heterogeneous group of inflammatory disorders affecting arteries and veins of different sizes. From the pathological viewpoint, they are characterized by inflammation of the vessels in the acute, subacute or chronic phase with or without granuloma formation (aggregates of macrophages and their derivates into nodular clumps in so-called granulomatous angiitis) and necrosis (necrotizing angiitis). These processes may lead to stenosis or occlusion of the vessel, thrombosis or dissection causing ischemia; otherwise they may manifest with aneurysm formation and hemorrhage. Angiitis may be distinguished as primary when they are the sole manifestation of the disease or secondary when they are a component of a more complex disease. The pathogenesis of angiitis is not completely understood, although an immunologic mechanism is the most widely accepted one. In this paragraph, we briefly describe some of the most common angiitis affecting large (aorta and its primary branches) and medium-sized arteries. All these type of angiitis are listed in Table 8.3.

Takayasu's arteritis

The first scientific presentation of this disease was given in 1905 by Takayasu (McKusick, 1962; Numano *et al.*, 2000). Takayasu's arteritis is a granulomatous vasculitis of unknown etiology involving primarily the thoracic and abdominal aorta and its branches, and occasionally the pulmonary artery. There is a strong predilection for young women. The majority of cases reported have been from Asia. From the pathological point of view, in early phases there are marked intimal fibrosis and fibrous scarring of the media, and mild perivascular lymphocyte infiltration in the media and adventitia with wall thickening of the vasa vasorum. Langhan's or foreign body type giant cells appear in the tunica media; however, they are fewer and differ in size and shape from those in giant cell arteritis. The histological features are not specific (Judge *et al.*, 1962; Vinijchaikul, 1967). In the chronic phase fibrous thickening of the vessel wall results in obliteration of the lumen. The occlusive changes of the large and medium size vessels cause characteristic symptoms such as absence of radial artery pulsation and various neurological symptoms such as subclavian steal syndrome. Renovascular hypertension often develops. Ischemic stroke and retinal ischemia may

Table 8.3 Angiitis affecting large and medium-sized arteries (modified from Hankey 1998).

Primary isolated angiitis of the central nervous system
    Isolated granulomatous angiitis of the central nervous
    system
Primary systemic granulomatous angiitis
    Takayasu's arteritis
    Giant cell (temporal) arteritis
Primary systemic necrotizing angiitides
    Polyarteritis nodosa
    Allergic angiitis and granulomatosis of Churg–Strauss
    Polyangiitis overlap syndrome
    Lymphomatoid granulomatosis
Angiitis associated with other systemic diseases
    Sarcoidosis
    Behcet's disease
    Relapsing polychondritis
    Inflammatory bowel disease
    Kohlmeier–Degos disease
Hypersensitivity angiitis associated with connective tissue
disease
    Systemic lupus erythematosus
    Mixed connective tissue disease
    Sneddon's syndrome
    Rheumatoid arthritis
    Sjogren's syndrome
    Sclerodermia
Others
    Eales' disease
    Radiation angiitis
    Infective angiitis

---

occur as a consequence of stenosis or occlusion of the extracranial carotid or vertebral arteries while the intracranial arteries are rarely involved (Ogata and Pantoni, in press).

Giant cell arteritis (also called temporal arteritis)

Giant cell arteritis is a systemic segmental angiitis involving large and medium-sized arteries in multiple locations even if the most commonly affected arteries are the branches of the external carotid (especially temporal artery), ophthalmic, posterior ciliary, vertebral, aorta, and its branches. It is a granulomatous angiitis characterized by intima proliferation, destruction of the internal elastic lamina, and thickening of the media. The inflammatory infiltrate consists of mononuclear cells, giant cells, and occasional eosinophils with granuloma formation. The granulomatous changes are considered typical for giant cell arteritis, although the presence of giant cells is not required for diagnosis. This is the most common angiitis causing ischemic stroke (Hankey, 1998).

Polyarteritis nodosa

Polyarteritis nodosa is a multi-system, multifocal, segmental necrotizing angiitis of small and medium-sized arteries with typical involvement of renal and visceral vessels. Peripheral and central nervous systems are commonly affected (Rosenberg *et al.*, 1990). In the acute phase, inflammation of the vessel wall and perivascular areas leads to intimal proliferation and wall degeneration. In a second phase, fibrinoid necrosis of the vessels develops leading to stenosis of the lumen. As the lesions heal, there is collagen deposition which may lead to further occlusion of the lumen. Typically, aneurysms occur along the involved arteries.

Allergic angiitis and granulomatosis of Churg–Strauss syndrome

This is a necrotizing arteritis, pathologically similar to polyarteritis nodosa, but capillaries, veins, and venules can be involved in addition to small and medium-sized arteries. There are granulomatous reactions associated with eosinophilic tissue infiltration. Any organ in the body may be affected, including the brain, but the lungs are involved predominantly (Hankey, 1998).

Lymphomatoid granulomatosis

Lymphomatoid granulomatosis is a rare lymphoproliferative multi-system disease, characterized by necrotizing angiocentric and angiodegenerative infiltrates within arteries, veins, and surrounding tissue. The histologic features are similar to those of a malignant lymphoreticular neoplasm and several authors believe that it represents an angiocentric T-cell malignant lymphoma (Katzenstein *et al.*, 1979; Kleinschmidt-DeMasters *et al.*, 1992).

Behcet's disease

Behcet's disease is a multi-system inflammatory disorder clinically characterized by recurrent oral and genital ulcerations and eye lesions. The neuropathological features are those of disseminated meningo-encephalomyelitis, with foci of necrosis and inflammation in the brain stem, deep gray nuclei, and spinal cord (neuro-Behcet). Small and medium-sized vessels may be affected by an inflammatory and rarely necrotizing angiitis (angio-Behcet) (Nishimura *et al.*, 1991; Serdaroglu, 1998).

Systemic lupus erythematosus (SLE)

SLE is a connective tissue disease with an accompanied multi-system angiitis whose etiology is unknown. Cerebral infarcts result from angiopathy, cardiac embolism, or hypercoagulability. The intracranial vessels present thickening of the intima and fibrinoid degeneration mostly of small vessels (Ellison *et al.*, 1993; Mitsias and Levine, 1994).

Moyamoya disease

Moyamoya disease is pathologically characterized by progressive stenosis or occlusion of the terminal portion of the bilateral internal carotid arteries and the proximal portions of the anterior and middle cerebral arteries. As a consequence, compensatory dilated and thin-walled collateral arteries (the moyamoya vessels) develop from the posterior portion of the circle of Willis. Intracranial aneurysms are frequently associated with this disease. The name derives from the typical angiographic picture (from the Japanese *moya-moya*, meaning puffs of smoke). Under the microscope, the intima

shows massive fibrocellular thickening. Lipid deposits are occasionally seen in the proliferative intima. The internal elastic lamina is preserved, but is often disrupted or triplicated, and the tunica media is thinned. Inflammation is absent, but thrombosis may occur (Ikezaki and Fukui, 2001; Masuda *et al.*, 1993; Masuda *et al.*, 2004; Ogata *et al.*, 1996). The pathogenesis of the disease is unknown; hereditary and some acquired factors may have a role, but data are controversial. A condition that is similar from the angiographic viewpoint is the moyamoya syndrome, where the vascular lesions are secondary to other disorders such as atherosclerosis or post-irradiation vasculopathy. While moyamoya disease is most common in Japan, the moyamoya syndrome is present also in Western countries. Ischemic and hemorrhagic strokes are associated with these conditions.

Pathogenesis of large-vessel vascular dementia

The pathogenesis of large-vessel VaD is complex and to some extent remains a matter of investigation. Patients with cognitive decline and co-existing multiple brain infarcts are often seen in clinical practice, but the notion that cognitive decline directly relates to the occurrence of brain infarcts is usually unproven. Efforts in defining diagnostic criteria are made in order to characterize patterns of brain infarction from which it is reliable to deduce the presence of dementia. Some of the most important pathophysiological mechanisms and factors implicated in large-vessel VaD are:
- volume of lesions,
- number of lesions,
- location of lesions,
- coexistence of other brain pathologies, particularly AD.

Probably, none of these factors is solely related to dementia, and in the majority of cases, several mechanisms contribute to the determination of dementia.

Volume of vascular lesions

It is of little conceptual difficulty understanding why patients with several hundred milliliters of cerebral softening become demented; what is more difficult is the definition of a threshold for volume tissue loss consequent to infarction to identify dementia cases. In a seminal paper, Tomlinson *et al.* emphasized the importance of the volume of infarcts in determining dementia due to vascular pathology (Tomlinson *et al.*, 1970). The authors compared 28 brains of non-demented old people with 50 brains of patients who were diagnosed with dementia during life, giving particular attention to features likely indicative of cerebral degeneration (such as brain weight, ventricular size, cerebral atrophy, senile plaques, neurofibrillary changes, and areas of softening). In terms of ischemic lesions, they found that mean volumes in the demented and in the control groups were, respectively, 48.9 and 13.2 ml. Softening of more than 20 ml was more common in the demented group (44% vs. 21%); only 2 out of the 28 non-demented patient brains showed more than 50 ml softening, whereas 16 of the 50 demented brain exceeded this amount, and softening greater than 100 ml was confined to the demented cases. In contrast to this study, where the comparison was between the morphological findings in unselected demented and non-demented patients, del Ser *et al.* studied a group of 40 patients who showed only vascular lesions on pathological examination (plaque count inferior to that needed for AD diagnosis), and compared those who were demented with those who were not (del Ser *et al.*, 1990). They found that the volume of the infarcts was significantly greater in the demented group, but also found an overlap between the groups, and, in the majority of the demented patients, the total infarct volume never reached 100 ml.

Other studies have also reported that smaller volumes, in the range of 1–40 ml, were associated with dementia (Erkinjuntti *et al.*, 1988; Liu *et al.*, 1992; Loeb *et al.*, 1988). Erkinjuntti *et al.* reported a series of 27 patients in whom VaD was diagnosed during life and whose brains were subsequently examined (clinical diagnosis confirmed in 23; Erkinjuntti *et al.*, 1988). The mean volume of infarction was only 40 ml, and 7 of the patients had volumes of infarction of less than 10 ml. Overall, it is believed to be very unlikely that a precise volume of infarcts able to predict VaD exists (Bowler *et al.*, 1999). Although the total volume is an important parameter, the volume of functional tissue loss might also be important, because it includes the effects of incompletely infarcted tissue, and deafferented cortex (Mielke *et al.*, 1992).

Number of vascular lesions

The number of lesions is probably not an independent factor being strictly related to volume, and only a few studies have addressed this problem. In the Cardiovascular Health Cognition Study (Kuller *et al.*, 2005), among the factors associated with the risk of developing dementia of the vascular type, there were the number of infarcts on MRI (silent and non-silent), together with a history of stroke. Schneider *et al.* quantified number and volume of old infarctions on post-mortem examination of 164 subjects who were clinically evaluated during life (Schneider *et al.*, 2003). Infarctions were associated with a twofold increase in odds of dementia, and the odds were higher if lesions were multiple and larger. In other studies, when the issue related to number of lesions was addressed, discrepant results emerged (Jellinger, 2005).

However, the hypothesis of the "synergistic" effect of multiple infarcts is indeed interesting. With the term synergistic it is implied that the effect of multiple lesions produces a pattern of clinical deficits different from what would be predicted by the simple sum of the effects of the single lesion. In the paradigmatic case reported by Wolfe and colleagues, a 66-year-old man was followed up with an extensive clinical and neuropsychological evaluation for 3.5 years, during which he suffered more than one cerebral infarction; as expected, the patient demonstrated a "classical" step-wise cognitive decline, but what was considered the most salient finding was the appearance of frontal symptoms after additional posterior cortical lesions (Wolfe *et al.*, 1994). Injury of multiple brain regions, each specific for certain cognitive functions, might lead to dementia simply on an additive basis, or, as proposed by Hachinski *et al.*, by a multiplicative mechanism where the cumulative effect of the lesions, each trivial in its clinical effects, might lead to dementia (Hachinski *et al.*, 1974).

Location of vascular lesions

Another major unsolved issue concerning patients with multiple brain infarcts is that the type of cognitive deficit may largely depend on the location of lesions. Some evidence exists suggesting that the left hemisphere might play an important role in the occurrence of VaD, compared with lesions affecting the right, non-dominant hemisphere (Liu *et al.*, 1992). Also, infarcts involving the territory of the middle cerebral artery and anterior cerebral artery (the anterior circulation) are usually considered more important compared with posterior lesions, particularly infra-tentorial lesions. However, it should be noted in this regard that, although current research criteria for VaD do not require infra-tentorial lesions to be present (Erkinjuntti *et al.*, 2000; Roman *et al.*, 1993), it has been reported recently that they may indeed be related to cognitive deficits, thus contributing to the clinical picture of VaD, probably by the interaction with supra-tentorial lesions (Bastos Leite *et al.*, 2006).

It is now well accepted that cognitive impairment due to vascular pathology may occur after the occurrence of a single infarct in a "strategic" region of the brain. According to the pathophysiological classification of VaD, single infarct strategic dementia is caused by a single strategically located infarct due to large- or small-vessel disease (Roman *et al.*, 1993). The regions involved are the medial temporal lobe, the frontal lobe, the angular gyrus, the head of the caudate, the thalamus, and the genu of the internal capsule. Clinical manifestations and time course in these cases may vary,

mostly depending on the affected region (Pantoni *et al.*, 2001; Tatemichi *et al.*, 1992, 1995).

Co-existence of other brain pathologies

When dealing with large-vessel VaD, and more in general with VaD, it is of undoubted importance to also take into account the possible role of co-existing degenerative processes such as AD, which is the most common form of dementia in the elderly. While vascular lesions need to be demonstrated in order to make a diagnosis of VaD, they are also often detected in subjects with AD, likely increasing and modulating the clinical course of the disease, and suggesting a synergistic effect of the two mechanisms (van der Flier and Scheltens, 2005).

It is usually thought that a definite diagnosis of the major types of dementia can be provided only post-mortem by pathological examination, although some criticism has been raised about it (Pantoni *et al.*, 2006). Over the last few years, many efforts have been made in order to find markers able to operate this distinction during lifetime. This issue is gathering particular importance as new drugs and treatments become available for the management of the different dementing diseases. In this respect, the identification of "markers" (clinical, neuroimaging, or laboratory-based) able to determine in vivo the etiology of dementia is nowadays considered fundamental. Among the investigated factors, neuroimaging plays a primary role, and it is becoming an indispensable tool in clinical practice. Structural imaging of the brain is not solely able to rule out the treatable causes of dementia (such as tumor, hematoma, or hydrocephalus), but may also add positive or negative predictive value to the diagnosis of the different types of dementia during life (Scheltens *et al.*, 2002). In fact, cortical atrophy, medial temporal lobe atrophy, as well as detection of vascular lesions, including white matter lesions, can be extensively evaluated, both by CT and MRI in clinical practice (see also Chapter 5).

What can be learned from studies on post-stroke dementia?

It is doubtless that stroke increases the risk of dementia but, as has been outlined in two recent reviews, the term post-stroke dementia encompasses all types of dementias that occur after a stroke, irrespective of their cause (Hénon *et al.*, 2006; Leys *et al.*, 2005). Vascular lesions of the brain can be the direct cause, may contribute, or only co-exist with cognitive changes, and thus the mechanisms related to vascular cognitive impairment are still a matter of discussion (Pasquier and Leys, 1997). Despite the fact that post-stroke dementia is not synonymous with large-vessel VaD, it is likewise true that post-stroke dementia is the commonest presentation of large-vessel VaD (Roman, 2003), and thus the study of determinants of post-stroke dementia may highlight some pathophysiological mechanisms involved in large-vessel VaD.

With this aim, a brief review of studies on post-stroke dementia will follow, focusing particularly on stroke-related features (stroke mechanism, size, location, and number of lesions) as determined both clinically and/or from the neuroimaging point of view, as well as on the pre-existing brain structural changes, which may raise the suspicion of the co-existence of other mechanisms, apart from stroke, as the cause of dementia. Studies on post-stroke dementia are here distinguished into: (1) case-control studies where dementia is prospectively evaluated in stroke patients compared to stroke-free subjects (Table 8.4); for our purposes, relevant information can be derived from the subgroup analysis of stroke patients; and (2) clinical stroke cohorts studies; main methodological aspects and results of clinical post-stroke dementia series published in the last 10 years are summarized in Tables 8.5 and 8.6.

From the analysis of these studies, it is quite clear that, due to the different types of assessment of stroke-related features, it is not easy to immediately grab which are the significant determinants of dementia related to large-vessel pathology. Only one study clearly demonstrated that large-vessel pathology, as opposed to other mechanisms of stroke, is a predictor of dementia (Desmond *et al.*, 2000). From other studies it can be extrapolated that large hemispheric infarcts are important determinants of post-stroke dementia, but it is not always clear if the mechanism is related to large-vessel pathology or to other mechanisms such as cardioembolism (Pohjasvaara *et al.*, 1998; Rasquin *et al.*, 2004). Also, Tang and colleagues distinguished between cerebral infarcts (cortical and subcortical) and lacunar strokes and found that dementia was related to cortical lesions and to the involvement of the middle cerebral artery vascular territory (Tang *et al.*, 2004). In another study, no significant differences were found between subjects with and without dementia in terms of the different ischemic stroke syndromes, although lacunar infarcts were more common among non-demented patients, and total anterior cerebral infarcts among the demented group (Inzitari *et al.*, 1998). Data from the community-based Framingham Study cohort revealed that among the stroke-related features, atherothrombotic strokes doubled the risk of developing dementia compared to cardioembolic stroke, but in the atherothrombotic group both lacunar and large-vessel strokes were included (Ivan *et al.*, 2004).

Relevant information regarding the main pathophysiological mechanisms and factors which have been outlined in the previous part of the chapter may derive from a closer look at the results of studies reported in Tables 8.4–8.6. A few comments might be necessary in order to clarify some important aspects. Considering the location of lesions, one major concern relates to the different approaches used for exclusion criteria. Many of the studies examined only a sub-sample of the patients registered in their clinical setting, as the subjects with aphasia (more or less severe), neglect, and severe disability were excluded for the difficulties that could have been encountered in their clinical and neuropsychological assessment. This kind of approach likely resulted in a major selection bias in terms of the role of the dominant hemisphere: it is plausible that left cortical infarctions

Table 8.4 Case-control studies evaluating post-stroke dementia. The reported data are related to the subgroup of patients with stroke.

Reference	Patient numbers	Characteristics of patients	Assessment of stroke-related features	Assessment of pre-existing brain structural changes	Predictors of post-stroke dementia
Desmond et al. (2002)	334	Ischemic stroke 60 years Excluded: pre-dementia and severe aphasia	Syndromes: major/minor; dominant/non-dominant; lacunar/hemispheral; brainstem/cerebellar Mechanism (according to TOAST) Location (R/L hemispheric, cerebellar, brainstem) Arterial vascular territory	–	Major hemispheral syndrome Prior stroke
Ivan et al. (2004)	217	Ischemic or hemorrhagic <95 years Excluded: pre-dementia	Mechanism: Hemorrhagic/ischemic Cardioembolic/atherothrombotic Location: R/L hemisphere, posterior fossa Number of infarcts (CT)	–	Athero-thrombotic stroke type
Sachdev et al. (2006)	169	Ischemic stroke 49–87 years Excluded: pre-dementia and severe aphasia	Mechanism (according to TOAST) Location (R/L, hemispheric, cerebellar, brainstem) Number and volume of infarcts (MRI, 101 patients)	Brain atrophy WMLs	Infarct volume Pre-stroke cognitive status

R/L: right/left; CT: computed tomography; MRI: magnetic resonance imaging.
TOAST: Trail of Org10172 in acute stroke treatment criteria (large-vessel atherosclerosis, cardioembolism, lacunar, other, undetermined).
WMLs: white matter lesions.

are predictors of multi-infarct dementia because the left hemisphere is the dominant one for what concerns language function. Indeed, the studies in which aphasic patients were not excluded more often found that left hemisphere and the presence of aphasia were predictors of dementia.

A second point relates to the impact that pre-existing brain structural changes may have in the occurrence of post-stroke dementia. These changes are related to different possible mechanisms responsible for the development of dementia, where brain atrophy and medial temporal lobe can underlie AD pathology, while white matter lesions underlie VaD of the subcortical type. As has been emphasized (Pantoni, 2003), there is an overlap between vascular and degenerative mechanisms responsible for the pathogenesis of VaD. Thus, the importance of the detection of the cognitive impairment eventually existing before stroke has been an emerging field of research over the last years; as a result of these efforts, the term "pre-stroke dementia" has been coined (Hénon, 2000; Hénon et al., 2001; Pohjasvaara et al., 1999). The status of pre-stroke cognitive functions has been

Table 8.5 Methodological aspects of stroke patients series evaluating post-stroke dementia.

Reference	Patient numbers	Inclusion criteria	Exclusion criteria	Prior strokes	Pre-cognitive status	Follow-up (months)[a]	Dementia criteria	Prevalence (%)
Altieri et al. (2004)	191	Ischemic or hemorrhagic >40 years >5 years education	Severe aphasia and neglect Pre-stroke dementia	Included	–	12, 24, 36, **48**	ICD-10	21.5
Barba et al. (2000)	251	Ischemic or hemorrhagic ≥18 years		Included	Assessed	**3**	DSM-IV	30.0 (10% pre-stroke dementia)
Censori et al. (1996)	146	First ever ischemic 40–79 years	Stroke history Pre-stroke dementia	Excluded	–	**3**	NINDS-AIREN	13.6
Cordoliani-Mackoviak et al. (2003)	144	Ischemic or hemorrhagic ≥40 years	Pre-stroke dementia	Included	–	6, 12, 24, **36**	ICD-10	23.6
Del Ser et al. (2005)	193	Ischemic or hemorrhagic ≥18 years	Pre-stroke dementia	Included	–	**3**, 6, 12, 24	DSM-IV	18.6
Desmond et al. (2000)	453	Ischemic ≥60 years	Severe aphasia	Included	Assessed	**3**	DSM-III-R	26.3
Hénon et al. (2001)	202	Ischemic or hemorrhagic >40 years		Included	Assessed	6, 12, 24, **36**	ICD-10	28.5
Inzitari et al. (1998)	339	Ischemic or hemorrhagic	Pre-stroke dementia	Included	–	3, **12**	ICD-10	16.8

Study	Patients (n)	Stroke type	Exclusion criteria	Pre-stroke dementia	Cognitive decline assessed[a]	Follow-up (months)	Criteria	Prevalence (%)
Lin et al. (2003)	283	Ischemic		Pre-stroke dementia Included	–	3	ICD-10	9.2
Madureira et al. (2001)	237	Ischemic or hemorrhagic	Aphasia, Severe disability, Pre-stroke dementia	Included	–	3	DSM-IV	6.0
Pohjasvaara et al. (1998)	337	Ischemic 55–85 years	Severe aphasia	Included	Assessed	3	DSM-III	31.8
Pohjasvaara et al. (2000a)	337	Ischemic 55–85 years	Severe aphasia	Included	Assessed	3	DSM-III	31.8
Pohjasvaara et al. (2000b)	273	First ever stroke 55–85 years	Severe aphasia	Excluded	Assessed	3	DSM III	28.9
Rasquin et al. (2004)	176	First ever ischemic stroke ≥ 40 years	Aphasia, posterior fossa lesions, Other neuro-psychiatric disorders	Excluded	–	1, 6, **12**	DSM-IV	9.0
Tang et al. (2004)	280	Ischemic or hemorrhagic ≥ 50 years		Included	Assessed	3	DSM-IV	20.0
Treves et al. (1997)	158	First ever ischemic stroke	Pre-stroke dementia	Excluded	–	12, **36**	DSM-III	34.0
Zhou et al. (2004)	434	Ischemic ≥ 55 years	Severe aphasia	Included	Assessed	3	DSM-IV	27.2

[a] Numbers in bold indicate the time when prevalence of dementia was assessed.

Table 8.6 Stroke patients series evaluating post-stroke dementia. Assessment of stroke-related features and of pre-existing brain structural changes, and main results of the stroke cohort studies.

| Reference | Stroke severity | Stroke-related features | | | | | Assessment of pre-existing brain structural changes | Post-stroke dementia predictors |
		Location	Infarct number	Size	Mechanism			
Altieri *et al.* (2004)	NIHSS mRS	L/R hemisphere; brainstem, cerebellum	Single vs. multiple	Infarction vs. lacuna	Ischemic vs. hemorrhagic		CT (*n*=104), MRI (*n*=87) Silent infarcts, WMLs, brain atrophy	Cortical atrophy Number of lesions
Barba *et al.* (2000)	CNS	Vascular territory: carotid (L/R ACA, MCA) vs. VB	Single vs. multiple	Lacunar vs. non-lacunar	Hemorrhagic Ischemic: embolic vs. thrombotic			Stroke severity Pre-stroke cognitive status
Censori *et al.* (1996)	NIHSS	OCSP criteria L/R hemisphere, VB		Volume (new and old lesions)	According to TOAST		CT Silent infarcts, WMLs, atrophy	TACI Stroke severity Aphasia Volume of new lesion
Cordoliani-Mackoviak *et al.* (2003)	Orgogozo Scale	–	–	–	Hemorrhagic Ischemic: according to TOAST		CT Silent infarcts, WMLs, brain atrophy, MTA	Pre-stroke cognitive status Stroke severity WMLs
Del Ser *et al.* (2005)	CNS	L/R carotid; VB Strategic areas	Single vs. multiple	Infarction vs. lacuna Volume	Hemorrhagic Ischemic: embolic, thrombotic		CT (167 pts) Silent infarcts, WMLs, Atrophy, MTA (102 pts)	Pre-stroke cognitive status

Study	Scale	Location	Number	Syndromes	Stroke type	Imaging	Predictors
Desmond et al. (2000)	SSS	L/R hemisphere; brainstem/cerebellum Vascular territory: ICA, ACA, MCA, PCA, VBA	–	Syndromes: major/minor dominant/non-dominant lacunar/hemispheral brainstem/cerebellar	Large-artery ATS Cardiac embolism; Lacunar, undetermined	–	Prior stroke Major dominant Hemisphere vs. brainstem/cerebellum ACA+PCA vs. other territories Large-artery ATS vs. other mechanism
Hénon et al. (2001)	Orgogozo Scale	L/R hemisphere, posterior fossa	–	–	Hemorrhagic Ischemic: according to TOAST	CT Silent infarcts, WMLs, Atrophy	Pre-stroke cognitive status Stroke severity WMLs Silent infarcts
Inzitari et al. (1998)	Assessed	OCSP criteria	–	–	Hemorrhagic Ischemic	–	Aphasia Stroke severity
Lin et al. (2003)	NIHSS	Cortical/subcortical L/R hemisphere; VB	Single vs. multiple	–	Lacunar, thrombotic, embolic	–	Left hemisphere Stroke severity Prior stroke
Madureira et al. (2001)	mRS	Cortical/subcortical L/R hemisphere	–	–	Ischemic Hemorrhagic	CT Atrophy, WMLs	Left-sided lesions (for cognitive impairment)

Table 8.6 (cont.)

Reference	Stroke severity	Stroke-related features				Assessment of pre-existing brain structural changes	Post-stroke dementia predictors
		Location	Infarct number	Size	Mechanism		
Pohjasvaara et al. (1998)	SSS NIHSS	R/L hemisphere Bilateral lesions Anterior/ posterior	–	Syndromes: major/minor dominant/non-dominant lacunar/ hemispheral brainstem/ cerebellar	According to TOAST	–	Prior stroke Left hemisphere Aphasia Major dominant syndrome
Pohjasvaara et al. (2000a)	–	Lobes Vascular territory Specific locations	Assessed	Volume	Lacunar vs. non-lacunar	MRI Silent infarcts, WMLs, atrophy, MTA	Volume of MCA lesions Number of lesions on the left MTA – WMLs
Pohjasvaara et al. (2000b)	–	Lobes Vascular territory Specific locations	Assessed	Volume	Lacunar vs. non-lacunar	MRI Silent infarcts, WMLs, atrophy, MTA	Volume and number of left lesions MTA WMLs
Rasquin et al. (2004)	–	R/L hemisphere		Lacunar/territorial	–	CT Silent infarcts, WMLs, atrophy	Territorial infarcts

	R/L side	Assessed	Lacunar vs. non-lacunar	Hemorrhagic, Ischemic: cortical/ subcortical, brainstem, cerebellar	CT	Stroke severity
Tang et al. (2004) NIHSS	Vascular territory ICA, ACA MCA, PCA, VBa			Hemorrhagic, Ischemic: cortical/ subcortical, brainstem, cerebellar	WMLs, atrophy	Number of lesions, MCA, Cortical and bilateral lesions, Pre-stroke cognitive decline, WMLs, Atrophy
Treves et al. (1997) Assessed	Carotid vs VB	–	–	–	–	Aphasia
Zhou et al. (2004) NIHSS	Vascular territory L/R carotid; VB	Single vs. multiple	–	Thrombotic Embolic, other	–	Prior stroke, Aphasia, Left carotid

NIHSS: National Institute of Health Stroke Scale; mRS modified Rankin Scale; CNS: Canadian Neurological Scale; SSS: Stroke Severity Scale. L/R: left/right; ICA: internal carotid artery; ACA: anterior cerebral artery; MCA: medial cerebral artery; PCA: posterior cerebral artery; VB: vertebro-basilar; OCSP Criteria: Oxfordshire Community Stroke Project; TACI: total anterior circulation infarct; PACI: partial anterior circulation infarct; LACI: lacunar infarcts; POCI: posterior circulation infarct; TOAST: trail of Org10-72 in acute stroke treatment criteria (large-vessel atherosclerosis, cardioembolism, lacunar, other, undetermined).

ATS: atherosclerosis; WMLs: white matter lesions; MTA: medial temporal lobe atrophy; pts: patients.

113

assessed only in some of the studies reported in Table 8.5, and in this case, it often resulted as a predictor of dementia.

Overall, from these data, it is not possible to find a single explanation for the development of dementia related to large-vessel pathology, as the etiology is probably multi-factorial, where stroke characteristics (size, location, and number), as well as host characteristics contribute to the risk independently. It is thus clear that there is not a single factor solely related to dementia, and in the majority of the cases, several mechanisms interact to exceed the critical threshold for normal cognition and dementia eventually supervenes.

Conclusions

In this chapter we have outlined some characteristics of VaD related to large-vessel diseases in terms of pathology, pathogenesis, and clinical aspects. As anticipated, the term *large-vessel VaD* encompasses a large spectrum of conditions that can be difficult to group and summarize. What is doubtless in our opinion is the fact that diseases affecting the large arteries and the consequent lesions of the parenchyma have a role in increasing the risk of dementia and, at least in a group of patients, play a direct role to cause dementia. The term large-vessel VaD is probably not the best one for clinical use given the heterogeneity of underlying conditions, and serves mainly to remind us of the role that large vessel diseases may play in the field of dementia, emphasizing the need for increasing awareness about this aspect and for reinforcing all the strategies able to reduce, through prevention, the burden of VaD.

REFERENCES

Adams HP Jr., Love BB, Jacoby MR. Arterial dissections. In: Ginsberg MD, Bogousslavsky J, eds. *Cerebrovascular Disease*. Oxford: Blackwell Science, 1998; 1430–46.

Adams RD, Vander Eecken HM. Vascular diseases of the brain. *Ann Rev Med* 1953; **4**: 213–52.

Altieri M, Di Piero V, Pasquini M *et al*. Delayed poststroke dementia: a 4-year follow-up study. *Neurology* 2004; **62**: 2193–7.

Amarenco P, Cohen A, Tzourio C, *et al*. Atherosclerotic disease of the aortic arch and the risk of ischemic stroke. *N Engl J Med* 1994; **331**: 1474–9.

Barba R, Martinez-Espinosa S, Rodriguez-Garcia E, *et al*. Poststroke dementia: clinical features and risk factors. *Stroke* 2000; **31**: 1494–501.

Bastos Leite AJ, van der Flier WM, van Straaten EC, *et al*. Infratentorial abnormalities in vascular dementia. *Stroke* 2006; **37**: 105–10.

Becker H, Desch H, Hacker H, Pencz A. CT fogging effect with ischemic cerebral infarcts. *Neuroradiology* 1979; **18**: 185–92.

Berger MS, Wilson CB. Intracranial dissecting aneurysms of the posterior circulation. Report of six cases and review of the literature. *J Neurosurg* 1984; **61**: 882–94.

Bowler JV, Steenhuis R, Hachinski V. Conceptual background to vascular cognitive impairment. *Alzheimer Dis Assoc Disord* 1999; **13** (Suppl 3): S30–7.

Brandt T, Orberk E, Weber R, *et al*. Pathogenesis of cervical artery dissections. Association with connective tissue abnormalities. *Neurology* 2001; **57**: 24–30.

Caplan LR. Dilatative arteriopathy (dolichoectasia). What is known and not known. *Ann Neurol* 2005; **57**: 469–71.

Censori B, Manara O, Agostinis C, *et al*. Dementia after first stroke. *Stroke* 1996; **27**: 1205–10.

Chalela JA, Kidwell CS, Nentwich LM, *et al*. Magnetic resonance imaging and computed tomography in emergency assessment of patients with suspected acute stroke: a prospective comparison. *Lancet* 2007; **369**: 293–8.

Chaves C, Estol C, Esnaola M, *et al*. Spontaneous intracranial internal carotid artery dissection. *Arch Neurol* 2002; **59**: 977–81.

Chuaqui R, Tapia J. Histologic assessment of the age of recent brain infarcts in man. *Neuropathol Exp Neurol* 1993; **52**: 481–9.

Cordoliani-Mackowiak MA, Hénon H, Pruvo JP, *et al*. Poststroke dementia: the influence of hippocampal atrophy. *Arch Neurol* 2003; **60**: 565–90.

del Ser T, Bermejo F, Portera A, *et al*. Vascular dementia. A clinicopathological study. *J Neurol Sci* 1990; **96**: 1–17.

del Ser T, Barba R, Morin M, *et al.* Evolution of cognitive impairment after stroke and risk factors for delayed progression. *Stroke* 2005; **36**: 2670–5.

del Zoppo GJ. Microvascular changes during cerebral ischemia and reperfusion. *Cerebrovasc Brain Metab Rev* 1994; **6**: 47–96.

Desmond DW, Moroney JT, Paik MC, *et al.* Frequency and clinical determinants of dementia after ischemic stroke. *Neurology* 2000; **54**: 1124–31.

Desmond DW, Moroney JT, Sano M, Stern Y. Incidence of dementia after ischemic stroke: results of a longitudinal study. *Stroke* 2002; **33**: 2254–60.

Eckert B, Zeumer H. Brain computed tomography. In: Ginsberg MD Bogousslavsky J, eds. *Cerebrovascular Disease.* Oxford: Blackwell Science, 1998; 1241–64.

Ellison D, Gatter K, Heryet A, Esiri M. Intramural platelet deposition in cerebral vasculopathy of systemic lupus erythematosus. *J Clin Pathol* 1993; **46**: 37–40.

Erkinjuntti T, Haltia M, Palo J, *et al.* Accuracy of the clinical diagnosis of vascular dementia: a prospective clinical and post-mortem neuropathological study. *J Neurol Neurosurg Psychiatry* 1988; **51**: 1037–44.

Erkinjuntti T, Inzitari D, Pantoni L, *et al.* Research criteria for subcortical vascular dementia in clinical trials. *J Neural Transm Suppl* 2000; **59**: 23–30.

Farrell MA, Gilbert JJ, Kaufmann JC. Fatal intracranial arterial dissection: clinical pathological correlation. *J Neurol Neurosurg Psychiatry* 1985; **48**: 111–21.

Fisher M, Fieman S. Geometric factors of the bifurcation in carotid atherogenesis. *Stroke* 1990; **21**: 267–71.

Garcia JH, Yoshida Y, Chen H, *et al.* Progression from ischemic injury to infarct following middle cerebral artery occlusion in the rat. *Am J Pathol* 1993; **142**: 623–35.

Garcia JH, Liu KF, Ho KL. Neuronal necrosis after middle cerebral artery occlusion in Wistar rats progresses at different time intervals in the caudoputamen and the cortex. *Stroke* 1995; **26**: 636–42.

Garcia JH, Anderson ML. Circulatory disorders and their effects on the brain. In: Davis RL and Robertson DM, eds. Textbook of Neuropathology. Baltimore: Williams & Wilkins, 1997; 715–822.

Hachinski VC, Lassen NA, Marshall J. Multi-infarct dementia. A cause of mental deterioration in the elderly. *Lancet* 1974; **2**: 207–10.

Hachinski VC, Iliff LD, Zilhka E, *et al.* Cerebral blood flow in dementia. *Arch Neurol* 1975; **32**: 632–7.

Hankey GJ. Necrotizing and granulomatous angiitis of the CNS. In: Ginsberg MD, Bogousslavsky J, eds. *Cerebrovascular Disease.* Oxford: Blackwell Science, 1998; 1647–83.

Hénon H. Pre-stroke dementia: prevalence and associated factors. *Cerebrovasc Dis* 2000; **10** (Suppl 4), 45–8.

Hénon H, Durieu I, Guerouaou D, *et al.* Poststroke dementia: incidence and relationship to prestroke cognitive decline. *Neurology* 2001; **57**: 1216–22.

Hénon H, Pasquier F, Leys D. Poststroke dementia. *Cerebrovasc Dis* 2006; **22**: 61–70.

Ikezaki K, Fukui M. Definition (guidelines). In: Ikezaki K, Loftus CM, eds. *Moyamoya Disease.* Illinois: American Association of Neurological Surgeons (AANS) Publications, 2001; 13–22.

Inzitari D, Di Carlo A, Pracucci G, *et al.* Incidence and determinants of poststroke dementia as defined by an informant interview method in a hospital-based stroke registry. *Stroke* 1998; **29**: 2087–93.

Ivan CS, Seshadri S, Beiser A, *et al.* Dementia after stroke: the Framingham study. *Stroke* 2004; **35**: 1264–68.

Jellinger KA. Understanding the pathology of vascular cognitive impairment. *J Neurol Sci* 2005; **229–230**: 57–63.

Jones EF, Kalman JM, Calafiore P, *et al.* Proximal aortic atheroma. An independent risk factor for cerebral ischemia. *Stroke* 1995; **26**: 218–24.

Judge RD, Currier RD, Gracie WA, Figley MM. Takayasu's arteritis and the aortic arch syndrome. *Am J Med* 1962; **32**. 379–92.

Katzenstein AL, Carrington CB, Liebow AA. Lymphomatoid granulomatosis: a clinicopathologic study of 152 cases. *Cancer* 1979; **43**: 360–73.

Khatri P, Wechsler LR, Broderick JP. Intracranial hemorrhage associated with revascularization therapies. *Stroke* 2007; **38**: 431–40.

Kleinschmidt-DeMasters BK, Filley CM, Bitter MA. Central nervous system angiocentric, angiodestructive T-cell lymphoma (lymphomatoid granulomatosis). *Surg Neurol* 1992; **37**: 130–7.

Kuller LH, Lopez OL, Jagust WJ, *et al.* Determinants of vascular dementia in the Cardiovascular Health Cognition Study. *Neurology* 2005; **64**: 1548–52.

Leys D, Henon H, Mackowiak-Cordoliani MA, Pasquier F. Poststroke dementia. *Lancet Neurol* 2005; **4**: 752–9.

Lin JH, Lin RT, Tai CT, *et al.* Prediction of poststroke dementia. *Neurology* 2003; **61**: 343–8.

Liu CK, Miller BL, Cummings JL, *et al.* A quantitative MRI study of vascular dementia. *Neurology* 1992; **42**: 138–43.

Loeb C, Gandolfo C, Bino G. Intellectual impairment and cerebral lesions in multiple cerebral infarcts. A clinical-computed tomography study. *Stroke* 1988; **19**: 560–5.

Lucas C, Moulin T, Deplanque D, et al. Stroke patterns of internal carotid artery dissection in 40 patients. *Stroke* 1998; **29**: 2646–48.

Madureira S, Guerreiro M, Ferro JM. Dementia and cognitive impairment three months after stroke. *Eur J Neurol* 2001; **8**: 621–7.

Masdeu JC, Irinia P, Asenbaum S, et al. EFNS guideline on neuroimaging in acute stroke. Report of an EFNS task force. *Eur J Neurol* 2006; **13**: 1271–83.

Masuda J, Ogata J, Butani C. Smooth muscle cell proliferation and localization of macrophages and T cells in the occlusive intracranial major arteries in moyamoya disease. *Stroke* 1993; **24**: 1960–67.

Masuda J, Ogata J, Yamaguchi T (2004). Moyamoya disease. In: JP Mohr, DW Choi, JC Grotta, B Weir, PA Wolf, eds. *Stroke: Pathophysiology, diagnosis, and management.* Philadelphia: Churchill Livingstone, 2004; 603–18.

McKusick VA. A form of vascular disease relatively frequent in the Orient. *Am Heart J* 1962; **63**: 57–64.

Mielke R, Herholz K, Grond M, et al. Severity of vascular dementia is related to volume of metabolically impaired tissue. *Arch Neurol* 1992; **49**: 909–13.

Mitsias P, Levine SR. Large cerebral vessel occlusive disease in systemic lupus erythematosus. *Neurology* 1994; **44**: 385–93.

Nishimura M, Satoh K, Suga M, Oda M. Cerebral angio- and neuro-Behcet's syndrome: neuroradiological and pathological study of one case. *J Neurol Sci* 1991; **106**: 19–24.

Numano F, Okawara M, Inomata H, Kobayashi Y. Takayasu's arteritis. *Lancet* 2000; **356**: 1023–5.

Ogata J, Masuda J, Nishikawa M, Yokota T. Sclerosed peripheral-artery aneurysm in moyamoya disease. *Cerebrovasc Dis* 1996; **6**: 248–9.

Ogata J, Pantoni L. Neuropathology of ischemic brain damage. In: Aminoff M, Boller F, Swaab D, eds. *Handbook of Clinical Neurology*, 3rd Series. Amsterdam: Elsevier. In press.

Pantoni L. Subtypes of vascular dementia and their pathogenesis: a critical overview. In: Bowler JV, Hachinski V, eds. *Vascular Cognitive Impairment-preventable Dementia.* New York: Oxford University Press, 2003; 217–29.

Pantoni L, Basile AM, Romanelli M, et al. Abulia and cognitive impairment in two patients with capsular genu infarct. *Acta Neurol Scand* 2001; **104**: 185–90.

Pantoni L, Sarti. C, Alafuzoff I, et al. Postmortem examination of vascular lesions in cognitive impairment.

A survey among neuropathological services. *Stroke* 2006; **37**: 1005–9.

Pasquier F, Leys D. Why are stroke patients prone to develop dementia? *J Neurol* 1997; **244**: 135–42.

Pohjasvaara T, Erkinjuntti T, Ylikoski R, et al. Clinical determinants of poststroke dementia. *Stroke* 1998; **29**: 75–81.

Pohjasvaara T, Mantyla R, Aronen HJ, et al. Clinical and radiological determinants of prestroke cognitive decline in a stroke cohort. *J Neurol Neurosurg Psychiatry* 1999; **67**: 742–8.

Pohjasvaara T, Mantyla R, Salonen O, et al. How complex interactions of ischemic brain infarcts, white matter lesions, and atrophy relate to poststroke dementia. *Arch Neurol* 2000a; **57**: 1295–300.

Pohjasvaara T, Mantyla R, Salonen O, et al. MRI correlates of dementia after first clinical ischemic stroke. *J Neurol Sci* 2000b; **181**: 111–7.

Rajamani K, Fisher M, Fisher M. In: Ginsberg MD, Bogousslavsky J, eds. *Cerebrovascular Disease.* Oxford: Blackwell Science, 1998; 308–18.

Rasquin SM, Verhey FR, van Oostenbrugge RJ, et al. Demographic and CT scan features related to cognitive impairment in the first year after stroke. *J Neurol Neurosurg Psychiatry* 2004; **75**: 1562–7.

Roman GC. Vascular dementia: distinguishing characteristics, treatment, and prevention. *J Am Geriatr Soc* 2003; **51**: S296–304.

Roman GC, Tatemichi TK, Erkinjuntti T, et al. Vascular dementia: diagnostic criteria for research studies. Report of the NINDS-AIREN International Workshop. *Neurology* 1993; **43**: 250–60.

Rosenberg MR, Parshley M, Gibson S, Wernick R. Central nervous system polyarteritis nodosa. *West J Med* 1990; **153**: 553–6.

Sachdev PS, Brodaty H, Valenzuela MJ, et al. Clinical determinants of dementia and mild cognitive impairment following ischaemic stroke: the Sydney Stroke Study. *Dement Geriatr Cogn Disord* 2006; **21**: 275–83.

Scheltens P, Fox N, Barkhof F, De Carli C. Structural magnetic resonance imaging in the practical assessment of dementia: beyond exclusion. *Lancet Neurol* 2002; **1**: 13–21.

Schievink WI. Spontaneous dissection of the carotid and vertebral arteries. *N Engl J Med* 2001; **344**: 898–906.

Schievink WI, Mokri B, Piepgras DG. Spontaneous dissections of cervicocephalic arteries in childhood and adolescence. *Neurology* 1994; **44**: 1607–12.

Schneider JA, Wilson RS, Cochran EJ, *et al.* Relation of cerebral infarctions to dementia and cognitive function in older persons. *Neurology* 2003; **60**: 1082–8.

Serdaroglu P. Behcet's disease and the nervous system. *J Neurol* 1998; **245**: 197–205.

Strong JP. Atherosclerotic lesions. Natural history, risk factors, and topography. *Arch Pathol Lab Med* 1992; **116**: 1268–75.

Tang WK, Chan SS, Chiu HF, *et al.* Frequency and determinants of poststroke dementia in Chinese. *Stroke* 2004; **35**: 930–5.

Tatemichi TK, Desmond DW, Mayeux R, *et al.* Dementia after stroke: baseline frequency, risks, and clinical features in a hospitalized cohort. *Neurology* 1992; **42**: 1185–93.

Tatemichi TK, Desmond DW, Prohovnik I. Strategic infarcts in vascular dementia. A clinical and brain imaging experience. *Arzneimittelforschung* 1995; **45**: 371–85.

Tomlinson BE, Blessed G, Roth M. Observations on the brains of demented old people. *J Neurol Sci* 1970; **11**: 205–42.

Treves TA, Aronovich BD, Bornstein NM, Korczyn AD. Risk of dementia after a first-ever ischemic stroke: a 3 year longitudinal study. *Cerebrovasc Dis* 1997; **7**: 48–52.

van der Flier WM, Scheltens P. Use of laboratory and imaging investigations in dementia. *J Neurol Neurosurg Psychiatry* 2005; **76** (Suppl. 5): v45–52.

Vinijchaikul K. Primary arteritis of the aorta and its major branches (Takayasu's arteriopathy). A clinicopathologic autopsy study of eight cases. *Am J Med* 1967; **43**: 15–27.

von Kummer R, Meyding-Lamade U, Forsting M, *et al.* Sensitivity and prognostic value of early CT in occlusion of the middle cerebral artery trunk. *Am J Neuroradiol* 1994; **15**: 9–15.

Warach S, Chien D, Li W, *et al.* Fast magnetic resonance diffusion-weighted imaging of acute human stroke. *Neurology* 1992; **42**: 1717–23.

Wolfe N, Babikian VL, Linn RT, *et al.* (1994). Are multiple cerebral infarcts synergistic? *Arch Neurol* **51**: 211–5.

Zhou DH, Wang JY, Li J, *et al.* Study on frequency and predictors of dementia after ischemic stroke: the Chongqing stroke study. *J Neurol* 2004; **251**: 421–7.

Zhou DH, Wang JY, Li J, *et al.* Frequency and risk factors of vascular cognitive impairment three months after ischemic stroke in China: the Chongqing stroke study. *Neuroepidemiology* 2005; **24**: 87–95.

9

Small-vessel diseases of the brain

Raj N. Kalaria and Timo Erkinjuntti

Introduction

A century ago, Alois Alzheimer and Emil Kraeplin, among other neuropsychiatrists, had formed an opinion that arteriosclerotic dementia resulting from gradual strangulation of the blood supply to the brain was the main cause of dementia (Berrios and Freeman, 1991). Otto Binswanger then introduced the notion of subclasses of vascular dementia (VaD). He described subcortical arteriosclerotic encephalopathy upon pathological verification of cerebral white matter disorder in a group of eight patients (Berrios and Freeman, 1991). These historical considerations have some implications for treatment strategies. Today we accept that cerebrovascular disease (CVD) causes the second most common form of age-related dementia. VaD, or rather vascular cognitive impairment, can, however, result from all forms of cerebrovascular changes that also include delayed dementia post-stroke (O'Brien et al., 2003; Roman, 2002; Roman et al., 2002). The challenge of defining the pathological substrates of VaD is complicated by the heterogeneous nature of CVD and the co-existence of other pathologies, including Alzheimer-type lesions. Blood vessel size, origin of vascular occlusion and genetic factors are critical factors in defining subtypes of VaD (Table 9.1). Multi-infarct dementia (MID) is thought to involve large vessels and wide territories predominantly due to athero-thrombotic and embolic events, which may cause up to 50% of all ischemic strokes, whereas Binswanger-type VaD involves subcortical regions including the white matter results from small-vessel changes. Subcortical ischemic VaD appears to be the most significant subtype of VaD. Other factors that may define the subtype and degree of impairment include multiplicity, size, anatomical location, laterality and age of the lesion. For the purposes of treatments and prevention strategies, it is imperative to recognize subtypes of VaD yet not devise numerous categories to make the task unnecessarily complicated (Roman et al., 1993).

Prevalence of small-vessel disease

Intracranial small-vessel disease is thought to cause 25% of infarcts (Kalimo et al., 2002a). Small-vessel alterations involve arteriosclerosis, hyalinosis, and are associated with lacunar infarcts and lacunes predominantly occurring in the subcortical structures. White matter disease or subcortical leukoencephalopathy with incomplete infarction and small-vessel disease are common pathological changes in CVD. Other features include border zone (watershed) infarctions, laminar necrosis and amyloid angiopathy (Table 9.2). Complicated angiopathies such as fibromuscular dysplasia, arterial dissections, granulomatous angiitis,

Vascular Cognitive Impairment in Clinical Practice, ed. Lars-Olof Wahlund, Timo Erkinjuntti and Serge Gauthier. Published by Cambridge University Press. © Cambridge University Press 2009.

Table 9.1. VaD subtypes defined by blood vessel size and pathological process.

- Large-vessel dementia (multiple infarcts)
- Small-vessel dementia (small-vessel disease and microinfarction)
- Strategic infarct dementia (infarcts in strategic locations)
- Hypoperfusive dementia
- Dementia related to angiopathies (hypertension, amyloid)*
- Haemorrhagic dementia
- Other causes of VaD (vasculitis)
- Hereditary VaD (CADASIL, CARASIL, HERNS, CRV, RVCL)

Notes: Hereditary forms of cerebral amyloid angiopathy involving ischemic strokes and intracerebral hemorrhages may also lead to cognitive impairment and stroke.
Abbreviations: CADASIL, cerebral autosomal dominant arteriopathy with subcortical infarcts and leukoencephalo-pathy; CARASIL, cerebral autosomal recessive arteriopathy with subcortical infarcts and leukoencephalopathy; CRV, cerebroretinal vasculopathy; HERNS, hereditary endo-theliopathy, retinopathy, nephropathy and stroke; RVCL, retinal vasculopathy with cerebral leukodystrophy.

Table 9.2 Main features to define the pathophysiology of SVD.

- Identify as ischaemic or hemorrhagic infarct(s)
- Presence of lacunes and lacunar infarcts: *état lacunaire* (gray) and *état crible* (white matter)
- Location of infarcts: white matter, basal ganglia, brainstem (pontine)
- Circulation involved: arterial territories – anterior, middle or posterior
- Laterality: right or left anterior and posterior
- Sizes and number of infarcts = dimension: 0–4 mm, 5–15 mm, 16–30 mm, 31–50 mm and >50 mm; if size <5 mm determine as small or microinfarcts
- Presence and location of small-vessel disease: lipohyalinosis; fibroid necrosis; CAA
- Presence of white matter disease: rarefaction or incomplete infarction
- Degree of gliosis: mild, moderate or severe
- Presence of Alzheimer pathology (incl. NFT and neuritic plaque staging). If degree >stage III, the case is mixed AD and VaD
- Presence of hippocampal sclerosis

For reporting purposes, each of the above features can be scored numerically to provide a summary. For example, 0 is absent and 1 means present. Less frequent lesions include watershed infarcts and laminar necrosis. Increasing numerical value may also be assigned to the infarcts.
Abbreviations: CAA, cerebral amyloid angiopathy; NFT, neurofibrillary tangles.

collagen vascular disease and giant-cell arteritis are rarer causes of CVD disease and VaD.

Previous studies have recorded ischemic, edema-tous and hemorrhagic lesions affecting the brain circulation or perfusion to be associated with VaD (Table 9.3). In four studies where VaD was diagnosed, 75% of the cases revealed cortical and subcortical infarcts, suggesting that other vascular pathologies involving incomplete infarction or border zone infarcts could be important factors. Among other lesions, 25% of the cases had cystic infarcts whereas 50% of the cases had lacunar infarcts or micro-infarcts. Lacunar infarcts, however, appear to be a common category of infarcts, and are currently rec-ognized as the most frequent cause of stroke. Severe amyloid angiopathy was present in 10% of the cases. Most interestingly, in one study, 55% of the cases revealed hippocampal atrophy (Vinters *et al.*, 2000). Ischemic vascular disease appears to correlate with widespread small ischemic lesions distributed throughout the CNS.

Subtypes of VaD and subcortical vascular syndrome

The main subtypes of VaD included in current classifications are cortical VaD or MID (also referred to as post-stroke VaD) and subcortical vascular dementia (SVD), or small-vessel disease related dementia (Brun, 1994; Cummings, 1994; Roman *et al.*, 1993; Wallin and Blennow, 1994). Strategic infarct dementia and hypoperfusive dementia resulting from global cerebrovascular insufficiency are less common types (Erkinjuntti and Kalaria, 2006). Further subtypes include hem-orrhagic dementia and hereditary vascular

Table 9.3 Importance of small-vessel disease in the spectrum of vascular cognitive impairment.

Pathological feature	Cases(%)
Complete infarctions (cortical and subcortical)	75
Lacunar infarcts (mostly WM and BG)	50
Small or microinfarcts	50
Cystic infarcts	25
Cerebral amyloid angiopathy	10
Intracerebral hemorrhages	7
Hippocampal atrophy and sclerosis	55

Data compiled from 70 cases reported in previous studies (Ballard *et al.*, 2000; Esiri *et al.*, 1997; Hulette *et al.*, 1997; Vinters *et al.*, 2000). Cases are averaged from two or more reported studies. Cystic infarcts (possibly also lacunar) with typically ragged edges were admixed in both cortical and subcortical structures.
Abbreviations: BG, basal ganglia; WM, white matter.

dementias. Cerebral autosomal dominant arteriopathy with subcortical infarcts and leukoencephalopathy (CADASIL) is probably the most common form of familial SVD (Kalimo and Kalaria, 2005).

Not surprisingly, the clinical presentation of cortical and subcortical forms of VaD show remarkable differences. Large-vessel occlusions resulting in large cortical infarcts produce cognitive and other deficits that depend on the location of the infarcts, while SVD may have a relatively characteristic neuropsychological profile that includes early impairment of attention and executive function, with slowing of motor performance and information processing (Erkinjuntti and Kalaria, 2006; O'Brien *et al.*, 2003; Roman, 2002; Roman *et al.*, 2002).

Clinically, SVD is characterized by pure motor hemiparesis, bulbar signs and dysarthria, gait disorder, variable depressive illness, emotional lability, and deficits in executive functioning (Babikian and Ropper, 1987; Wallin and Blennow, 1994). The early phase of SVD includes episodes of mild upper motor neuron signs (drift, reflex asymmetry, incoordination), gait disorder (apractic–atactic or small-stepped), imbalance and falls, urinary frequency and incontinence, dysarthria, and dysphagia, as well as extrapyramidal signs such as hypokinesia and rigidity (O'Brien, 2006). However, these focal neurological signs are often subtle (Desmond *et al.*, 1999). Upon imaging, patients with SVD have multiple lacunes and extensive WMLs and often reveal clinical history of "prolonged or multiple TIAs", which mostly are small strokes without residual symptoms and only mild focal findings (e.g. drift, reflex asymmetry, gait disturbance). This also emphasizes the need for neuroimaging in the criteria (Erkinjuntti *et al.*, 1999).

The early cognitive features of SVD are characterized by a dysexecutive syndrome with slowed information processing, usually mild memory deficit and behavioral symptoms (Roman *et al.*, 2002). The dysexecutive syndrome includes impairment in goal formulation, initiation, planning, organizing, sequencing, executing, set-shifting and set-maintenance, as well as in abstraction (Cummings, 1994; Desmond *et al.*, 1999). The memory deficit in SVD is usually milder than in AD, and is specified by impaired recall, relative intact recognition, less severe forgetting and better benefit from cues. Episodic memory may be relatively spared, compared with AD. There is more learning impairment that can be partially corrected by providing salient cues to encourage learning and promote recognition (Pillon *et al.*, 1993). Therefore, memory deficits in VaD appear to be caused by problems in retrieval of information (Kertesz and Clydesdale, 1994; Sachdev *et al.*, 2004; Traykov *et al.*, 2002), whereas memory retrieval deficits are due to aberrant fronto-subcortical circuits. In contrast, in AD, involvement of the hippocampus by neurofibrillary tangles (Braak Stage III) prevents storage of new information, causing amnesic mild cognitive impairment (AMCI). The SVD syndrome may be readily confused with AD in view of the neuronal loss and co-existing vascular factors. The onset can be variable as suggested previously (Babikian and Ropper, 1987). Sixty percent of the patients had a slow, less abrupt onset, and only 30% an acute onset of cognitive symptoms. The course was gradual without (40%) and with (40%) acute deficits, and fluctuating in only 20%.

Behavioral and psychological symptoms in SVD include depression, personality change, emotional lability, loss of volition (apathy) (O'Brien, 2006), incontinence, as well as inertia, emotional bluntness, and psychomotor retardation (Mahler and Cummings, 1991). These may include greater tendencies of aggression and agitation. Such symptomatology is attributed to damage to the prefrontal subcortical circuits (Cummings, 1993).

SVD versus mixed dementia

In a previous neuropathological series, the sensitivity of the NINDS-AIREN criteria for probable and possible VaD was determined to be 58%, and the specificity 80% (Gold et al., 1997). The criteria successfully excluded AD in 91% of cases, and the proportion of mixed cases misclassified as probable VaD was 29%. Interestingly, compared to the ADDTC criteria (Chui et al., 1992), the NINDS-AIREN criteria were more specific and better in excluding mixed cases (54% vs. 29%). Despite these limitations, the frequencies of VaD in autopsy series have been reported to be as low as 0.03% and as high as 58%, with an overall mean rate of 17% (Jellinger, 2007), which is consistent with estimates from clinical studies. In cases where currently accepted criteria have been applied, the frequencies are even lower, with a mean of 7%, whereas the incidence of VaD cases in Japan was reported to be 35% and 22% (Akatsu et al., 2002). Taking these into account, the worldwide frequency of VaD in autopsy-verified cases might be estimated to be between 10 and 15%.

Clinical and pathological evidence indicates that combined neurodegenerative and vascular pathologies worsen the presentation and outcome of dementia (Esiri et al., 1997, 1999; Rossi et al., 2004; Snowdon et al., 1997). A high proportion of individuals fulfilling the neuropathological diagnosis of AD have significant cerebrovascular lesions including silent infarcts upon imaging and extensive white matter disease (Heyman et al., 1998; Kalaria and

Ballard, 1999; Premkumar et al., 1996). Conversely, clinically diagnosed VaD patients frequently show extensive AD-type neuropathological changes (Erkinjuntti et al., 1988; Hulette et al., 1997). Nolan et al. (1999) reported that 87% of patients clinically diagnosed by the NINDS-AIREN criteria were found to have AD either alone (58%) or in combination with CVD (42%) at post-mortem (Figure 9.1). Others (Hulette et al., 1997) have reported that "pure" VaD is very uncommon, because VaD cases without co-existing neuropathological evidence of AD are rarely found. Therefore, current clinical diagnostic criteria serve to detect pathology but not "pure" pathology. Early validation studies indicated that while mixed dementia could be distinguished from AD, it could not be separated from VaD (Rosen et al., 1980). Recent studies suggest that 30–50% of mixed AD and VaD cases are misclassified as VaD (Gold et al., 1997, 2002) and the neuroimaging component of the NINDS-AIREN criteria does not distinguish between people with and without dementia in the context of CVD. The potential overlap of pathologies is therefore complex, with different types of cerebrovascular lesions including subcortical infarction and small-vessel disease (Ballard et al., 2000; Rossi et al., 2004), and accompanying neurodegenerative changes including tau, amyloid and α-synuclein pathology (Figure 9.1). While evidence based pathological criteria for the diagnosis of mixed dementia remains to be perfected, the diagnosis (Erkinjuntti et al., 2002; Kalaria and Ballard, 2001) should be made when a primary neurodegenerative disease known to cause dementia exists with one or more of the pathological lesions defining the VaD subtypes (Table 9.1). The diagnosis of mixed dementia (AD and VaD, or less frequently dementia with Lewy bodies and VaD), particularly among the oldest old (>85, years of age), therefore also remains a challenge.

Pathophysiology of sporadic SVD

SVD incorporates two entities "the lacunar state" and "Binswanger's disease" (Roman et al., 2002).

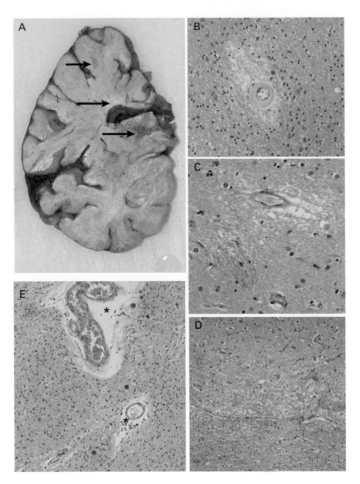

Figure 9.1 Pathological lesions associated with SVD. *A*, recent infarct (arrow) in the thalamus and lacunes (short arrows) in the white matter of a 78-year-old man with cognitive impairment. *B*, hyalinized vessel with severe demyelination in white matter. Moderate gliosis in the perivascular region is also evident. *C* and *D*, microinfarcts and perivascular rarefaction in the basal ganglia. *E*, dilated perivascular spaces (*) in small vessels in the subcortical white matter. See Figure 9.1 in the color plate section. Magnification bar: A=2 cm; B=50 μm; C–D=100 μm; E=200 μm.

SVD is accredited to small-vessel disease and is characterized by lacunar infarcts, focal and diffuse ischemic WMLs, and incomplete ischemic injury (Kalaria *et al.*, 2004). Small vessels including intracerebral end-arteries and arterioles undergo progressive age-related changes (Kalaria *et al.*, 2004; Lammie, 2000), which may result in lacunar infarcts and microinfarcts. These range from wall thickening by hyalinosis, reduction or increment of the intima,

to severe arteriosclerosis and fibroid necrosis. Uncomplicated hyalinosis is characterized by almost complete degeneration of vascular smooth muscle cells (becoming acellular) with concentric accumulation of extracellular matrix components such as the collagens and fibroblasts. The changes are most common in the small vasculature of the white matter (Figure 9.1B). Small-vessel changes likely promote occlusion or progressive stenosis with consequent acute or chronic ischemia of the tissue behind it (Kalimo *et al.*, 2002a). Alternatively, arteriosclerotic changes located in small vessels in the deep white matter and basal ganglia (lenticulostriate) may lose their elasticity to dilate and constrict in response to variations of systemic blood pressure or loss of auto-regulation. This in turn causes fluctuations in blood flow response and changes in cerebral perfusion. The deep cerebral structures would be rendered most vulnerable because the vessels are end-arteries almost devoid of anastomoses. Small-vessel pathology could also lead to edema and damage of the blood–brain barrier (BBB) with chronic leakage of fluid and macromolecules in the white matter (Ho and Garcia, 2000).

Lacunes (or empty spaces) are formed from remnants of small infarcts that may measure up to 15 mm in diameter (Table 9.2; Figure 9.1A) and can be readily quantified by neuroimaging methods, principally MRI (see Chapter 5). Most lacunar infarcts occur in the territory of the deep penetrating arteries including the lenticulostriate branches of the middle cerebral artery, the anterior striate and Heubner arteries, anterior choroidal artery, paramedian branches of the basilar artery and thalamic branches of the posterior cerebral artery. The penetrating vessels that feed lacunar infarcts are 100–400 μm in diameter. Upon gross examination at autopsy, lacunes are largely confined to the white matter (centrum semiovale) and subcortical structures including the thalamus, basic ganglia and brainstem (pons). Lacunar infarcts occasionally occur in the cerebellum and spinal cord but are rare in the gray matter of the cerebral surface and corpus callosum. Most lacunes (*état lacunaire*) are detected in the cystic or chronic stage with no viable central tissue, which may have liquefied and resorbed, but could have perifocal regions with incomplete infarction, particularly in the white matter. A few lacunar may represent healed or be re-absorbed as minute or petechial hemorrhages. Microlacunes have also been described, which should essentially be thought of as large cystic microinfarcts. To distinguish perivascular cavities, it has been suggested that lacunes be classified into three subtypes: lacunar infarcts,

lacunar hemorrhages, and dilated perivascular spaces (Benhaiem-Sigaux *et al.*, 1987). Lacunar infarcts usually result from progressive small-vessel changes manifested as hypertensive angiopathy that may involve stenosis caused by hyalinosis. Small-vessel disease in a perforating artery, for example, may also reveal regions of incomplete infarction, attenuation, or rarefaction, usually recognized by pallor upon microscopic examination. However, lacunar lesions can also be caused by infections and neoplasms. Lacunes may be associated with small perivascular cavities up to 2 mm in diameter frequently found in the basal ganglia and the white matter (Kalaria *et al.*, 2004). Dilated perivascular spaces or *état criblé*, translated as tissue riddled with holes (Figure 9.1E), can be numerous in the white matter of older subjects (Kalaria and Hedera, 1995).

Microinfarcts have been variably described but are widely thought to be small ischemic lesions visible only upon light microscopy (Figures 9.1C and D). These lesions of up to 5 mm diameter may or may not involve a small vessel at its center, but are foci with pallor, neuronal loss, axonal damage (white matter) and gliosis. Sometimes these may include regions of incomplete infarction or rarefied (subacute) change. Microinfarcts have also been described as attenuated lesions of indistinct nature occurring in both cortical and subcortical regions. Microinfarcts and lacunar infarcts appear central to the most common cause of VaD and predict poor outcome in the elderly (Benhaiem-Sigaux *et al.*, 1987; Vinters *et al.*, 2000). Interestingly, in the autopsied older Japanese-American men, the importance of microvascular lesions as a likely explanation for dementia was nearly equal to that of Alzheimer lesions (White *et al.*, 2002). Microinfarction in the subcortical structures has been emphasized as substrate of cognitive impairment, and correlated with increased Alzheimer-type pathology, but cortical microinfarcts also appear to contribute significantly to the progression of cognitive deficits in brain aging (Kovari *et al.*, 2004). Furthermore, microinfarcts even in border zone (watershed) regions may aggravate the degenerative process, as indicated by worsening impairment in AD (Suter *et al.*, 2002). Thus multiple microinfarction appears strongly correlated with dementia indicated by several studies (Jellinger, 2002).

White matter changes (or subcortical leukoencephalopathy) incorporating myelin loss are considered a consequence of vascular disease. The frequency of white matter changes is increased in patients with CVD and those at risk for vascular disease including arterial hypertension, cardiovascular disease and diabetes mellitus (O'Brien *et al.*, 2003). Lesions in the deep white matter have been correlated with dementia including VaD (Kalaria and Ballard, 1999). Conflicting data with respect to periventricular lesions may depend on the definition of the boundaries between the periventricular and deep white matter if the coursing of the fibers are used as markers. Lacunar infarcts are produced when the ischemic damage is focal and of sufficient severity to result in a small area of necrosis, whereas diffuse white matter change is considered a form of rarefaction or incomplete infarction where there may be selective damage to some cellular components. While the U-fibers are usually spared, white matter disease comprises several patterns of alterations including pallor or swelling of myelin, loss of oligodendrocytes, axons and myelin fibers, cavitations with or without the presence of macrophages and areas of reactive astrogliosis, where the astrocytic cytoplasm and cell processes may be visible with standard stains. Lesions in the white matter (WML) also include spongiosis, i.e. vacuolization of the white matter structures and widening of the perivascular spaces (Kalaria *et al.*, 2004).

Ischemic WMLs associated with lipohyalinosis and narrowing of the lumen of the small perforating arteries and arterioles, which nourish the deep white matter, often occur in AD and are common in VaD. Upon MRI, these correspond best with deep white matter hyperintensities (WMH), which may increase the likelihood of correct diagnosis (Greenberg, 2002). In a few studies, biopsy-proven CAA was associated with extensive diffuse hyperintensities presenting as multi-focal non-hemorrhagic leukoariosis (Greenberg *et al.*, 2004; White *et al.*, 2002).

Pathological studies also supported the robust relationship between CAA and WMLs irrespective of the presence of Alzheimer-type pathology (Haglund and Englund, 2002; Sarazin *et al.*, 2002).

Cerebral amyloid angiopathies as SVDs (see also Chapter 11)

Cerebral amyloid angiopathy (CAA) also falls into the category of small-vessel diseases and contributes to the SVD syndrome. CAA is most common in AD and consistently present in Down syndrome (Premkumar *et al.*, 1996); it also occurs in elderly subjects with CVD in the general absence of Alzheimer lesions (Cohen *et al.*, 1997). Current evidence shows age rather than gender, history of hypertension or other vascular disease to be the strongest risk factor for sporadic occurrence of CAA (Greenberg, 2002; Vinters, 1987). Several familial forms of CAA presenting with ischemic and hemorrhagic infarcts or oligemia are perhaps the most studied among the hereditary cerebrovascular disorders (Kalaria, 2001). The clinical features comprise focal neurological signs including spasticity, ataxia, facial paralysis, occasional seizures, and cognitive impairment often leading to dementia (Bornebroek *et al.*, 1999; Greenberg *et al.*, 2004; Haan *et al.*, 1990). CAA is an important cause of intracerebral and lobar hemorrhages leading to profound ischemic damage (Vonsattel *et al.*, 1991). CAA also appears to be causally related to white matter changes described by subcortical leukoencephalopathy in patients with CAA, who lacked changes characteristic of AD (Lammie, 2000). Genetic factors such as the *APOE ε*4 allele associated with the severity of CAA may modify or attenuate the perfusion of the white matter (Kalaria, 2001).

Consideration of the hereditary cerebral hemorrhage with amyloidosis of the Dutch type (HCHWA-D) disease provides certain clues to a link between CAA and stroke. It is thought that the first stroke-like episode triggers multiple cerebral bleeds, which may be preceded by diffuse white matter changes that in turn lead to rapid decline of cognitive functions (Greenberg, 2002; Natte *et al.*, 2001). The degree of CAA is strongly correlated with the presence or absence of dementia, while this was not true for diffuse plaques or neurofibrillary tangles. This suggests that CAA alone causes dementia in HCHWA-D (Bornebroek *et al.*, 1999), a notion likely to be the case in other hereditary amyloid angiopathies. However, cognitive impairment is also a consistent feature in sporadic CAA cases in the absence of other pathologies, as verified by MRI and neuropathological assessment (Greenberg, 2002).

CADASIL and related small-vessel diseases causing dementia

Early reports suggest the existence of several familial stroke disorders unrelated to atherosclerotic disease. Most of these disorders may be classed as SVD involving small vessels of the subcortical structures (Kalimo *et al.*, 2002b). CADASIL is the most common form of hereditary small-vessel diseases leading to cognitive decline and dementia (Chabriat *et al.*, 1995; Dichgans *et al.*, 1998; Opherk *et al.*, 2004). It is difficult to estimate the world-wide prevalence of CADASIL, but in western countries approximately 5 CADASIL cases occur in 100,000. There are estimated to be at least 600, CADASIL families world-wide, suggesting that this disorder is much more common than familial AD (Kalimo *et al.*, 2002b). CADASIL begins with migraine as the first symptom in up to 40% of the patients (Chabriat *et al.*, 1995; Dichgans *et al.*, 1998). The age of onset is usually ascribed by the age at which the first ever stroke occurs, rather than the migraine attack. CADASIL may be manifest well before the first stroke on the basis of characteristic WMHs upon MRI (Chabriat *et al.*, 1998; Singhal *et al.*, 2004). Migraine, usually with aura, may begin even before the age of 10 years, but more commonly during the third decade. More severe manifestations including TIAs, recurrent strokes and

depressive illness follow quickly. Motor deficits, an ataxic hemiparesis, hemianopsia, and dysarthria may accompany these principal events. Other features include seizures, incomplete cerebellar ataxia, pseudobulbar palsy and unexplained coma. Neocortical strokes are rare and they usually do not cover a wide territory (Chabriat *et al.*, 1998). Large artery infarcts such as those of the middle or posterior cerebral artery are uncommon. Dichgans and colleagues (Opherk *et al.*, 2004) have suggested that men are at greater risk for early immobilization and death. However, smoking and high homocysteine (>15 μmol l^{-1}) can increase the risk for more strokes and migraine (Singhal *et al.*, 2004). There is no clear consensus for genotype–phenotype correlations, and the apolipoprotein E ε4 allele does not influence disease progression (Singhal *et al.*, 2004; van den Boom *et al.*, 2006).

Pathological features include severe arteriopathy with the presence of granular osmiophilic material in the arterial walls of both the brain and systemic organs (Lesnik Oberstein *et al.*, 2001). Loss of brain vascular smooth muscle cells leads to wall thickening and fibrosis in small and medium-sized penetrating arteries. This would reduce both cerebral blood flow and blood volume in affected white matter, with effects on the haemodynamic reserve by decreasing the vasodilatory response. Affected vessels presumably progress to obliteration or thrombose, as evident by the appearance of lacunar infarcts, mainly in the basal ganglia and frontotemporal white matter (Lesnik Oberstein *et al.*, 2001). These pathologies initiate cognitive deficits, which progress to dementia of the subcortical vascular type.

CADASIL is caused by single missense mutations or exon deletions in the *NOTCH3* gene (Ruchoux and Maurage, 1997). The gene encodes a type 1 transmembrane protein (Notch3), which is essential during development and regulating cellular differentiation. In adults, NOTCH3 appears to be expressed only in vascular smooth muscle cells, and may promote cell survival by inhibiting apoptosis, but the exact function remains to be elucidated (Kalimo *et al.*, 2002b). *NOTCH 3* mutations consistently result in either a gain or loss of one (or more odd number of) cysteine residue(s) in one of the 34 epidermal growth factor-like repeats in the amino-terminal region of the molecule (Ruchoux *et al.*, 1995). It is not entirely clear which step in the Notch signaling pathway leads to the characteristic vascular pathology of CADASIL. The clinical diagnosis of CADASIL relies upon positive family history and hyperintense lesions upon T2 MRI, particularly in the temporal pole as confirmed by *NOTCH*3 gene screening, or the presence of granular osmophilic material (GOM) in skin or nerve–muscle biopsies (Kalimo *et al.*, 2002b).

In the last 60 years, several CADASIL-like disorders of the brain that do not involve the *NOTCH3* gene have been reported. In addition to the disorders described by Sourander and Walinder (1977) and Colmant (Hagel *et al.*, 2004), an autosomal recessive disorder similar to CADASIL was described in Japan as the Maeda syndrome, or more descriptively as cerebral autosomal recessive arteriopathy with subcortical infarcts and leukoencephalopathy (CARASIL). The normotensive affected subjects exhibit not only severe arteriopathy, leukoencephalopathy and lacunar infarcts, but also spinal anomalies and alopecia. Strokes lead to step-wise deterioration, with most subjects becoming demented in older age.

Hereditary retinopathies and other small-vessel diseases

Small-vessel diseases of the brain may also manifest in progressive visual impairment (Kalimo and Kalaria, 2005). Hereditary endotheliopathy with retinopathy, nephropathy and stroke (HERNS), cerebroretinal vasculopathy (CRV) and hereditary vascular retinopathy (HVR) were reported independently, but are different phenotypes in the same disease spectrum (Jen *et al.*, 1997; Ophoff *et al.*, 2001; Terwindt *et al.*, 1998). They are now described as autosomal dominant retinal vasculopathy with cerebral leukodystro-

phy (RVCL). The RVCL group of small-vessel diseases are caused by C-terminal truncations in the human *TREX1* gene, encoding DNA-specific 3′–5′ exonuclease DNA III (Richards *et al.*, 2007). Renal disease appears to be restricted to HERNS and CRV, whereas HVR is associated with Raynaud phenomenon. The retinopathy involves capillary tortuosity, aneurysms and telangiectasias that begin in the third and fourth decades with increasing migraine-like episodes. Neurological complications of CRV and HERNS usually lead to death before the age of 55 years, whereas HVR patients live longer.

Cerebral small-vessel disease has also been described in association with pseudoxanthoma elasticum, a hereditary connective tissue disorder with abnormalities in the skin and eye and multiple lacunar infarcts in deep white matter and pons (Pavlovic *et al.*, 2005). The disease trait co-segregates with mutations in the ATP-binding cassette transporter gene, ABCC6, located on chromosome 16p13.1. Other recently discovered SVDs include hereditary infantile hemiparesis, retinal arteriolar tortuosity, and leukoencephalopathy (Gould *et al.*, 2006; Vahedi *et al.*, 2003), and a novel autosomal dominant SVD of the brain in a large Portuguese–French family. Chabriat and colleagues (Verreault *et al.*, 2006) reported that this SVD was not fully penetrant and distinguished by motor hemiplegia, memory deficits, executive dysfunction, and white matter changes upon MRI in the general absence of vascular risk.

Conclusions

Small-vessel disease related to subcortical dementia is one of the main subtypes of the VaD syndrome. SVD is clinically characterized by pure motor hemiparesis, bulbar signs and dysarthria, gait disorder, variable depressive illness, emotional lability, and deficits in executive functioning. The pathological features of SVD involve small-vessel degeneration, lacunes, multiple microinfarcts in the subcortical structures, and white matter lesions extending into the deep white matter. CADASIL and CARASIL are examples of familial SVD that present with recurrent subcortical strokes and slowly progressing course leading to dementia. The SVD syndrome may be readily confused with AD in view of the neuronal loss and co-existing vascular factors. However, the symptomatology in SVD is attributed to damage to the frontal–subcortical neuronal circuits.

ACKNOWLEDGMENTS

Our work has been supported by grants from the Medical Research Council (UK), the EC grant QLK6-CT-1999–02112, the B Overstreet fund of the Alzheimer's Association (USA), the Alzheimer's Research Trust (UK) and the CADASIL Trust (UK).

REFERENCES

Akatsu H, Takahashi M, Matsukawa N, *et al*. Subtype analysis of neuropathologically diagnosed patients in a Japanese geriatric hospital. *J Neurol Sci* 2002; **196**: 63–9.

Babikian V, Ropper AH. Binswanger's disease: a review. *Stroke* 1987; **18**: 2–12.

Ballard C, McKeith I, O'Brien J, *et al*. Neuropathological substrates of dementia and depression in vascular dementia, with a particular focus on cases with small infarct volumes. *Dementia Geriatr Cogn Disord* 2000; **11**: 59–65.

Benhaiem-Sigaux N, Gray F, Gherardi R, Roucayrol AM, Poirier J. Expanding cerebellar lacunes due to dilatation of the perivascular space associated with Binswanger's subcortical arteriosclerotic encephalopathy. *Stroke* 1987; **18**: 1087–92.

Berrios GE, Freeman HL. Alzheimer and the dementia. In: Berrios GE, ed. *Eponymists in Medicine Series*. London: Royal Society of Medicine Services, 1991; 69–76.

Bornebroek M, Haan J, Roos RA. Hereditary cerebral hemorrhage with amyloidosis–Dutch type (HCHWA-D): a review of the variety in phenotypic expression. *Amyloid* 1999; **6**: 215–24.

Brun A. Pathology and pathophysiology of cerebrovascular dementia: pure subgroups of obstructive and hypoperfusive etiology. *Dementia* 1994; **5**: 145–7.

Chabriat H, Vahedi K, Iba-Zizen MT, *et al*. Clinical spectrum of CADASIL: a study of 7 families. Cerebral autosomal dominant arteriopathy with subcortical infarcts and leukoencephalopathy. *Lancet* 1995; **346**: 934–9.

Chabriat H, Levy C, Taillia H, *et al*. Patterns of MRI lesions in CADASIL. *Neurology* 1998; **51**: 452–7.

Chui HC, Victoroff JI, Margolin D, Jagust W, Shankle R, Katzman R. Criteria for the diagnosis of ischemic vascular dementia proposed by the State of California Alzheimer's Disease Diagnostic and Treatment Centers. *Neurology* 1992; **42**: 473–80.

Cohen DL, Hedera P, Premkumar DR, Friedland RP, Kalaria RN. Amyloid-beta protein angiopathies masquerading as Alzheimer's disease? *Ann NY Acad Sci* 1997; **826**: 390–5.

Cummings JL. Frontal–subcortical circuits and human behavior. *Arch Neurol* 1993; **50**: 873–80.

Cummings JL. Vascular subcortical dementias: clinical aspects. *Dementia* 1994; **5**: 177–80.

Desmond DW, Erkinjuntti T, Sano M, *et al*. The cognitive syndrome of vascular dementia: implications for clinical trials. *Alzheimer Dis Assoc Disord* 1999; **13** (Suppl 3): S21–9.

Dichgans M, Mayer M, Uttner I, *et al*. The phenotypic spectrum of CADASIL: clinical findings in 102 cases. *Ann Neurol* 1998; **44**: 731–9.

Erkinjuntti T, Haltia M, Palo J, Sulkava R, Paetau A. Accuracy of the clinical diagnosis of vascular dementia: a prospective clinical and post-mortem neuropathological study. *J Neurol Neurosurg Psychiatry* 1988; **51**: 1037–44.

Erkinjuntti T, Bowler JV, DeCarli CS, *et al*. Imaging of static brain lesions in vascular dementia: implications for clinical trials. *Alzheimer Dis Assoc Disord* 1999; **13** (Suppl 3): S81–90.

Erkinjuntti T, Kurz A, Gauthier S, Bullock R, Lilienfeld S, Damaraju CV. Efficacy of galantamine in probable vascular dementia and Alzheimer's disease combined with cerebrovascular disease: a randomised trial. *Lancet* 2002; **359**: 1283–90.

Erkinjuntti T, Kalaria R. Vascular cognitive impairment. In: Growdon J, Rossor M, eds. *The Dementias*. Oxford: Elsevier, 2006.

Esiri MM, Wilcock GK, Morris JH. Neuropathological assessment of the lesions of significance in vascular dementia. *J Neurol Neurosurg Psychiatry* 1997; **63**: 749–53.

Esiri MM, Nagy Z, Smith MZ, Barnetson L, Smith AD. Cerebrovascular disease and threshold for dementia in the early stages of Alzheimer's disease. *Lancet* 1999; **354**: 919–20.

Gold G, Giannakopoulos P, Montes-Paixao Junior C, *et al.* Sensitivity and specificity of newly proposed clinical criteria for possible vascular dementia. *Neurology* 1997; **49**: 690–4.

Gold G, Bouras C, Canuto A, *et al.* Clinicopathological validation study of four sets of clinical criteria for vascular dementia. *Am J Psychiatry* 2002; **159**: 82–7.

Gould DB, Phalan FC, van Mil SE, *et al.* Role of COL4A1 in small-vessel disease and hemorrhagic stroke. *N Engl J Med* 2006; **354**: 1489–96.

Gould DB, Cerebral amyloid angiopathy and vessel dysfunction. *Cerebrovasc Dis* 2002; **13** (Suppl 2): 42–7.

Gould DB, Gurol ME, Rosand J, Smith EE. Amyloid angiopathy-related vascular cognitive impairment. *Stroke* 2004; **35**: 2616–19.

Haan J, Lanser JB, Zijderveld I, van der Does IG, Roos RA. Dementia in hereditary cerebral hemorrhage with amyloidosis-Dutch type. *Archives of Neurology* 1990; **47**: 965–7.

Hagel C, Groden C, Niemeyer R, Stavrou D, Colmant HJ. Subcortical angiopathic encephalopathy in a German kindred suggests an autosomal dominant disorder distinct from CADASIL. *Acta Neuropathol (Berl)* 2004; **108**: 231–40.

Haglund M, Englund E. Cerebral amyloid angiopathy, white matter lesions and Alzheimer encephalopathy – a histopathological assessment. *Dementia Geriatr Cogn Disord* 2002; **14**: 161–6.

Heyman A, Fillenbaum GG, Welsh-Bohmer KA, *et al.* Cerebral infarcts in patients with autopsy-proven Alzheimer's disease: CERAD, part XVIII. Consortium to Establish a Registry for Alzheimer's Disease. *Neurology* 1998; **51**: 159–62.

Ho K-L, Garcia JH. Neuropathology of the small blood vessels in selected disease of the cerebral white matter. In: Pantoni L, Inzitari D, Wallin A, eds. *The Matter of White Matter*, Vol 10. Utrecht: The Netherlands Academic Pharmaceutical Productions, 2000; 247–73.

Hulette C, Nochlin D, Mckeel D, *et al.* Clinical–neuropathologic findings in multi-infarct dementia: a report of six autopsied cases. *Neurology* 1997; **48**: 668–72.

Jellinger KA. Vascular–ischemic dementia: an update. *J Neural Transm Suppl* 2002; **62**: 1–23.

.Jellinger KA. The enigma of vascular cognitive disorder and vascular dementia. *Acta Neuropathol (Berl)* 2007; **113**: 349–88.

Jen J, Cohen AH, Yue Q, *et al.* Hereditary endotheliopathy with retinopathy, nephropathy, and stroke (HERNS). *Neurology* 1997; **49**: 1322–30.

Kalaria RN. Advances in molecular genetics and pathology of cerebrovascular disorders. *Trends Neurosci* 2001; **24**: 392–400.

Kalaria RN, Hedera P. Differential degeneration of the cerebral microvasculature in Alzheimer's disease. *Neuroreport* 1995; **6**: 477–80.

Kalaria RN, Ballard C. Overlap between pathology of Alzheimer disease and vascular dementia. *Alzheimer Dis Assoc Disord* 1999; **13** (Suppl 3): S115–23.

Kalaria RN, Ballard C. Stroke and cognition. *Curr Atherosclerosis Rep* 2001; **3**: 334–9.

Kalaria RN, Kenny RA, Ballard CG, Perry R, Ince P, Polvikoski T. Towards defining the neuropathological substrates of vascular dementia. *J Neurol Sci* 2004; **226**: 75–80.

Kalimo H, Kaste M, Haltia M. Vascular diseases. In: Graham DI, Lantos PL, eds. *Greenfield's Neuropathology*. London: Arnold 2002a; 281–355.

Kalimo H, Ruchoux MM, Viitanen M, Kalaria RN. CADASIL: a common form of hereditary arteriopathy causing brain infarcts and dementia. *Brain Pathol* 2002b; **12**: 371–84.

Kalimo H, Kalaria RN. Hereditary forms of vascular dementia. In: Kalimo H, ed. *Cerebrovascular Diseases, Pathology & Genetics*, Vol 5. Basel: ISN Neuropath Press, 2005: 324–84.

Kertesz A, Clydesdale S. Neuropsychological deficits in vascular dementia vs Alzheimer's disease. Frontal lobe deficits prominent in vascular dementia. *Arch Neurol* 1994; **51**: 1226–31.

Kovari E, Gold G, Herrmann FR, *et al.* Cortical microinfarcts and demyelination significantly affect cognition in brain aging. *Stroke* 2004; **35**: 410–4.

Lammie GA. Pathology of small vessel stroke. *Br Med Bull* 2000; **56**: 296–306.

Lesnik Oberstein SA, van den Boom R, van Buchem MA, *et al.* Cerebral microbleeds in CADASIL. *Neurology* 2001; **57**: 1066–70.

Mahler ME, Cummings JL. Behavioral neurology of multi-infarct dementia. *Alzheimer Dis Assoc Disord* 1991; **5**: 122–30.

Natte R, Maat-Schieman ML, Haan J, Bornebroek M, Roos RA, van Duinen SG. Dementia in hereditary cerebral hemorrhage with amyloidosis-Dutch type is associated with cerebral amyloid angiopathy but is independent of plaques and neurofibrillary tangles. *Ann Neurol* 2001; **50**: 765–72.

Nolan KA, Lino MM, Seligmann AW, Blass JP. Absence of vascular dementia in an autopsy series from a dementia clinic. *J Am Geriatr Soc* 1998; **46**: 597–604.

O'Brien JT. Vascular cognitive impairment. *Am J Geriatr Psychiatry* 2006; **14**: 724–33.

O'Brien JT, Erkinjuntti T, Reisberg B, *et al.* Vascular cognitive impairment. *Lancet Neurol* 2003; **2**: 89–98.

Opherk C, Peters N, Herzog J, Luedtke R, Dichgans M. Long-term prognosis and causes of death in CADASIL: a retrospective study in 411 patients. *Brain* 2004; **127**: 2533–9.

Ophoff RA, DeYoung J, Service SK, *et al.* Hereditary vascular retinopathy, cerebroretinal vasculopathy, and hereditary endotheliopathy with retinopathy, nephropathy, and stroke map to a single locus on chromosome 3p21.1-p21.3. *Am J Hum Genet* 2001; **69**: 447–53.

Pavlovic AM, Zidverc-Trajkovic J, Milovic MM, *et al.* Cerebral small vessel disease in pseudoxanthoma elasticum: three cases. *Can J Neurol Sci* 2005; **32**: 115–18.

Pillon B, Deweer B, Agid Y, Dubois B. Explicit memory in Alzheimer's, Huntington's, and Parkinson's diseases. *Arch Neurol* 1993; **50**: 374–9.

Premkumar DR, Cohen DL, Hedera P, Friedland RP, Kalaria RN. Apolipoprotein E-epsilon4 alleles in cerebral amyloid angiopathy and cerebrovascular pathology associated with Alzheimer's disease. *Am J Pathol* 1996; **148**: 2083–95.

Roman GC. Vascular dementia revisited: diagnosis, pathogenesis, treatment, and prevention. *Med Clin North Am* 2002; **86**: 477–99.

Roman GC, Tatemichi TK, Erkinjuntti T, *et al.* Vascular dementia: diagnostic criteria for research studies. Report of the NINDS-AIREN International Workshop. *Neurology* 1993; **43**: 250–60.

Roman GC, Erkinjuntti T, Wallin A, Pantoni L, Chui HC. Subcortical ischaemic vascular dementia. *Lancet Neurol* 2002; **1**: 426–36.

Richards A, van den Maagdenberg AM, Jen JC, *et al.* C-terminal truncations in human 3′-5′ DNA exonuclease TREX1 cause autosomal dominant retinal vasculopathy with cerebral leukodystrophy. *Nat Genet* 2007; **39**: 1068–70.

Rosen WG, Terry RD, Fuld PA, Katzman R, Peck A. Pathological verification of ischemic score in differentiation of dementias. *Ann Neurol* 1980; **7**: 486–8.

Rossi R, Joachim C, *et al.* Association between subcortical vascular disease on CT and neuropathological findings. *Int J Geriatr Psychiatry* 2004; **19**: 690–5.

Ruchoux MM, Guerouaou D, Vandenhaute B, Pruvo JP, Vermersch P, Leys D. Systemic vascular smooth muscle cell impairment in cerebral autosomal dominant arteriopathy with subcortical infarcts and leukoencephalopathy. *Acta Neuropathol (Berl)* 1995; **89**: 500–12.

Ruchoux MM, Maurage CA. CADASIL: cerebral autosomal dominant arteriopathy with subcortical infarcts and leukoencephalopathy. *J Neuropathol Exp Neurol* 1997; **56**: 947–64.

Sachdev PS, Brodaty H, Valenzuela MJ, *et al.* The neuropsychological profile of vascular cognitive impairment in stroke and TIA patients. *Neurology* 2004; **62**: 912–9.

Sarazin M, Amarenco P, Mikol J, Dimitri D, Lot G, Bousser MG. Reversible leukoencephalopathy in cerebral amyloid angiopathy presenting as subacute dementia. *Eur J Neurol* 2002; **9**: 353–8.

Singhal S, Bevan S, Barrick T, Rich P, Markus HS. The influence of genetic and cardiovascular risk factors on the CADASIL phenotype. *Brain* 2004; **127**: 2031–8.

Snowdon DA, Greiner LH, Mortimer JA, Riley KP, Greiner PA, Markesbery WR. Brain infarction and the clinical expression of Alzheimer disease. The Nun Study. *JAMA* 1997; **277**: 813–17.

Sourander P, Wallnder J. Hereditary multi-infarct dementia. Morphological and clinical studies of a new disease. *Acta Neuropathol (Berl)* 1977; **39**: 247–54.

Suter O-C, Sunthorn T, Kraftsik R, *et al.* Cerebral hypoperfusion generates cortical watershed microinfarcts in Alzheimer disease. *Stroke* 2002; **33**: 1986–92.

Terwindt GM, Haan J, Ophoff RA, *et al.* Clinical and genetic analysis of a large Dutch family with autosomal dominant vascular retinopathy, migraine and Raynaud's phenomenon. *Brain* 1998; **121** (Pt 2): 303–16.

Traykov L, Baudic S, Thibaudet M-C, Rigaud A-S, Smagghe A, Boller F. Neuropsychological deficit in early subcortical vascular dementia: comparison to Alzheimer's disease. *Dementia Geriatr Cogn Disord* 2002; **14**: 26–32.

Vahedi K, Massin P, Guichard JP, *et al.* Hereditary infantile hemiparesis, retinal arteriolar tortuosity, and leukoencephalopathy. *Neurology* 2003; **60**: 57–63.

van den Boom R, Lesnick Oberstein SA, van den Berg-Huysmans AA, Ferrari MD, van Buchem MA, Haan J.

Cerebral autosomal dominant arteriopathy with sub-cortical infarcts and leukoencephalopathy: structural MR imaging changes and apolipoprotein E genotype. *Am J Neuroradiol* 2006; **27**: 359–62.

Verreault S, Joutel A, Riant F, *et al.* A novel hereditary small vessel disease of the brain. *Ann Neurol* 2006; **59**: 353–7.

Vinters HV. Cerebral amyloid angiopathy. *A critical review.* Stroke 1987; **18**: 311–24.

Vinters HV, Ellis WG, Zarow C, *et al.* Neuropathologic substrates of ischemic vascular dementia. *J Neuropathol Exp Neurol* 2000; **59**: 931–45.

Vonsattel JP, Myers RH, Hedley-Whyte ET, Ropper AH, Bird ED, Richardson EP, Jr. Cerebral amyloid angiopathy without and with cerebral hemorrhages: a comparative histological study. *Ann Neurol* 1991; **30**: 637–49.

Wallin A, Blennow K. The clinical diagnosis of vascular dementia. *Dementia* 1994; **5**: 181–4.

White L, Petrovitch H, Hardman J, *et al.* Cerebrovascular pathology and dementia in autopsied Honolulu–Asia Aging Study participants. *Ann NY Acad Sci* 2002; **977**: 9–23.

10

White matter changes

Franz Fazekas, Christian Enzinger, Stefan Ropele and Reinhold Schmidt

Introduction

For a long time, views regarding the role of white matter changes (WMC) in relation to the development of vascular cognitive impairment (VCI) have been quite controversial. One could even say that fervent believers in a significant impact of WMC on cerebral functioning opposed harsh sceptics of such a concept.

The believers have built their reasoning along the lines of Binswanger's disease, or subcortical arteriosclerotic encephalopathy (SAE) (Binswanger, 1894; Pantoni and Garcia, 1995). They assumed that ill-defined, patchy or diffuse areas of hypodensity without cortical involvement on CT were clear evidence for diffuse ischemic brain damage and representative for SAE. Support for this assumption came from histopathologic data, which indicated rarefaction of myelin as a morphologic substrate of such CT findings – an observation which led to the introduction of the descriptive term *leukoaraiosis* (Hachinski *et al.*, 1987). Earlier studies had linked SAE with cognitive impairment, gait disorders, and urinary disturbances, and hence it appeared quite obvious that leukoaraiosis should be associated with these clinical symptoms in a similar way (Steingart *et al.*, 1987). Consequently, more severe WMC were readily included in a set of criteria for vascular dementia (VaD) despite the absence of solid data which would have supported

a certain threshold beyond which WMC could be confidently expected to exert cognitive impairment (Chui *et al.*, 1992; Roman *et al.*, 1993).

The sceptics were overwhelmed by the enormously high prevalence of WMC, even in the normal elderly population, which was noted with the advent of magnetic resonance imaging (MRI) (Brust, 1988). At least half of individuals around the age of 50 years show some spots of signal abnormality of the white matter. These have descriptively been termed as "white matter hyperintensities" (WMH) as they appear hyperintense on T_2-weighted images. With advancing age, these numbers further increase and reach a proportion of up to 90% in octogenarians (Schmidt *et al.*, 1988). As a consequence, it was felt that such a high proportion of focal signal changes could not be consistent with a "true" and clinically relevant pathologic process. Support for such an attitude came with increasing appreciation of the limited specificity of conventional MRI regarding the etiology of underlying tissue changes. Many pathologies ranging from edema over demyelination to infarction and even neoplastic processes may all appear hyperintense on T_2-weighted MRI. So it was reasoned that WMC observed with aging were a rather unspecific phenomenon not truly suggestive of vascular damage, and therefore unlikely to be associated with clinical consequences.

Vascular Cognitive Impairment in Clinical Practice, ed. Lars-Olof Wahlund, Timo Erkinjuntti and Serge Gauthier. Published by Cambridge University Press. © Cambridge University Press 2009.

The last two decades have witnessed increasing research efforts into age-related WMC and their possible association with clinical deficits. In addition to cross-sectional investigations on representative numbers of individuals, more and more information has come from longitudinal studies. Furthermore, novel analysis and imaging techniques have enabled us to obtain an ever-more sensitive and specific view of the range of WMC and the correlation with other morphologic abnormalities. As a consequence, it appears timely to try to mitigate and reconcile the arguments of both believers and sceptics regarding the potential impact of WMC on cognitive functioning,

Etiology and progression of age-related WMC

Several reviews including a book chapter in this series have already summarized the abundant evidence of a predominantly vascular etiology of WMC in the elderly (Fazekas and Englund, 2002; Fazekas et al., 1998a; Pantoni and Garcia, 1995). Such evidence includes histopathologic data which confirm increasing rarefaction of myelin in association with small-vessel disease (SVD) as a predominant pathologic substrate of more widespread areas of hypodensity on CT or hyperintensity on MRI. More recently, probabilistic lesion mapping has confirmed a quite consistent preponderance of WMC in the watershed regions of the brain (Enzinger et al., 2006). Clear associations of the severity of WMC not only with increasing age, but to a variable extent also with cerebrovascular risk factors (Jeerakathil et al., 2004) and with cerebrovascular disorders like stroke and intracerebral hemorrhage have been documented repeatedly. Furthermore, WMC are commonly associated with other signs of SVD, such as lacunes and past microbleeds (Van Dijk et al., 2002; Wardlaw et al., 2006) (Figure 10.1). The latter are focal deposits of iron resulting from the extravasation of minimal amounts of blood through leaking blood vessels

and underline the potentially complex consequences of SVD (Fazekas et al., 1999). From all these data, it can be assumed quite confidently that the majority of WMC are a consequence of vascular disturbances in a broader sense – which means that they need not result from true ischemia but may also be caused by other pathomechanisms in association with diseased blood vessels (Fazekas et al., 1998b).

Research over the past few years has also provided increasing evidence regarding the rate of progression of WMC. Careful long-term follow-up studies of up to almost 2000 individuals have shown a quite pronounced accumulation of WMC in some individuals. This fact has been substantiated both by visual rating as well as by quantitative measurements (Longstreth et al., 2005; Schmidt et al., 2003; Ten Dam et al., 2005; Whitman et al., 2001). Unfortunately, difficulties in the comparison of measurement methods employed as well as between populations investigated still prohibit indication of a "normal range" of WMC progression with aging, as summarized in a recent review (Table 10.1) (Enzinger et al., 2007). Lesion progression has been related primarily to age and baseline lesion load, while cerebrovascular risk factors per se appear to play a minor role, at least over the relatively short times of follow-up. In the absence of other plausible causative factors, this argues for an important role of our genetic disposition towards the development of WMC. All sceptics who bring into account that MRI might possibly overestimate WMC progression due to its high sensitivity should consider that a rather rapid development of WMC can also be seen with CT in some elderly individuals. Analyzing the follow-up CT scans of those 596 participants in the North American Symptomatic Carotid Endarterectomy Trial who were without leukoaraiosis at baseline, 18% had developed at least some extent of WMC after a mean follow-up of 6.1 years, while 3% showed widespread leukoaraiosis (Streifler et al., 2003). Also interesting in the context of dementia, WMC progression itself does not appear to be favored by specific degenerative processes of the brain. An investigation of several smaller groups of different types of dementia,

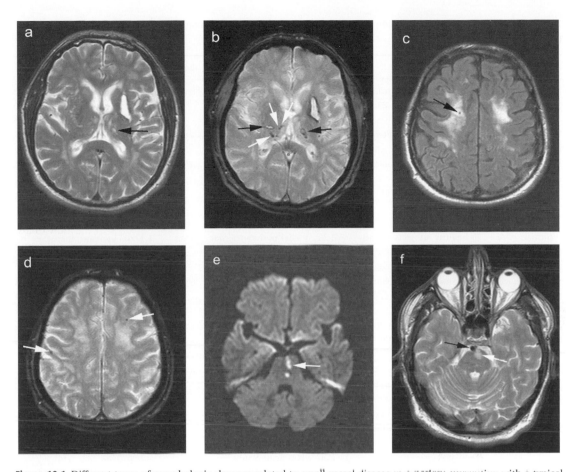

Figure 10.1 Different types of morphologic damage related to small vessel disease in a patient presenting with a typical lacunar stroke, i.e with acute onset of a dysarthria/clumsy hand syndrome. (a) Besides a defect from infarction in the left putamen T2-weighted MRI shows multiple lacunar lesions and a cribriform state in the thalami and basal ganglia bilaterally. Confluent WMH is noted adjacent to the posterior horns. (b) Gradient-echo T2*-weighted MRI shows a rim of hemosiderin around the infarct and lacunes (black arrows) as well as several additional focal areas of hemosiderin deposition consistent with past microbleeds (white arrows). (c) The FLAIR image shows confluent WMH to extend up to the centrum semiovale and a small lacune (arrow). Strictly subcortical white matter tracts are spared from the signal changes. (d) Corresponding gradient-echo T2*-weighted MRI shows additional cortico-subcortical remnants of microbleeds. (e) Diffusion-weighted MRI shows an acute pontine infarct from occlusion of a long perforating artery. (f) T2-weighted MRI shows corresponding signal changes within the pons and an ectatic basilar artery which indicates vascular damage at all levels.

including Alzheimer's disease, dementia with Lewy bodies and Parkinson disease dementia, failed to show differences in the rate of WMC progression both between dementia subtypes and in comparison to controls (Burton *et al.*, 2006). Beyond lesion volume, however, spatial differences in the distribution of WMC may be a further modifying aspect which needs to be considered in the complex interaction of WMC with cognitive functioning (Yoshita *et al.*, 2006).

Table 10.1 Studies on the progression of cerebral white matter lesions in non-demented elderly subjects (from Ten Dam *et al.* 2005).

Author	Cohort	Method	Length	Results
Wahlund *et al.* (1996)	13 healthy subjects (mean age 79 yrs, range 75–85)	0.02T and 0.5T; semi-quantitative rating scale (Scheltens Scale)	5 yrs	12/13 increase (mean value at baseline: 2.3, at follow-up: 6.9)
Veldink *et al.* (1995)	14 normal and cognitively impaired subjects	0.6T; semi-quantitative rating scale (Scheltens Scale)	2 yrs	8/14 increase
Schmidt *et al.* (1999)	273 community-dwelling subjects (mean age 60±6 yrs, range 50–75)	1.5T; 3 independent raters, progression: minor (+1–4 punctate); marked (>4 punctate or transition to early confluent or confluent)	3 yrs	17.9% any and 8.1% marked progression
Whitman *et al.* (2001)	70 healthy subjects (mean age 79 yrs, range 74–88)	1.5T; 3 axial periventricular slices point grid volume estimate	4 yrs	1.1 cm^3 increase; increase greater in subjects with marked WML at baseline
Schmidt *et al.* (2003)	296 community-dwelling subjects (range 50–75)	1.5T; semiautomatic measurement of lesion volume	6 yrs	Increase dependent on scored lesion severity at baseline
Taylor *et al.* (2003)	117 community-dwelling subjects (mean age 69±7 yrs)	1.5T; semiautomatic measurement of lesion volume	2 yrs	27% volume increase (1.4 cm^3); greater increase in subjects with greater initial lesion volumes
Prins *et al.* (2004)	20 healthy subjects (mean age 72 yrs, range 61–88); randomly selected from population-based study by WMH grade	1.5T; semiautomatic measurement of lesion volume	3.3 yrs	0.28 ml yr^{-1} mean increase (periventricular: 0.42 ml yr^{-1}; subcortical: 0.15 ml yr^{-1})
Van Dijk *et al.* (2005)	636 subjects, population-based (mean age 71 yrs, range 60–90 yrs)	1.5T; subjective rating by 2 raters on scale based on Rotterdam Scan Study	3.3 yrs	periventricular: 27% WML progression (9% marked); subcortical: 32% WML progression (10% marked)
Longstreth *et al.* (2005)	1919 community-dwelling subjects (age 65 yrs)	1.5T; subjective rating using a library of templates, change score	5 yrs	28% any progression (85% by 1 grade)
Ten Dam *et al.* (2005)	535 subjects with a history of or increased risk for vascular disease (mean age 75±3 yrs, range 70–82)	1.5T; semiautomatic measurement of lesion load	2.8 yrs	0.9 cm^3 increase in placebo and 1.0 cm^3 in pravastatin treated group
Garde *et al.* (2005)	26 non-demented octogenarians	1.5T; semiautomatic measurement of lesion volume	3.8 yrs	0.63 ml yr^{-1} increase (0–6.8); correlated with decline in verbal IQ

Morphologic correlates of WMC

Signal hyperintensity on MRI or hypodensity on CT both do not adequately allow insight into the actual severity of tissue damage. This is an important drawback, as it appears quite obvious that functional consequences will depend not only on the volume of the brain that is affected by vascular damage, but also on the grade of structural abnormalities which are caused by such a process. In order to provide such information, quantitative MRI techniques have been increasingly used for defining tissue composition and integrity. As shown in CADASIL (cerebral autosomal dominant arteriopathy with subcortical infarcts and leukoencephalopathy), measurements of mean diffusivity and fractional anisotropy by diffusion tensor imaging (DTI) hold great promise to show a better correlation between grades of tissue destruction and clinical consequences such as cognitive impairment than conventional MRI (Chabriat *et al.*, 1999). In a simplified manner, increases in mean diffusivity, i.e. a higher mobility of water protons, may be taken as evidence for a decrease in the structural organization of the brain. Fractional anisotropy, in turn, is an indicator for the directionality of the movement of water protons along intact fiber tracts. Therefore, disorganization of the brain or a destruction of pathways will be recognized by a drop in fractional anisotropy, and there is increasing evidence that such measures will add functionally relevant information (Moller *et al.*, 2007).

Our group has used magnetization transfer imaging (MTI) to probe changes in tissue composition with ageing of the brain. It is assumed that the magnetization transfer ratio (MTR) is proportional to the amount of bound protons that mainly reside in myelin (Filippi, 2003). Consequently, MTR is highest in areas with abundant white matter tracts such as the corpus callosum. Focal age-related WMC were shown to have a lower MTR than normal white matter, but this reduction was only around 10%. This attests to relatively little tissue damage associated with WMC in a normal elderly population as investigated in the setting of the Austrian Stroke Prevention Study (ASPS). For comparison, more pronounced reductions of the MTR of 20% or more have been observed in lesions of multiple sclerosis (Fazekas *et al.*, 2002; Gass *et al.*, 1994). We also did not see effects on the MTR of normal appearing white matter (NAWM) in relation to WMC, except for a relationship between the NAWM of the frontal lobes with WMC volume.

Interestingly, MTR values of this region were also associated with measures of fine motor dexterity. This led us to speculate on a possible distant effect of WMC regarding especially the frontal areas and their functionality (Fazekas *et al.*, 2005). A different situation may exist in individuals with more pronounced WMC. Investigating participants of the "Leukoaraiosis and Disability" (LADIS) study, we observed MTR changes of the entire NAWM which were related to the severity of WMC (Ropele *et al.*, 2007). This argues for gradual differences in the impact of WMC depending both on their extent and the entire clinical situation (Prins *et al.*, 2005).

WMC and cognition

Several cross-sectional studies have provided evidence for some impact of WMC on neuropsychologic functioning, although the effects were often less striking and consistent than expected. Consistent with prevailing subcortical damage, deficits were seen primarily in the speed of motor and cognitive processing and regarding executive function (Roman *et al.*, 2002). In these investigations, an impact on cognitive performance was better demonstrable in non-demented individuals, although extensive WMC were also judged to make a (small) contribution to the cognitive impairment in Alzheimer's disease. While such cross-sectional data lack a clear relation in time, more recent longitudinal observations support such an association. In an analysis of the Cardiovascular Health Study, a subcohort of 1919 elderly participants underwent MRI scans separated by 5 years and 28% of these participants showed worsening WMC. These individuals also experienced a greater decline on the modified Mini-Mental State Examination and the Digit Single Substitution Test when compared to participants who showed no progression of WMC (Longstreth *et al.*, 2005).

Evolution of WMC as determined by a semi-automated segmentation method was also correlated with cognitive functioning over a period of

6 years in 329 participants of the ASPS (Schmidt *et al.*, 2005). Parallel to progression of WMC, there was a significant decline in the performance on tests assessing memory, conceptualization, visual practical skills, attention, and speed. Importantly, this association between lesion load and cognitive function was no longer significant when adding change in brain volume to the model. This suggests that cognitive decline was related rather to loss of brain volume than to the progression of lesion burden. Interestingly, study participants without evidence for brain atrophy but with coalescent white matter lesions at baseline showed significantly more loss of brain parenchyma during the 6 years of follow-up than did those with minor WMC suggesting a secondary effect of WMC on brain volume. Such an association has also been reported regionally regarding an association of WMC with progression of temporal lobe atrophy (de Leeuw *et al.*, 2006).

Conclusions

Over the past few years we have accumulated quite convincing evidence for a vascular etiology of at least the majority of age-related WMC. There is also an indication for an association between the severity of WMC and neuropsychologic dysfunction of the subcortical type from both cross-sectional and longitudinal studies. However, these associations are relatively weak and may disappear when considering other types of morphologic change, such as increasing brain atrophy, simultaneously. Importantly, it must not be overlooked that WMC are only one element of brain damage related to SVD. Other types of SVD-related morphologic changes, such as lacunar infarcts especially, are certainly also of importance for the development of cognitive dysfunction (Van der Flier *et al.*, 2005). Discrepancies in findings regarding the individual and combined weight of these abnormalities are likely to come from differences in study populations and from still existing limits of the quantification of WMC (and other SVD

morphologies), which probably should include not only quantitative metrics like lesion volume but also lesion severity and location. Modern imaging and analysis techniques will help to address these issues in the future. With this armamentarium, time has come for probing the clinical effects of delaying WMC (and SVD) progression in appropriate treatment trials (Bowler and Gorelick, 2007; Schmidt *et al.*, 2004).

REFERENCES

Binswanger O. Die Abgrenzung der allgemeinen progressiven Paralyse. *Berl Klin Wochenschr* 1894; **31**: 1103–05, 1137–9, 1180–6.

Bowler J, Gorelick P. Advances in vascular cognitive impairment 2006. *Stroke* 2007; **38**: 241–4.

Brust J. Vascular dementia is overdiagnosed. *Arch Neurol* 1988; **45**: 799–801.

Burton E, McKeith I, Burn D, *et al.* Progression of white matter hyperintensities in Alzheimer disease, dementia with Lewy bodies, and Parkinson disease dementia: a comparison with normal aging. *Am J Geriatr Psychiatry* 2006; **14**: 842–9.

Chabriat H, Pappata S, Poupon C, *et al.* Clinical severity in CADASIL related to ultrastructural damage in white matter: in vivo study with diffusion tensor MRI. *Stroke* 1999; **30**: 2637–43.

Chui H, Victoroff J, Margolin D, *et al.* Criteria for the diagnosis of ischemic vascular dementia proposed by the State of California Alzheimer's Disease Diagnostic and Treatment Centers. *Neurology* 1992; **42**: 473–80.

de Leeuw F, Korf E, Barkhof F, Scheltens P. White matter lesions are associated with progression of medial temporal lobe atrophy in Alzheimer disease. *Stroke* 2006; **37**: 2248–52.

Enzinger C, Smith S, Fazekas F, *et al.* Lesion probability maps of white matter hyperintensities in elderly individuals: results of the Austrian stroke prevention study. *J Neurol* 2006; **253**: 1064–70.

Enzinger C, Fazekas F, Ropele S, Schmidt R. Progression of cerebral white matter lesions – clinical and radiological considerations. *J Neurol Sci* 2007; **257**: 5–10.

Fazekas F, Englund E. White matter lesions. In: Erkinjuntti T, Gauthier S, eds. *Vascular Cognitive Impairment*. London: Martin Dunitz, 2002; 135–43.

Fazekas F, Schmidt R, Kleinert R, *et al.* The spectrum of age-associated brain abnormalities: their measurement and histopathological correlates. *J Neural Transm* 1998a; **53** (Suppl): S31–9.

Fazekas F, Schmidt R, Scheltens P. Pathophysiologic mechanisms in the development of age-related white matter changes of the brain. *Dement Geriatr Cogn Disord* 1998b; **9**(Suppl 1): 2–5.

Fazekas F, Kleinert R, Roob G, *et al.* Histopathologic analysis of foci of signal loss in gradient-echo T2*-weighted MR images in patients with spontaneous intracerebral hemorrhage: evidence of microangiopathy-related microbleeds. *Am J Neuroradiol* 1999; **20**: 637–42.

Fazekas F, Ropele S, Enzinger C, *et al.* Quantitative magnetization transfer imaging of pre-lesional white-matter changes in multiple sclerosis. *Mult Scler* 2002; **8**: 479–84.

Fazekas F, Ropele S, Enzinger C, *et al.* MTI of white matter hyperintensities. *Brain* 2005; **128**: 2926–32.

Filippi M. Magnetization transfer MRI in multiple sclerosis and other central nervous system disorders. *Eur J Neurol* 2003; **10**: 3–10.

Garde E, Lykke Mortensen E, Rostrup E, Paulson O. Decline in intelligence is associated with progression in white matter hyperintensity volume. *J Neurol Neurosurg Psychiatry* 2005; **76**: 1289–91.

Gass A, Barker G, Kidd D, *et al.* Correlation of magnetization transfer ratio with clinical disability in multiple sclerosis. *Ann Neurol* 1994; **36**: 62–7.

Hachinski V, Potter P, Merskey H. Leuko-araiosis. *Arch Neurol* 1987; **44**: 21–3.

Jeerakathil T, Wolf P, Beiser A, *et al.* Stroke risk profile predicts white matter hyperintensity volume: the Framingham Study. *Stroke* 2004; **35**: 1857–61.

Longstreth W, Arnold A, Beauchamp N, *et al.* Incidence, manifestations, and predictors of worsening white matter on serial cranial magnetic resonance imaging in the elderly: the Cardiovascular Health Study. *Stroke* 2005; **36**: 56–61.

Moller M, Frandsen J, Andersen G, *et al.* Dynamic changes of corticospinal tracts after stroke detected by fiber tracking. *J Neurol Neurosurg Psychiatry* 2007; **78**: e-pub.

Pantoni L, Garcia J. The significance of cerebral white matter abnormalities 100 years after Binswanger's report: a review. *Stroke* 1995; **26**: 1293–301.

Prins N, van Straaten E, van Dijk E, *et al.* Measuring progression of cerebral white matter lesions on MRI: visual rating and volumetrics. *Neurology* 2004; **62**: 1533–39.

Prins N, Van Dijk E, den Heijer T, *et al.* Cerebral small-vessel disease and decline in information processing speed, executive function and memory. *Brain* 2005; **128**: 2034–41.

Roman G, Tatemichi T, Erkinjuntti T, *et al.* Vascular dementia: diagnostic criteria for research studies. Report of the NINDS-AIREN International Work Group. *Neurology* 1993; **43**: 250–60.

Roman G, Erkinjuntti T, Wallin A, *et al.* Subcortical ischaemic vascular dementia. *Lancet Neurol* 2002; **1**: 426–36.

Ropele S, Seewann A, Gouw A, *et al.* Quantitation of brain tissue changes associated with white matter hyperintensities by diffusion-weighted and magnetization transfer imaging: the LADIS (Leukoaraiosis and Disability in the Elderly) study. *J Magn Reson Imaging* 2008, in press.

Schmidt R, Fazekas F, Offenbacher H, *et al.* Prevalence and risk factors for white matter damage. In: Fazekas F, Schmidt R, Alavi A, eds. *Neuroimaging of Normal Ageing and Uncommon Causes of Dementia.* Dordrecht: ICG Publications, 1998; 11–25.

Schmidt R, Fazekas F, Kapeller P, *et al.* MRI white matter hyperintensities: three year follow-up of the Austrian Stroke Prevention Study. *Neurology*, 1999; **53**: 132–9.

Schmidt R, Enzinger C, Ropele S, *et al.* Progression of cerebral white matter lesions: 6-year results of the Austrian Stroke Prevention Study. *Lancet* 2003; **361**: 2046–8.

Schmidt R, Scheltens P, Erkinjuntti T, *et al.* White matter lesion progression: a surrogate endpoint for trials in small-vessel disease. *Neurology* 2004; **63**: 139–44.

Schmidt R, Ropele S, Enzinger C, *et al.* White matter lesion progression, brain atrophy, and cognitive decline: the Austrian Stroke Prevention Study. *Ann Neurol* 2005; **58**: 610–16.

Steingart A, Hachinski V, Lau C, *et al.* Cognitive and neurological findings in subjects with diffuse white matter lucencies on computed tomographic scan (leuko-araiosis). *Arch Neurol* 1987; **44**: 32–3.

Streifler J, Eliasziw M, Bonavente O, *et al.* Development and progression of leukoaraiosis in patients with brain ischemia and carotid artery disease. *Stroke* 2003; **34**: 1913–17.

Taylor W, MacFall J, Provenzale J, *et al.* Serial MR imaging of volumes of hyperintense white matter lesions in elderly patients: correlation with vascular risk factors. *Am J Roentgenol* 2003; **181**: 571–6.

Ten Dam V, van den Heuvel D, van Buchem M, *et al.* Effect of pravastatin on cerebral infarcts and white matter lesions. *Neurology* 2005; **64**: 1807–09.

Van der Flier W, Van Straaten E, Barkhof F, *et al.* Small vessel disease and general cognitive function in non-disabled elderly: the LADIS study. *Stroke* 2005; **36**: 2116–20.

Van Dijk E, Prins N, Vermeer S, *et al.* Frequency of white matter lesions and silent lacunar infarcts. *J Neural Transm* 2002; **25** (Suppl): 25–39.

Van Dijk E, Prins N, Vermeer S, *et al.* C-reactive protein and cerebral small-vessel disease: the Rotterdam Scan Study. *Circulation* 2005; **112**: 900–05.

Veldink J, Scheltens P, Jonker C, Launer LJ. Progression of cerebral white matter hyperintensities on MRI is related to diastolic blood pressure. *Neurology* 1998; **51**: 319–20.

Wahlund L, Almkvist O, Basun H, Julin P. MRI in successful ageing, a 5-year follow-up study from eighth to ninth decade of life. *Magn Res Imag* 1996; **14**: 601–08.

Wardlaw J, Lewis S, Keir S, *et al.* Cerebral microbleeds are associated with lacunar stroke defined clinically and radiologically, independently of white matter lesions. *Stroke* 2006; **37**: 2633–6.

Whitman G, Tang T, Lin M, Baloh R. A prospective study of cerebral white matter abnormalities in older people with gait dysfunction. *Neurology* 2001; **57**: 990–4.

Yoshita M, Fletcher E, Harvey D, *et al.* Extent and distribution of white matter hyperintensities in normal aging, MCI, and AD. *Neurology* 2006; **67**: 2192–8.

11

Hereditary forms of cerebrovascular amyloidosis

Agueda Rostagno and Jorge Ghiso

The generic term "amyloidosis" describes a wide spectrum of protein misfolding diseases characterized by the intra- and/or extracellular deposition of normally soluble proteins in the form of Congo red positive fibrillar structures in different tissues and organs. Once formed, these fibrils are resistant to proteolytic degradation and poorly antigenic, characteristics that impair their effective physiologic removal by macrophages. Accumulation of fibrils and/or of their intermediate structural assemblies leads to cell damage, organ dysfunction and, eventually, death. Twenty-six unrelated proteins and more than 100 genetic variants have been so far identified as the main constituents of systemic and localized amyloid deposits in humans. In spite of this biochemical diversity, all types of amyloid share common physical, tinctorial and structural properties: (i) with few exceptions, deposited amyloid subunits are in the 4–30 kDa mass range, exhibit a wide range of post-translational modifications and typically display high heterogeneity at the amino- and/or carboxyl-terminal ends; (ii) in general, amyloid molecules are rich in β-pleated sheet secondary structure, a conformation largely responsible for their high tendency to aggregate and polymerize as well as for their tinctorial characteristics following Congo red or thioflavin S staining; and (iii) regardless of their biochemical composition, all known amyloid molecules self-assemble into poorly soluble structures

exhibiting long, unbranched, ~8 nm wide, twisted fibrillar morphology under the electron microscope (reviewed in Ghiso and Frangione (2002) and Rostagno and Ghiso (2003)).

Cerebral amyloidoses

The most frequent forms of amyloidoses are those localized to the central nervous system (CNS). Only about one-third of amyloid proteins known to be linked to disease in humans produce fibrillar deposits in the CNS which, in turn, translate into cognitive deficits, dementia, stroke, cerebellar and extrapyramidal signs, or a combination thereof. Classical lesions in the CNS are usually found in the form of (i) parenchymal pre amyloid deposits, amorphous non fibrillar structures negative under Congo red or thioflavin S staining, which are visualized by their diffuse immunoreactivity with specific antibodies, and are extractable by treatment with aqueous buffers in the presence of mild detergents; (ii) parenchymal fibrillar amyloid lesions, usually in the form of compact plaques exhibiting extensive Congo red/thioflavin S staining, which are immunoreactive with specific antibodies and poorly soluble, requiring the use of either chaotropes (e.g. 6 M guanidine–HCl) or strong acids (e.g. formic acid) to be retrieved from the lesions; and (iii) cerebral amyloid angiopathy

Vascular Cognitive Impairment in Clinical Practice, ed. Lars-Olof Wahlund, Timo Erkinjuntti and Serge Gauthier. Published by Cambridge University Press. © Cambridge University Press 2009.

(CAA), Congo red/thioflavin S-positive fibrillar deposits affecting the media and adventitia of medium and small cerebral arteries and arterioles as well as many cerebral capillaries. In general terms, stroke – either ischemic or hemorrhagic – is the most common clinical manifestation of amyloid deposition primarily restricted to cerebral vessel walls, whereas widespread distribution throughout brain parenchymal areas is concomitantly associated with dementia.

Late-onset (sporadic) Alzheimer's disease (AD) is the most common form of dementia in humans above the age of 65. In this disorder, intraneuronal neurofibrillary tangles (deposits of hyperphosphorylated protein tau in the form of paired helical filaments) co-exist with diffuse pre-amyloid lesions and parenchymal amyloid deposits in the form of neuritic plaques. The cerebrovascular dysfunction, always present in AD and often neglected as an active player in the mechanism of neurodegeneration, is now being recognized as a major contributor to the disease pathogenesis (Bailey *et al.*, 2004; de la Torre, 2004; Gorelick, 2004; Farkas and Luiten, 2001; Petty and Wettstein, 2001). Although the relationship CAA–dementia is complex and probably encompasses a range of different pathogenic mechanisms, it is clear that the presence of CAA translates in reduction of the cerebral blood flow, hypoxia, breakdown of the blood–brain barrier (BBB) , detrimental metabolic conditions and cell stress; features that, in time, contribute to the impaired cognition characteristic of the disease.

Both vascular and parenchymal amyloid lesions in AD are composed of self-aggregates of the Aβ peptide, a processing product of a larger precursor protein (APP) codified by a single gene located on chromosome 21. The 39–42 residues-long Aβ peptide is generated by proteolytic cleavage of APP by the so-called β and γ secretases (Ghiso and Frangione, 2002; Kang *et al.*, 1987; Masters *et al.*, 1985). For reasons still poorly understood, Aβ42 is the main component of the parenchymal deposits, whereas Aβ40 is the predominant constituent of vascular amyloid lesions. This structural segregation of the Aβ deposits is also typical in normal aging, in Down syndrome and in sporadic CAA, the reasons for this selectivity as well as its importance for disease pathogenesis being still unknown. Whereas cognitive impairment and vascular amyloid deposits commonly co-exist, it is puzzling that the majority of patients diagnosed with CAA-related intracerebral hemorrhage do not have pre-existing symptoms of AD. Similarly, only a minority of AD cases demonstrate hemorrhages suggestive of advanced CAA (reviewed in Zhang-Nunes *et al.* (2006)). Although the exact factors predisposing Aβ40 to deposit primarily in vessels and not in brain parenchyma remain to be determined, Aβ genetic variants with specific vasculotropic tendency provide interesting insights into the pathways leading to advanced CAA.

Early-onset (<60 years) familial forms of AD account for less than 5% of the total cases and are linked to mutations in three different genes codifying for APP, presenilin 1 (PS1), and presenilin 2 (PS2). PS1 and PS2 mutations affect the levels of Aβ production, whereas nucleotide changes in the APP molecule have a differential effect depending on the location of the mutated residue (Figure 11.1). Substitutions at residues flanking the Aβ region in close proximity with the secretases cleavage sites modulate the rate of enzymatic processing of APP (Selkoe, 1999). The Swedish double mutation (K670N/M671L) flanks the β-secretase cleavage site (Mullan *et al.*, 1992) and its presence increases the production of Aβ40 and Aβ42 (Cai *et al.*, 1993; Citron *et al.*, 1992). In contrast, the numerous mutations occurring in close proximity to the γ-secretase cleavage sites are typically associated with increased production of Aβ42 in a similar manner to the effect caused by mutations in the presenilin genes (Cai *et al.*, 1993; Suzuki *et al.*, 1994). A complete list of all reported APP genetic variants as well as the pertinent references may be found at the Alzheimer Disease & Frontotemporal Dementia Mutation Database (http://www.molgen.ua.ac.be/ADMutations/).

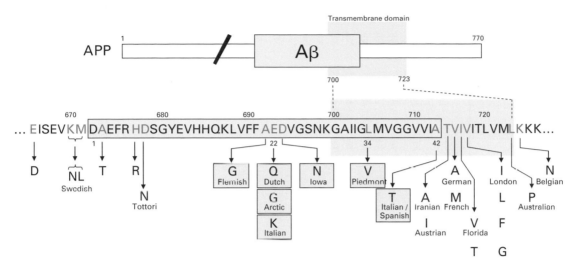

Figure 11.1 Schematic representation of the APP molecule and location of known mutations in exons 16 and 17. The APP sequence 665–728 is indicated in one-letter code. Amino acid residues highlighted in red are found in the wild-type molecule, whereas the corresponding mutation(s) for each position are indicated in black letters. Aβ genetic variants primarily associated with CAA are shown in yellow squares. Whenever available, the given name of the mutation is specified. Location of the transmembrane domain (residues 700–723) is indicated by a green box. See Figure 11.1 in the color plate section.

Aβ cerebral amyloidosis associated with CAA

Mutations located within the Aβ sequence are, with few exceptions (Wakutani *et al.*, 2004), associated with vascular compromise (Figure 11.1). In particular, genetic variants at residues 21–23 and, as more recently described at positions 34 and 42, produce Aβ variants that preferentially associate with CAA, hemorrhagic strokes and dementia (Grabowski *et al.*, 2001; Hendriks *et al.*, 1992; Levy *et al.*, 1990a; Miravalle *et al.*, 2000; Rossi *et al.*, 2004). These mutations, their clinical phenotypes as well as their associated neuropathological abnormalities, whenever available, are described below and listed in Table 11.1.

Flemish mutation

The Flemish mutation is a C to G transversion at codon 692 of APP resulting in a Gly for Ala substitution at position 21 of Aβ and leading to a form of

AD with prominent amyloid angiopathy. The presence of the mutation which correlates with early onset of the disease and death occurring at a mean age of 53 has been reported in 2 kindreds, a 4-generation Dutch family with 17 affected members (Hendriks *et al.*, 1992), and a British family with 5 affected individuals (Brooks *et al.*, 2004). Whereas some of the cases presented with lobar intracerebral hemorrhage, other members in both pedigrees developed pre-senile dementia. Neuropathologically, affected brains demonstrate diffuse cortical atrophy and an abundance of vascular and parenchymal Aβ deposits, primarily ending at position 40, together with neurofibrillary tangles. Vascular amyloid, present in cortical and leptomeningeal vessel walls, accumulate in the basement membrane of small vessels and capillaries. Although diffuse plaques are present, there is a predominance of mature plaques, typically surrounded by tau-reactive dystrophic neurites and which exhibit atypically large cores that may

Table 11.1 Familial Aβ and non-Aβ cerebrovascular amyloidoses.

	Protein	Nucleotide change/codon	Amyloid mutation	Chromosome	Onset (years)	Dementia	CAA	Clinical phenotype			
								Plaques	NFTs	Stroke / hemorrhage	Systemic deposits
Aβ cerebrovascular amyloidoses	APP	C > G 692	AβA21G	21	35–60	Yes	Massive	Perivascular	Yes	Yes	NR
	APP	G > C 693	AβE22Q	21	30s–40s	Yes	Massive	Diffuse	No	Yes	NR
	APP	G > A 693	AβE22K	21	50s–60s	Mild	Massive	Diffuse	No	Yes	NR
	APP	A > G 693	AβE22G	21	55–60	Yes	Scarce	Compact	Yes	No	NR
	APP	G > A 694	AβD23N	21	50s–60s	Rare	Massive	Diffuse	Yes	Yes	NR
	APP	C > G 705	AβL34V	21	50s–70s	Yes	Massive	No	No	Yes	NR
	APP	G > A 713	AβA42T	21	58–68	Yes	Massive	Yes	Yes	Yes	NR
Non-Aβ cerebrovascular amyloidoses	Cystatin C	T > A 68	ACysL68Q	20	30s–40s	Late onset	Massive	No	No	Yes	Yes
	Gelsolin	G > A 187	AGelD187N	9	30s–40s	Mild	Extensive	No	No	No	Yes
	Gelsolin	G > T 187	AGelD187Y	9	40s	Mild	Extensive	No	No	No	Yes
	TTR	G > A 18	ATTRD18G	18	35–50	Yes	Extensive	No	No	NR	Yes
	TTR	G > T 30	ATTRV30G	18	45–55	Yes	Extensive	No	No	NR	Yes
	TTR	T > C 30	ATTRV30M	18	28	No	Massive	No	No	Yes	Yes
	PrP	T > G 145	PrPY145Stop	20	38	Yes	Extensive	Perivascular	Yes	No	Yes
	Bri2	T > A 266	ABri	13	30s–40s	Severe	Massive	Perivascular & diffuse	Yes	Rare	Yes
	Bri2	TTTAATTTGT 265	ADan	13	20s	Severe	Massive	Perivascular & diffuse	Yes	Rare	Yes

N.R. = not reported

account for up to 48% of the entire plaque size (Cras *et al.*, 1998). Remarkably, these plaques are mostly of perivascular or vasocentric nature, appearing to radiate from the affected vessel, a feature which suggests that the AD pathology might be a secondary consequence to CAA (Brooks *et al.*, 2004; Kumar-Singh *et al.*, 2002).

In contrast to other mutations occurring within the Aβ sequence, the Flemish variant peptides display increased in vitro solubility and a decreased rate of protofibrillar structure formation in comparison with the wild-type counterparts (Walsh *et al.*, 1997). Although Flemish homologs exhibit a time-dependent increase in thioflavin-T binding correlating with the formation of β-sheet-containing assemblies, there is an overall poor fibrillization tendency (van Nostrand *et al.*, 2001). Moreover, once formed, fibrils exhibit morphological differences with the wild-type structures. Electron-microscopic studies revealed variations in the diameter of the filaments, the extent and density of the lateral filament associations as well as the helicity of the fibrils with respect to wild-type fibrils. These structural differences have been claimed to potentially alter the thermodynamic stability of the fibrils, and their ability to be metabolized or degraded, features that could explain the aggressiveness of the disease in spite of the higher solubility of the synthetic homologues (Walsh *et al.*, 2001).

Dutch mutation

The first mutation described in the APP gene, and undoubtedly the most studied, was found in a condition known as hereditary cerebral hemorrhage with amyloidosis – Dutch type (HCHWA-Dutch), an autosomal dominant disorder clinically defined by recurrent strokes, vascular dementia, and fatal cerebral bleeding in the fifth to sixth decades of life. The first stroke episode is fatal in about one-third of the patients, and survivors typically develop a succession of recurrent strokes that lead to severe disability (Bornebroek *et al.*, 1999). Dementia is the second most common symptom of HCHWA-D.

Cognitive deterioration generally manifests after the first stroke, but in some cases it is the first symptom of the disease and may develop even before the appearance of focal lesions on brain imaging. Histologically, the disease is characterized by a massive amyloid deposition in the walls of leptomeningeal and cortical arteries and arterioles, as well as in vessels in the brainstem and cerebellum, a phenotype recapitulated in transgenic mice carrying the mutation although at old age (Herzig *et al.*, 2004). In addition to the vascular involvement, a moderate number of parenchymal amyloid deposits resembling the diffuse pre-amyloid plaques seen in AD are also observed in Dutch familial cases, while dense-core plaques and neurofibrillary tangles are limited or even completely absent. The non-fibrillar diffuse plaques, variably associated with reactive astrocytes and activated microglia (Maat-Schieman *et al.*, 2004), seem to evolve into more fibrillar, dense lesions which are more abundant in older patients. Nevertheless, the degree of dementia appears to be independent of plaque involvement and neurofibrillary degeneration, and correlates contrastingly with the severity of CAA (Natte *et al.*, 2001).

The amyloid subunit in HCHWA-D is homologous to Aβ, bearing a single amino acid substitution (Gln for Glu) at position 22 as a result of a single nucleotide change (G to C) at codon 693 of APP. The mutation confers the molecule a higher tendency to adopt a β-sheet structure and form oligomeric and fibrillar assemblies in comparison to the wild-type Aβ peptide (Miravalle *et al.*, 2000). These conformational properties correlate, in turn, with the enhanced activity of Dutch-Aβ to induce in vitro deleterious effects on vessel wall cells, which may correlate with the early onset phenotype of the disease (Davis *et al.*, 1999; Melchor and van Nostrand, 2000; Miravalle *et al.*, 2000).

Italian mutation

A G to A substitution at codon 693 resulting in a Lys for Glu amino acid change at position 22, the same site of the Dutch mutation, was found in three apparently unrelated Italian families (Miravalle *et al.*, 2000). This genetic variant, although much less studied than the Dutch, is also linked to familial CAA with cerebral hemorrhage. The disease, associated with early onset and death between the ages of 65 and 75, is clinically characterized by a 10–20-year progression of recurrent strokes and mild cognitive decline. The neuropathological findings also appear to resemble those in the Dutch kindred, with extensive Aβ deposits in the walls of leptomeningeal and cortical vessels. The parenchymal compromise is limited to diffuse thioflavin S-negative deposits with the absence of mature plaques and neurofibrillary tangles. Immunochemical studies with C-terminal specific antibodies indicate that, as is most common in CAA pathology including that associated with the Dutch variant (Maat-Schieman *et al.*, 2000), Aβ40 species predominate in the vascular deposits and Aβ42 in the parenchyma.

The Italian variant exhibits in vitro a predominantly unordered secondary structure and a low fibrillization tendency, resulting in the formation of atypical fibrils – short and straight, without the distinctive twisted pattern characteristic of most amyloid molecules – and at an even lower rate than the Aβ40 wild-type counterpart (Miravalle *et al.*, 2000). These conformational properties correlate well with the predominantly thioflavin S-negative fluorescence of the parenchymal and vascular deposits observed in the Italian kindred, as well as with the lack of toxicity for vessel wall cells exhibited by synthetic homologues of the genetic variant. The lower capacity of Italian-Aβ to induce apoptosis in cerebrovascular endothelial cells in comparison to the Dutch variant may, in turn, reflect the later onset of the disease in contrast with the early-onset of the Dutch familial cases.

Arctic mutation

A form of AD affecting a family of northern Sweden and spanning four generations is characterized by a different genetic substitution: A to G also at codon 693, known as the Arctic mutation, and which results in the substitution of Gly for Glu at position 22 of Aβ. The phenotypic manifestation of the disease is memory impairment at early onset – mean age 57 years – with progressive cognitive decline rather than stroke (Nilsberth *et al.*, 2001). The clinical history is typical of AD but without the severe amyloid angiopathy that characterizes the other mutations within the Aβ sequence. The disease shows a slow, insidious progression and a decline in short-term memory as the first presenting symptoms, with no signs of strokes or significant vascular involvement found in the cases that were subjected to neuroimaging studies. The parenchymal compromise is recapitulated in transgenic mice carrying the Arctic mutation, which show an aggressive formation of plaque deposits in association with dystrophic neurites and in the absence of vascular involvement (Cheng *et al.*, 2004). One possibly related Swedish patient with the same mutation demonstrated moderate to severe CAA in cortical and leptomeningeal vessels as well as senile plaques and neurofibrillary tangles (Kamino *et al.*, 1992).

In vitro, the Arctic mutation induces a dramatic increase in the rate and capacity to form protofibrils in comparison to the wild-type counterpart (Nilsberth *et al.*, 2001), significantly enhancing the peptide insolubility, a phenomenon likely correlating with the accelerated disease initiation and progression observed in vivo. Notably, carriers of the Arctic mutation show lower levels of both Aβ42 and Aβ40 than healthy family members, a feature observed even in very young mutation carriers – 20–30 years before the expected onset of the disease – suggesting a long period of biochemical abnormality before the clinical onset. The decreased levels of Aβ peptides observed in the Arctic cases were also reproduced in transfected cell lines and have been claimed to reflect an altered APP processing induced by the mutation (Stenh *et al.*, 2002).

Iowa mutation

The Iowa genetic variant shows, among all mutations located within the Aβ sequence, the closest biological relationship to the Dutch mutant, perhaps reflecting the similar characteristics of the amino acid substitution. The Iowa mutation is a G to A substitution at codon 694 of APP, resulting in the change of Asp for Asn at residue 23 of Aβ, a loss of a negatively charged residue as in the Dutch substitution, occurring at the immediate location of the molecule. The genetic variant was identified in an Iowa family of German descent (Grabowski *et al.*, 2001; Zhang-Nunes *et al.*, 2006). Patients of the Iowa kindred develop progressive, early onset AD-like memory impairment and personality changes with cerebral atrophy, leukoencephalopathy, and occipital lesions neuropathologically identified as calcified, amyloid-laden meningeal vessels. Although small hemorrhages could be identified by MRI and post-mortem examination, there were no reported episodes of clinically manifest intracerebral hemorrhage. Of note, a second family from Spain carrying the identical mutation presents cerebral hemorrhage in the majority of the cases, suggesting that the mutation may or not produce major hemorrhagic episodes under different settings (Greenberg *et al.*, 2003; Iglesias *et al.*, 2000). The neuropathological features of the Iowa variant consist of a predominant vascular compromise co-existing with scattered pre-amyloid deposits, abundant neurofibrillary tangles and dystrophic neurites in the presence of remarkably few mature plaques (Grabowski *et al.*, 2001). A wide range of CAA-associated changes have been described in the Iowa cases, including luminal narrowing, wall thickening, and occluded small vessels, together with loss of smooth muscle cells, microbleeds, and presence of perivascular inflammatory cells (Shin *et al.*, 2002). An interesting feature of the Iowa amyloid deposits is the presence of post-translationally modified Iso-Asp residues, not only at the position of the mutation, residue 23, but also in the Asp residue at position 7. Puzzlingly, the former modification appears to be specific for vascular deposits, while Iso-Asp 7 is a component of both parenchymal and vascular lesions (Shin *et al.*, 2003).

Synthetic homologs bearing the Iowa mutation, in similar manner to the Dutch variant and in contrast to the Flemish, rapidly assemble in solution to form fibrils consistent with their high content in β-sheet secondary structure indicated by circular dichroism (van Nostrand *et al.*, 2001). This conformational tendency for fibrillization appears to confer, in turn, enhanced toxicity for smooth muscle cells in vitro with a concomitant decrease in the cells α-actin expression (Davis *et al.*, 1999; Miravalle *et al.*, 2000).

Piedmont mutation

The most recently identified mutation associated with CAA and recurrent cerebral hemorrhages is also located within the Aβ sequence, but apart from the 21–23 cluster. The C to G transversion at codon 705 leads to a replacement of Leu at position 34 by a Val residue (Obici *et al.*, 2005). The mutation occurs in a three-generation family from the Piedmont region in Italy and presents with early onset, usually ranging between 50 and 72 years of age. The clinical features of the disease include recurrent hemorrhagic strokes, weakness and parasthesias together with confusional states. Cognitive impairment is infrequent as a presenting symptom, but is observed after various episodes of intracerebral hemorrhages.

Neuropathological examination of the few available cases showed severe CAA with compromise of small and medium-sized arteries as well as capillaries in all lobes of the brain, particularly the occipital and cerebellar regions. The vascular involvement includes vessel-within-the-vessel configurations, microhemorrhages, microaneurysms, microthrombi, and lymphocytic infiltration of the vessel walls. Diffuse and dense-cored plaques as well as neurofibrillary pathology were notably absent (reviewed in Zhang-Nunes *et al.*, 2006).

At the present time and due to the recent discovery of the mutation, no in vitro data are available characterizing the biophysical or biological properties of the Piedmont variant peptides.

New Italian/Spanish mutation

A mutation at codon 713 of APP (G to A transition) resulting in an Ala for Thr substitution at position 42 of the Aβ molecule was recently described in an Italian family of 54 members spanning four generations (Rossi *et al.*, 2004). Notably, this mutation had been previously described in a single individual from France (Carter *et al.*, 1992), but no clear-cut relation with the disease pathogenesis could be demonstrated at that time. The mutation, of unknown penetrance since most healthy carriers are below the age of onset, is unique in view of the fact that, although located within the Aβ sequence, it is also adjacent to the γ-secretase cleavage site. The affected kindred present an autosomal dominant form of dementia with clinical symptoms of AD, severe CAA, and multiple infarcts. Clinical manifestations include early age of onset – between 52 and 68 years – progressive cognitive decline, and stroke-like episodes including monoparesis and language disturbances. Neuropathologic examination revealed the presence of the hallmark lesions of AD, senile plaques, CAA, neurofibrillary tangles and neuropil threads. CAA was particularly severe with the presence of 8–10 nm fibrils within and around the vessel walls. Leptomeningeal arteries and small parenchymal vessels in the cerebral hemisphere and cerebellum were severely affected by amyloid deposition. The normal architecture of the compromised vessels was disrupted by amyloid deposition presenting thickening and double barreling of the walls, loss of smooth muscle cells, and narrowing of the lumina.

Presenilin mutations

PS mutations correlate, as described above, with the presence of familial forms of AD. The majority of the PS genetic variants induce accelerated Aβ production and early onset of the disease. Of the many PS1 and PS2 mutations described, only a few correlate with the presence of CAA. Specifically, mutations located after codon 200 appear to result in a particularly severe vascular compromise. In cases with Δ9 and ΔI83/ΔM84 mutations of the *PS1* gene, the clinical phenotype includes spastic paraparesis and cotton wool plaques together with extensive and severe CAA (Steiner *et al.*, 2001). The predominance of cotton wool plaques is not, however, unique to these mutations, as they have also been described in association with a number of other *PS1* genetic variants. CAA was also identified as a prominent feature in a Volga–German family characterized by the change of Asn for Ile at position 141 in the PS2 gene. The mutation was also associated with cerebral hemorrhage in at least one case in the family (Nochlin *et al.*, 1998).

Non-Aβ cerebral amyloidosis associated with CAA

Disorders correlating with Aβ deposition, as described above, constitute undoubtedly the most frequent forms of cerebral amyloidosis. However, a variety of other non-Aβ subunits have also been identified, composing brain amyloid deposits in disorders presenting with predominant cerebrovascular compromise (Table 11.1). In many of them, the vascular involvement is overwhelming, although, notably, some entities correlate with cerebral hemorrhagic episodes, while in others the predominant clinical phenotype is cognitive impairment without any signs of stroke or hemorrhage, even in the presence of comparable vascular amyloid load.

Cystatin C-related cerebral amyloidosis

Hereditary cerebral hemorrhage with amyloidosis, Icelandic-type (HCHWA-Icelandic), is an autosomal dominant disorder described in individuals from small rural communities of Western Iceland (Gudmundsson *et al.*, 1972). The disease is associated with a T to A point mutation (Levy *et al.*, 1989), translating into a Leu for Gln change at position 68 of cystatin C, a ubiquitously expressed inhibitor of cysteine proteases codified by a single gene on chromosome 20. The 110-residue-long amyloid subunit constituting the amyloid deposits in HCHWA-Icelandic not only bears the mutated amino acid residue, but is also degraded at the N terminus, starting at position 11 of the normal cystatin C (Ghiso *et al.*, 1986a, 1986b). The main clinical hallmark of the disease is cerebral hemorrhage with fatal outcome in the third to fourth decade of life in approximately 50% of the cases. Strokes are rare after the age of 50, and cognitive decline followed by dementia may occur in those cases that survive the hemorrhagic episodes. Neuropathologically, the mutation is associated with massive amyloid deposition within small arteries and arterioles of leptomeninges, cerebral cortex, basal ganglia, brainstem, and cerebellum. Although brain involvement is the main clinicopathologic feature, silent amyloid deposits have also been described in peripheral tissues, such as skin, lymph nodes, spleen, salivary glands, and seminal vesicles.

The biochemical and structural properties of the variant form of cystatin C have been studied extensively. The mutated residue is located within the hydrophobic core of the protein and the amino acid substitution affects the stability of the molecule destabilizing alpha-helical structures, yielding a more unfolded molecule with higher tendency to form dimeric assemblies compared with the wild-type counterpart (reviewed in Levy *et al.*, 2006). The crystal structure of the molecule revealed that dimerization occurs through three-dimensional domain swapping (Janowski *et al.*, 2001) and, in turn, through dimer association, results in the formation of larger amyloid-like structures with involvement of intermolecular β-sheet interactions (Janowski *et al.*, 2005). The N-terminal truncation of the molecule found in vivo in the amyloid deposits of the Icelandic patients seems not to be crucial for the overall domain-swapped dimer formation; however, the absence of the N-terminal decapeptide appears to facilitate the subsequent association of the protein via β-sheet interactions through intermolecular contacts (Janowski *et al.*, 2004).

Gelsolin-related cerebral amyloidosis

Gelsolin-related amyloidosis, also known as familial amyloidosis Finnish type (FAF), is an autosomal dominant condition of systemic compromise characterized by ophthalmologic, dermatologic, and neurological symptoms with common cerebral amyloid deposition (reviewed in Revesz *et al.*, 2003). Although the majority of FAF patients have been reported in Finland with a marked geographic clustering of cases in the southeastern part of the country, the disease has world-wide distribution (Kiuru, 1998). Two different mutations at codon 187 of gelsolin, an actin-binding protein, co-segregate with the disease. The first mutation, described in Finnish, Dutch, American, and Japanese families, results from a single G to A transition at position 654, the first nucleotide of codon 187, and translates in an Asp for Asn change (Ghiso *et al.*, 1990; Haltia *et al.*, 1990a, 1990b; Levy *et al.*, 1990b). A different amino acid substitution at the same codon is present in patients of Danish and Czech origin suffering from the same disorder (Kiuru, 1998). In these cases, a transition of G to T results in the presence of a Tyr instead of the normally occurring Asp.

Clinical manifestations result from the compromise of multiple organs and include peripheral neuropathy, facial palsy, dry and itchy skin, intermittent proteinuria, and cardiac symptoms. Patients have typical faces with droopy eyelids and protruding lips. Lattice corneal dystrophy, a lace-like deposition of amyloid within the stroma, is the earliest clinical finding of the syndrome. Amyloid deposition in the spinal and cerebral blood vessel walls, meninges, spinal nerve roots and sensory ganglia are critical features of this systemic amyloidosis contributing to the CNS symptoms. Amyloid deposition in basement membranes and vessels is common to most of the organs, in addition to the CNS (Kiuru, 1998).

Biochemical analysis of the deposits revealed that the amyloid fibrils are formed by a 7-kDa internal degradation product of the gelsolin molecule. This amyloid subunit is located in a repetitive motif with actin-binding activity – highly conserved among species – and spanning from position 173 to residue 243 of the gelsolin molecule (Ghiso *et al.*, 1990).

Transthyretin-related cerebral amyloidosis

Familial transthyretin-related (TTR) amyloidosis is usually associated with peripheral neuropathy and involvement of visceral organs, with only exceptional cases presenting with CNS compromise. Three unrelated families have been reported carrying different point mutations in the chromosome 18-TTR gene and showing abundant cerebral amyloid deposition in the presence of rare hemorrhagic episodes. The Hungarian kindred, consisting of 56 members spanning 4 generations, is associated with a single A for G miss-sense mutation at codon 18, resulting in the presence of Gly instead of Asp (Garzuly et al., 1996; Vidal et al., 1996). The onset of symptoms varies between 36 and 53 years, with death occurring between the ages of 51 and 60. The major clinical symptoms include short-term memory decline, hearing loss, cerebellar dysfunction with ataxia, and bilateral pyramidal dysfunction with progressive spasticity. Most patients show temporary disorientation, and migraine-like headache with vomiting, and tremor. Neuropathological studies revealed extensive amyloid deposition in meningeal vessels as well as in subarachnoid, subpial, and subependymal cerebrospinal regions, and spinal ganglia. Although not associated with any clinical symptoms, small systemic deposits were also present in kidney, skin, ovaries, and peripheral nerves.

A different mutation, T for G at codon 30 resulting in the substitution of Val for Gly and also presenting with CNS compromise, was identified in a large Ohio family of German ancestry consisting of 59 members spanning four generations (Petersen et al., 1997). The main clinical symptoms are slowly progressive dementia, seizures, ataxia, hemiparesis, decreased vision, and mutism. The age of onset is between 46 and 56 years, with the duration of disease varying between 3 and 26 years. The histopathologic hallmark is the presence of amyloid deposits in the subependymal region, the leptomeninges, the choroid plexus, and in the wall of the subarachnoid blood vessels. Small and medium-sized vessels are the most severely affected by amyloid, even though, notably, the vascular compromise is absent once the vessels penetrate into the brain parenchyma. Although not a frequent finding, vascular amyloid has also been described affecting vessels of virtually all visceral organs, skin, and skeletal muscle (reviewed in Frangione et al., 2000).

More recently, a different mutation in the TTR gene was linked to lethal CAA and cerebral hemorrhage in a single case in Japan (Sakashita et al., 2001). The point mutation associated with the disease also takes place at codon 30 and results in the substitution of Val for Met. This mutation is the most common genetic variation related to the TTR-associated form of amyloidosis known as familial amyloidotic polyneuropathy (FAP), which typically presents with massive amyloid deposition in the peripheral nervous and vascular systems as well as in systemic organs, but with uncommon cerebral compromise. The case, belonging to a typical FAP pedigree, presented with renal dysfunction as the starting symptom followed by cardiac involvement and death by complications of the heart condition. Histopathologic studies at autopsy disclosed, in addition to the systemic compromise, massive intracerebral hemorrhages in the absence of neurofibrillary tangles and senile plaques. Cerebral amyloid formation was apparent not only in the choroid plexus and leptomeninges, but also in dilated small arteries in the cerebral cortex. The case presents a striking difference with typical FAP phenotypes associated with the identical mutation, in which amyloid accumulation in cerebrocortical vessels is not only significantly lower than the systemic deposition, but has never been associated with hemorrhagic complications.

Prion-related cerebral amyloidosis

A unique category in amyloid disorders is constituted by prion-related diseases, in which the etiology is thought to be related to the conversion, by a post-translational process, of the normal prion protein PrP^C into an infectious and pathogenic form PrP^{SC}. The infectious etiological agent is devoid of nucleic acids, and was called "prion" to denote its proteinaceous nature and distinguish it from viruses and viroids (Pan *et al.*, 1993). The infective protein PrP^{SC} differs from its normal counterpart only in the conformational folding, in which the higher β-sheet content of the disease-associated form translates into enhanced propensity to aggregation and resistance to proteolysis. This group of diseases includes, among others, Creutzfeldt–Jakob disease (CJD), kuru, Gerstmann–Sträussler–Scheinker disease (GSS), and fatal familial insomnia in humans, as well as scrapie and bovine spongiform encephalopathy (BSE) in animals. Extensive cortical spongiform change, gliosis, and neuronal loss are common although not invariable features of these disorders. On the contrary, amyloid angiopathy is rare and has been documented in a single pedigree caused by a T to G mutation occurring at codon 145 and resulting in a premature stop codon and the production of a 70-amino acids long N- and C-terminally truncated PrP peptide. In this genetic variant, the main neuropathological finding is PrP-immunoreactive-CAA in leptomeningeal and parenchymal blood vessels together with prominent perivascular amyloid deposition and neurofibrillary tangle pathology (Ghetti *et al.*, 1996).

BRI2 gene-related dementias

This novel group of hereditary disorders, also known as chromosome 13 dementias, and composed of familial British and Danish dementias (FBD and FDD, respectively), presents with severe CAA as one of the main defining pathological hallmarks (reviewed in Rostagno *et al.*, 2005 and Ghiso *et al.*, 2000). Both diseases share many features with Alzheimer's disease, including the presence of neurofibrillary tangles, parenchymal pre-amyloid and amyloid deposits, extensive cerebral amyloid angiopathy and a variety of amyloid-associated proteins and inflammatory components. These early onset conditions, as described below, are linked to specific mutations at or near the stop codon of the chromosome 13 gene *BRI2* that cause the generation of longer-than-normal protein products.

Familial British dementia

This hereditary disorder, originally reported in 1933, is the first described cerebral amyloidosis in the western world (Worster-Drought *et al.*, 1933) and affects an extensive pedigree of British origin which spans over nine generations (reviewed in Rostagno *et al.*, 2005). The disease presents with early onset, typically around the fifth decade of life, its earliest manifestations being personality changes – with patients becoming irritable or depressed – followed by cerebellar ataxia and spastic paralysis more severe than that seen in atypical forms of AD or in GSS. Pseudobulbar palsy and dysarthria are universal, and all patients progress to a chronic vegetative state, becoming mute, unresponsive, quadriplegic, and incontinent. Neuropathologically, FBD cases exhibit severe and widespread amyloid angiopathy of the brain and spinal cord and characteristic perivascular changes that include vessel-associated amyloid plaques and white matter changes resembling Binswanger's leukoencephalopathy. Notably, despite the extensive amyloid deposition in the vasculature, large intracerebral hemorrhage is a rare feature. Neuritic and non-neuritic amyloid plaques affect cerebellum, hippocampus, amygdala, and occasionally, cerebral cortex. Neurofibrillary degeneration is indistinguishable from that observed in AD cases. As it occurs in other forms of non-Aβ cerebral amyloidosis described above, FBD presents systemic thioflavin T-positive deposits in many organs, including the pancreas, adrenal gland, lung, myocardium, liver, spleen, and skeletal muscle (Ghiso *et al.*, 2001). Nevertheless, this systemic deposition appears to be asymptomatic, since clinical phenotypes of all described cases are only related to the cerebral compromise.

The disease is associated with a T to A substitution at codon 267 of the *BRI2* gene, which results in the presence of an Arg residue in place of the stop codon normally occurring in the wild-type precursor molecule, and a longer open-reading frame of 277 amino acids instead of 266 (Vidal *et al.*, 1999). Furin-like processing of this longer precursor releases a 34-amino acids long C-terminal fragment, named ABri, which is found constituting the characteristic cerebral and systemic deposits in FBD (Ghiso *et al.*, 2001; Vidal *et al.*, 1999).

ABri synthetic homologs recapitulate in vitro the aggregation/fibrillization propensity observed in vivo in the tissue deposits by forming spontaneous β-sheet rich structures and exhibiting fast aggregation kinetics. In fact, ABri molecules demonstrate an even higher tendency to form high-ordered oligomeric assemblies than Alzheimer's Aβ42. Consistent with the behavior of other amyloid-forming proteins, ABri aggregation kinetics is favored by slightly acidic conditions, which result in the formation of protofibrils as intermediate structures during fibril maturation (reviewed in Rostagno *et al.*, 2005).

Familial Danish dementia

Familial Danish dementia (FDD), also known as heredopathia ophthalmo-oto-encephalica, is an early onset autosomal dominant disorder originating in the Djursland peninsula in Denmark, and also associated with a genetic mutation in the *BRI2* gene (Vidal *et al.*, 2000). The disease, identified in a single family and spanning three generations, is characterized clinically by the development of cataracts, hearing loss, and progressive cerebellar ataxia before the age of 40, with subsequent paranoid psychosis and dementia. Death occurs in most patients during their fifth or sixth decade. The disease is characterized by diffuse brain atrophy with a severe involvement of the cerebellum, cerebral cortex, and white matter. Neuropathological characteristics, similarly to those seen in FBD, include widespread amyloid angiopathy in the blood vessels of the cerebrum, choroid plexus, cerebellum, spinal cord, and retina. Neurofibrillary pathology is severe in the limbic structures, and it is also present in neocortical areas where it is more pronounced than in FBD. Abnormal neurites, as seen in some other forms of CAA, mainly cluster with the vascular deposits and are absent around non-fibrillar diffuse parenchymal lesions (Holton *et al.*, 2001).

An interesting feature observed in FDD cases is the deposition of variable amounts of Aβ in blood vessels and, to a lesser extent, in brain parenchyma in the form of pre-amyloid deposits, either in combination with ADan or in isolated lesions (Holton *et al.*, 2002). Biochemical analysis of brain-extracted amyloid revealed that CAA-deposited Aβ is an N-terminal truncated form of Aβ42, a surprising finding in view of the prevalence of Aβ ending at position 40 in vascular deposits observed in sporadic and familial AD, Down syndrome, and normal aging (Tomidokoro *et al.*, 2005). Detailed mass spectrometry analysis of extracted brain amyloids revealed that the deposited ADan species, similarly to the ABri counterparts, are post-translationally modified at the N-terminus (Ghiso *et al.*, 2001; Tomidokoro *et al.*, 2005). The glutamate to pyroglutamate modification, involving the loss of one molecule of water, is notably not present in the circulating ADan or ABri counterparts, indicative of in situ generation. Similar modifications have been described in Aβ deposits (Russo *et al.*, 1997; Saido *et al.*, 1995) and appear to convey in vitro high insolubility and aggregation proclivity to the peptides, with significant changes in the oligomerization kinetics and enhanced toxicity (Russo *et al.*, 2002). It has been proposed that the presence of pGlu, even in minor concentrations, may act as potential seeding species for aggregate formation in vivo and even contribute to the formation of mixed aggregates such as those observed in FDD and composed of ADan and Aβ subunits (Schilling *et al.*, 2006).

Concluding remarks

Recent epidemiologic, clinical, and pathologic studies have emphasized the importance of the microvascular system for the functional integrity of the neurovascular unit, revealing a strong association between cognitive decline, microvessel abnormalities, and cerebrovascular dysfunction. The presence of amyloid deposits in cerebral vessels is perhaps one of the most frequent conditions associated with focal ischemia, cerebral hemorrhage and neurovascular dysfunction, compromising not only medium and small-size cerebral arteries and arterioles, but also the capillary endothelium, producing endothelial degeneration, decreased cerebral blood flow and ischemic metabolic changes. The prevalence of CAA, which increases dramatically with age, constitutes the major cause of cerebral hemorrhage in the elderly. Among the many amyloid subunits producing CAA, Aβ is by far the most common. However, the presence of familial forms of CAA, either related to genetic variants of Aβ or to non-Aβ CAA proteins, provides unique paradigms to examine the role of amyloid in the mechanism of disease pathogenesis, and to dissect the link between vascular and parenchymal amyloid deposition and their differential contribution to neurodegeneration. The striking neuropathological similarities among some of the CAA-related entities, in spite of differences in the amyloid subunits, are suggestive of common mechanistic pathways leading to cell toxicity, cellular dysfunction and death.

REFERENCES

Bailey TL, Rivara CB, Rocher AB, Hof PR. The nature and effects of cortical microvascular pathology in aging and Alzheimer's disease. *Neurol Res* 2004; **26**: 573–8.

Bornebroek M, Haan J, Roos N. Hereditary cerebral hemorrhage with amyloidosis–Dutch type (HCHWA-D): a review of the variety in phenotypic expression. *Amyloid* 1999; **6**: 215–24.

Brooks WS, Kwok JB, Halliday GM, *et al.* Hemorrhage is uncommon in new Alzheimer family with Flemish amyloid precursor protein mutation. *Neurology* 2004; **63**: 1613–17.

Cai XD, Golde, TE, Younkin S. Release of excess amyloid β protein from a mutant amyloid β protein precursor. *Science* 1993; **259**: 514–16.

Carter DA, Desmarais E, Bellis M, *et al.* More missense in amyloid gene. *Nature Genet*, 1992; **2**: 255–6.

Cheng IH, Palop JJ, Esposito LA, Bien-Ly N, Yan F, Mucke, L. Aggressive amyloidosis in mice expressing human amyloid peptides with the Arctic mutation. *Nat Med* 2004; **10**: 1190–2.

Citron M, Oltersdorf T, Haass C, *et al.* Mutation of the β-amyloid precursor protein in familial Alzheimer's disease increases β-protein production. *Nature* 1992; **360**: 672–4.

Cras P, Van Harskamp F, Hendriks L, *et al.* Presenile Alzheimer dementia characterized by amyloid angiopathy and large amyloid core type senile plaques in the APP 692Ala →Gly mutation. *Acta Neuropathol* 1998; **96**: 253–60.

Davis JB, Cribbs DH, Cotman CW, Van Nostrand WE. Pathogenic amyloid beta-protein induces apoptosis in cultured human cerebrovascular smooth muscle. *Amyloid Int J Exp Clin Invest* 1999; **6**: 157–64.

De La Torre JC. Alzheimer's disease is a vasocognopathy: a new term to describe its nature. *Neurol Res* 2004; **26**: 517–24.

Farkas E, Luiten PGM. Cerebral microvascular pathology in aging and Alzheimer's disease. *Progr Neurobiol* 2001; **64**: 575–611.

Frangione B, Vidal R, Rostagno A, Ghiso J. Familial cerebral amyloid angiopathies and dementia. *Alz Dis Assoc Disord* 2000; **14**: S25–30.

Garzuly F, Vidal R, Wisniewski T, Brittig F, Budka H. Familial meningocerebrovascular amyloidosis, Hungarian type, with mutant transthyretin (TTR Asp18Gly). *Neurology* 1996; **47**: 1562–7.

Ghetti B, Piccardo P, Spillantini MG, *et al.* Vascular variant of prion protein cerebral amyloidosis with tau-positive neurofibrillary tangles: the phenotype of the stop codon 145 mutation in PRNP. *Proc Natl Acad Sci USA* 1996; **93**: 744–8.

Ghiso J, Jensson O, Frangione, B. Amyloid fibrils in hereditary cerebral hemorrhage with amyloidosis of Icelandic type is a variant of gamma-trace basic protein (cystatin C). *Proc Natl Acad Sci USA* 1986a; **83**: 2974–8.

Ghiso J, Pons-Estel B, Frangione B. Hereditary cerebral amyloid angiopathy: the amyloid contains a protein which is a variant of cystatin C, an inhibitor of lysosomal cysteine proteases. *Biochem Biophys Res Comm* 1986b; **136**: 548–54.

Ghiso J, Haltia M, Prelli F, Novello J, Frangione B. Gelsolin variant (Asn-187) in familial amyloidosis, Finnish type. *Biochem J* 1990; **272**: 827–30.

Ghiso J, Holton J., Miravalle L, *et al.* Systemic amyloid deposits in Familial British Dementia. *J Biol Chem* 2001; **276**: 43, 909–14.

Ghiso J, Frangione B. Amyloidosis and Alzheimer's disease. *Adv Drug Delivery Rev* 2002; **54**: 1539–51.

Ghiso J, Vidal R, Rostagno A, *et al.* Amyloidogenesis in Familial British Dementia is associated with a genetic defect on chromosome 13. In: Growdon J, Wurtman R, Corkin S, Nitsch R, eds. *Molecular Basis of Dementia.* New York: New York Academy of Sciences, 2000.

Gorelick PB. Risk factors for vascular dementia and Alzheimer's disease. *Stroke* 2004; **35**: 2620–7.

Grabowski TJ, Cho HS, Vonsattel JPG, Rebeck GW, Greenberg SM. A novel APP mutation in an Iowa family with dementia and severe cerebral amyloid angiopathy. *Ann Neurol* 2001; **49**: 697–705.

Greenberg SM, Shin Y, Grabowski TJ, *et al.* Hemorrhagic stroke associated with the Iowa amyloid precursor protein mutation. *Neurology* 2003; **60**: 1020–2.

Gudmundsson G, Hallgrimsson J, Jonasson T, Bjarnason O. Hereditary cerebral hemorrhage with amyloidosis. *Brain* 1972; **95**: 387–404.

Haltia M, Ghiso J, Prelli F, *et al.* Amyloid in familial amyloidosis, Finnish type, is antigenically and structurally related to gelsolin. *Am J Pathol* 1990a; **136**: 223–8.

Haltia M, Prelli F, Ghiso J, *et al.* Amyloid protein in familial amyloidosis (Finnish type) is homologous to gelsolin, an actin-binding protein. *Biochem Biophys Res Comm* 1990b; **176**: 927–32.

Hendriks L, Van Duijn CM, Cras P, *et al.* Presenile dementia and cerebral hemorrhage linked to a mutation at codon 692 of the beta-amyloid precursor protein gene. *Nat Genetics* 1992; **1**: 218–21.

Herzig MC, Winkler DT, Burgermeister P, *et al.* Aβ is targeted to the vasculature in a mouse model of hereditary cerebral hemorrhage with amyloidosis. *Nature Neurosci* 2004; **7**: 954–60.

Holton J, Ghiso J, Lashley T, *et al.* Regional distribution of fibrillar and non-fibrillar ABri deposition and its association with neurofibrillary degeneration in Familial British Dementia. *Am J Pathol* 2001; **158**: 515–26.

Holton J, Lashley T, Ghiso J, *et al.* Familial Danish Dementia: a novel form of cerebral amyloidosis associated with deposition of both amyloid-Dan and amyloid-beta. *J Neuropathol Exp Neurol* 2002; **61**: 254–67.

Iglesias S, Chapon F, Baron JC. Familial occipital calcifications, hemorrhagic strokes, leukoencephalopathy, dementia, and external carotid dysplasia. *Neurology* 2000; **55**: 1661–7.

Janowski R, Abrahamson M, Grubb A, Jaskolski M. Domain swapping in N-truncated cystatin C. *J Mol Biol* 2004; **341**: 151–60.

Janowski R, Kozak M, Abrahamson M, Grubb A, Jaskolski M. 3D domain-swapped human cystatin C with amyloid-like intermolecular-sheets. *Structure Funct Bioinform* 2005; **61**: 570–8.

Janowski R, Kozak M, Jankowska E, *et al.* Human cystatin C, an amyloidogenic protein, dimerizes through three-dimensional domain swapping. *Nat Struct Biol* 2001; **8**: 316–20.

Kamino K, Orr HT, Payami H, *et al.* Linkage and mutational analysis of familial Alzheimer disease kindreds for the APP gene region. *Am J Hum Genet* 1992; **51**: 998–1014.

Kang I, Lemaire HG, Unterbeck A, *et al.* The precursor of Alzheimer's disease amyloid A4 protein resembles a cell-surface receptor. *Nature* 1987; **325**: 733–6.

Kiuru S. Gelsolin-related familial amyloidosis, Finnish type (FAF), and its variants found worldwide. *Amyloid* 1998; **5**: 55–66.

Kumar-Singh S, Cras P, Wang R, *et al.* Dense-core senile plaques in the Flemish variant of Alzheimer's disease are vasocentric. *Am J Pathol* 2002; **161**: 507–20.

Kumar-Singh S, Lopez-Otin C, Ghiso J, Geltner D, Frangione B. Stroke in Icelandic patients with hereditary amyloid angiopathy is related to a mutation in the cystatin C gene, an inhibitor of cysteine proteases. *J Exp Med* 1989; **169**: 1771–8.

Kumar-Singh S, Carman MD, Fernandez Madrid IJ, *et al.* Mutation of the Alzheimer's disease amyloid gene in hereditary cerebral hemorrhage, Dutch type. *Science* 1990a; **248**: 1124–6.

Kumar-Singh S, Haltia M, Fernandez-Madrid I, *et al.* Mutation in gelsolin gene in Finnish hereditary amyloidosis. *J Exp Med* 1990b; **172**: 1865–7.

Kumar-Singh S, Jascolski M, Grubb A. The role of cystatin C in cerebral amyloid angiopathy and stroke: cell biology and animal models. *Brain Pathol* 2006; **16**: 60–70.

Maat-Schieman M, Yamaguchi H, Van Duinen S, Natte R, Roos RA. Age-related plaque morphology and C-terminal heterogeneity of amyloid β in Dutch-type hereditary cerebral hemorrhage with amyloidosis. *Acta Neuropathol* 2000; **99**: 409–19.

Maat-Schieman M, Yamaguchi H, Hegeman-Kleinn IM, *et al.* Glial reactions and the clearance of amyloid β protein in the brains of patients with hereditary cerebral hemorrhage with amyloidosis-Dutch type. *Acta Neuropathol* 2004; **107**: 389–98.

Masters CL, Simms G, Weinman NA, Multhaup G, Mcdonald BL, Beyreuther K. Amyloid plaque core protein in Alzheimer disease and Down syndrome. *Proc Natl Acad Sci USA* 1985; **82**: 4245–9.

Melchor JP, Van Nostrand WE. Charge alterations of E22 enhance the pathogenic properties of the amyloid beta-protein. *J Biol Chem* 2000; **275**: 9782–91.

Miravalle L, Tokuda T, Chiarle R, *et al.* Substitution at codon 22 of Alzheimer's Aβ peptide induces diverse conformational changes and apoptotic effects in human cerebral endothelial cells. *J Biol Chem* 2000; **275**: 27, 110–16.

Mullan M, Crawford F, Axelman K, *et al.* A pathogenic mutation for probable Alzheimer's disease in the APP gene at the N-terminus of β-amyloid. *Nature Genet* 1992; **1**: 345–7.

Natte R, Maat-Schieman M, Haan J, Bornebroek M, Roos R, Van Duinen S. Dementia in hereditary cerebral hemorrhage with amyloidosis-Dutch type is associated with cerebral amyloid angiopathy but is independent of plaques and neurofibrillary tangles. *Ann Neurol* 2001; **50**: 765–72.

Nilsberth C, Westlind-Danielsson A, Eckman CB, *et al.* The 'Arctic' APP mutation (E693G) causes Alzheimer's disease by enhanced Abeta protofibril formation. *Nat Neurosci* 2001; **4**: 887–93.

Nochlin D, Bird TD, Nemens E, Ball MJ, Sumi SM. Amyloid angiopathy in a Volga German family with Alzheimer's disease and a presenilin-2 mutation (N141I). *Ann Neurol* 1998; **43**: 131–5.

Obici L, Demarchi A, De Rosa G, *et al.* A novel AbetaPP mutation exclusively associated with cerebral amyloid angiopathy. *Ann Neurol* 2005; **58**: 639–44.

Pan KM, Baldwin M, Nguyen J, *et al.* Conversion of alpha-helices into beta-sheets features in the formation of the scrapie prion proteins. *Proc Natl Acad Sci USA* 1993; **90**: 10962–6.

Petersen RB, Goren H, Cohen M, *et al.* Transthyretin amyloids: a new mutation associated with dementia. *Ann Neurol* 1997; **41**: 307–13.

Petty MA, Wettstein JG. Elements of cerebral microvascular ischaemia. *Brain Res Rev* 2001; **36**: 23–34.

Revesz T, Ghiso J, Lashley T, *et al.* Cerebral amyloid angiopathies: a pathologic, biochemical, and genetic view. *J Neuropathol Exp Neurol* 2003; **62**: 885–98.

Rossi G, Giaccone G, Maletta R, *et al.* A family with Alzheimer disease and strokes associated with

A713T mutation of the APP gene. *Neurology* 2004; **63**: 910–12.

Rostagno A, Ghiso J. Amyloidosis. In: Aminoff M, Daroff R, eds. *Encyclopedia of Neurological Sciences.* San Diego: Academic Press, 2003.

Rostagno A, Tomidokoro Y, Lashley T, *et al.* Chromosome 13 dementias. *Cell Mol Life Sci* 2005; **62**: 1814–25.

Russo C, Saido TC, Debusk LM, Tabaton M, Gambetti P, Teller JK. Heterogeneity of water-soluble amyloid b-peptide in Alzheimer's disease and Down's syndrome brains. *FEBS Lett* 1997; **409**: 411–16.

Russo C, Violani E, Salis S, *et al.* Pyroglutamate-modified amyloid β-peptides – AβN3(pE) – strongly affect cultured neuron and astrocyte survival. *J Neurochem* 2002; **82**: 1480–9.

Saido T, Iwatsubo T, Mann DM, Shimada H, Ihara Y, Kawashima S. Dominant and differential deposition of distinct β-amyloid peptide species, $Aβ_{N3(pE)}$, in senile plaques. *Neuron* 1995; **14**: 457–66.

Sakashita N, Ando Y, Jinnouchi K, *et al.* Familial amyloidotic polyneuropathy (ATTR Val30Met) with widespread cerebral amyloid angiopathy and lethal cerebral hemorrhage. *Pathol Int* 2001; **51**: 476–80.

Schilling S, Lauber T, Schaupp M, *et al.* On the seeding and oligomerization of pGlu-amyloid peptides (*in vitro*). *Biochemistry* 2006; **45**: 12394–9.

Selkoe D. Translating cell biology into therapeutic advances in Alzheimer's disease. *Nature* 1999; **399**: 23–31.

Shin Y, Cho HS, Rebeck GW, Greenberg BD. Vascular changes in Iowa-type hereditary cerebral amyloid angiopathy. *Ann NY Acad Sci* 2002; **977**: 245–51.

Shin Y, Cho HS, Fukumoto H, *et al.* Abeta species, including IsoAsp23 Abeta, in Iowa-type familial cerebral amyloid angiopathy. *Acta Neuropathol* 2003; **105**: 252–8.

Steiner H, Revesz T, Neumann M, *et al.* A pathogenic presenilin-1 deletion causes abberrant Abeta 42 production in the absence of congophilic amyloid plaques. *J Biol Chem* 2001; **276**: 7233–39.

Stenh C, Nilsberth C, Hammarback J, Engvall B, Naslund J, Lannfelt L. The Arctic mutation interferes with processing of the amyloid precursor protein. *Neuro Report* 2002; **13**: 1857–60.

Suzuki N, Cheung TT, Cai XD, *et al.* An increased percentage of long amyloid beta protein secreted by familial amyloid beta protein precursor (APP717) mutants. *Science* 1994; **264**: 1336–40.

Tomidokoro Y, Lashley T, Rostagno A, *et al.* Familial Danish dementia: co-existence of ADan and Aβ amyloid subunits in the absence of compact plaques. *J Biol Chem* 2005; **280**: 36883–94.

Wakutani Y, Watanabe K, Adachi Y, *et al.* Novel amyloid precursor protein gene missense mutation (D678N) in probable familial Alzheimer's disease. *J Neurol Neurosurg Psychiatry* 2004; **75**: 1039–42.

Walsh DM, Lomakin A, Benedek GB, Condron MM, Teplow D. Amyloid β-protein fibrillogenesis. Detection of a protofibrillar intermediate. *J Biol Chem* 1997; **272**: 22364–72.

Walsh DM, Hartley DM, Condron MM, Selkoe DJ, Teplow DB. In vitro studies of amyloid b-protein fibril assembly and toxicity provide clues to the aetiology of Flemish variant (Ala^{692} → Gly) Alzheimer's disease. *Biochem J* 2001; **355**: 869–77.

Van Nostrand WE, Melchor JP, Cho HS, Greenberg SM, Rebeck GW. Pathogenic effects of D23N Iowa mutant amyloid β-protein. *J Biol Chem* 2001; **276**: 32860–6.

Vidal R, Garzuly F, Budka H, *et al.* Meningocerebrovascular amyloidosis associated with a novel transthyretin mis-sense mutation at codon 18 (TTRD 18G). *Am J Pathol* 1996; **148**: 351–4.

Vidal R, Frangione B, Rostagno A, Mead S, Revesz T, Plant G, Ghiso J. A stop-codon mutation in the *BRI* gene associated with familial British dementia. *Nature* 1999; **399**: 776–81.

Vidal R, Ghiso J, Revesz T, *et al.* A decamer duplication in the 3′ region of the *BRI* gene originates a new amyloid peptide that is associated with dementia in a Danish kindred. *Proc Natl Acad Sci USA* 2000; **97**: 4920–5.

Worster-Drought C, Hill T, McMenemey W. Familial presenile dementia with spastic paralysis. *J Neurol Psychopathol* 1933; **14**: 27–34.

Zhang-Nunes SX, Maat-Schieman M, Van Duinen S, Roos R, Frosch MP, Greenberg SM. The cerebral β-amyloid angiopathies: Hereditary and sporadic. *Brain Pathol* 2006; **16**: 30–9.

12

Role of vascular risk factors in dementia

Chengxuan Qiu and Laura Fratiglioni

Introduction

Dementia is a common disorder in older people, affecting approximately 5–8% of those aged 65 years and older (Fratiglioni *et al.*, 2008). Vascular dementia (VaD), caused by different types of cerebrovascular disease or vascular lesions, is the second most common form of dementia after Alzheimer's disease (AD). Epidemiological studies have explored the potential risk factors for different dementing disorders widely. As a history or sign of a recent stroke is one of the items in the diagnostic criteria for VaD, risk factors for this type of dementia are supposed to be similar to those of cerebrovascular disease. In addition, increasing evidence suggests that vascular lesions in the brain also play an important role in the clinical manifestation of Alzheimer's dementia, such that neurodegenerative lesions may interact with cerebrovascular damage to enhance the likelihood of the clinical expression of the dementia syndrome. In fact, the mixed dementia resulting from co-existence of neurodegenerative changes and cerebrovascular lesions becomes more common with increasing age (Agüero-Torres *et al.*, 2006; Langa *et al.*, 2004).

This chapter provides an overview of the current knowledge on vascular risk factors for dementia including mixed dementia, as well as risk factors for post-stroke dementia; most of these vascular factors may play a role also in AD, which will be fully addressed elsewhere in this book. As most vascular risk factors and disorders are modifiable or treatable, understanding the role of vascular risk factors in dementia may provide a great potential for the prevention and treatment of these dementing disorders.

Vascular risk factors in dementia

The main vascular risk factors for dementia are summarized in Table 12.1.

Vascular disorders and conditions

Genetic factors

Several studies have confirmed the existence of hereditary forms of vascular dementia, such as autosomal dominant hereditary cerebral hemorrhage with amyloidosis, and cerebral autosomal dominant arteriopathy with subcortical infarct and leukoencephalopathy (CADASIL) (Qiu *et al.*, 2002; Viitanen and Kalimo, 2000). In addition, some studies have suggested that the ε4 allele of apolipoprotein E gene (APOE) may be a susceptibility gene for vascular dementia or stroke-related dementia (Qiu *et al.*, 2002). This may be plausible, as APOE genotypes have been associated with cardiovascular and cerebrovascular disease.

Vascular Cognitive Impairment in Clinical Practice, ed. Lars-Olof Wahlund, Timo Erkinjuntti and Serge Gauthier. Published by Cambridge University Press. © Cambridge University Press 2009.

Table 12.1 Putative vascular risk factors in dementia.

Vascular disorders and conditions
  Cerebrovascular disease: clinical stroke, cerebral emboli,
  silent brain infarcts, white matter lesions, and cerebral
  amyloid angiopathy
  Cardiovascular disease: arterial fibrillation, myocardial
  infarction, and heart failure
  Diabetes mellitus
  Hypertension
  Hyperlipidemia
  Overweight and obesity
  Systemic inflammation: serum inflammatory markers,
  and use of non-steroidal anti-inflammatory drugs as a
  protective factor
Lifestyles and habits
  Cigarette smoking
  Alcohol consumption
  Physical exercise
  Dietary/nutritional factors: fats, fish, polyunsaturated
  fatty acids, antioxidants, vitamin B_{12}, folic acid, and high
  serum homocysteine
Clustering of vascular risk factors
  The metabolic syndrome
  Vascular risk factor profile: aggregation of multiple
  vascular risk factors such as hypertension, diabetes, and
  heart disease

However, the observed association of APOE $\varepsilon4$ allele with vascular dementia should be interpreted with caution, because the $\varepsilon4$ allele is a well-established genetic risk factor for AD, and in most studies vascular dementia diagnoses were made based only on clinical examination. Thus, the common co-occurrence of CVD with Alzheimer-type pathology in older people may explain at least part of the association.

Cerebrovascular disease

Cerebrovascular disease is by definition the cause of vascular dementia, although it may also play a key role in the development and clinical expression of AD and mixed dementia (Onyike, 2006). Growing evidence has suggested that different types of cerebrovascular lesions, even in the absence of

clinical symptoms such as stroke, may lead to cognitive impairment and dementia.

Vascular dementia may occur after multiple infarctions in the brain, but a relatively small and strategically located infarction (such as in the thalamus or in the caudate nucleus) may also lead to dementia. The Cardiovascular Health Study reported a linear relation between incidence of vascular dementia and number of brain infarcts, as well as the severity of ventricular atrophy (Kuller et al., 2005). Spontaneous cerebral emboli and even silent brain infarcts detected with brain imaging are also associated with an increased risk of dementia and cognitive decline (Purandare et al., 2006; Vermeer et al., 2003). This is in accord with the observation that a considerable proportion of patients with pathological evidence of vascular dementia had no history of clinically recognized stroke. Finally, evidence is accumulating that white matter lesions (WMLs) increase the risk of cognitive decline and dementia. Population-based cross-sectional as well as longitudinal studies show that older individuals with more severe WMLs have a more than twofold increased risk of dementia (Kuller et al., 2005; Vermeer et al., 2003). Recently, the LADIS Study of non-disabled elderly people showed that cerebral white matter hyperintensities were associated with mild cognitive impairment (van der Flier et al., 2005), and that individuals with more severe age-related white matter changes were at considerable risk of global functional dependence, owing mostly to motor and cognitive deterioration (Inzitari et al., 2007). There is also evidence indicating that progression of WMLs is accompanied by significant decline in cognitive performance (Longstreth et al., 2005), supporting an etiological role of white matter changes in cognitive disturbance. White matter hyperintensities and lacunar infarcts are markers of small-vessel disease and microvascular lesions in the brain; their frequency increases dramatically with increasing age and in the presence of long-term high blood pressure and diabetes.

Cerebral amyloid angiopathy (CAA) (see also Chapter 11), caused by deposition of amyloid β

peptides in the cerebrovasculature, is correlated with WMLs, cortical infarctions, and cerebral micro-hemorrhages (Selnes and Vinters, 2006). CAA is strongly associated with AD, such that almost all Alzheimer patients have some degree of CAA. Sporadic CAA contributes significantly to cognitive decline and vascular dementia in older people, as shown by a series of clinicopathologic studies reporting the presence of severe CAA in a large proportion of vascular dementia cases with only mild Alzheimer-type pathology (Haglund et al., 2006). These studies suggest that cortical microinfarcts associated with severe CAA may be the primary pathological substrates of vascular dementia.

Cardiovascular disease

The Cardiovascular Health Study reported an association between increased risk of dementia and cardiovascular disorders, especially peripheral arterial disease, suggesting that extensive peripheral atherosclerosis may be an indicator of an increased risk of dementia. In the Cache County Study, a history of coronary artery bypass graft surgery, but not myocardial infarction, was associated with substantially increased risk of vascular dementia. In addition, other heart diseases such as atrial fibrillation and heart failure may be independently related to the risk of dementia. For instance, the Rotterdam Study showed that atrial fibrillation was associated with vascular dementia independent of a history of clinical stroke. In the Kungsholmen Project, heart failure was associated with a more than 80% increased risk of dementia, but proper use of antihypertensive drugs (83% diuretics) might partially counteract this increased risk (Qiu et al., 2006).

Diabetes mellitus

Long-term diabetes mellitus is a major risk factor for cardiovascular and cerebrovascular disease. Thus, it is not surprising that the increased risk of dementia, and of vascular dementia in particular, among persons with diabetes has been reported

repeatedly in longitudinal studies, and confirmed by a systematic review (Biessels et al., 2006). In the Rotterdam cohort, both cross-sectional and longitudinal studies showed an association of diabetes mellitus with increased risk of both vascular and degenerative types of dementia. In the Kungsholmen Project, diabetes mellitus as well as borderline diabetes or impaired glucose tolerance was also linked to an increased risk of dementia (Xu et al., 2007). It is well known that diabetes can cause micro- and macrovascular complications, but the association of diabetes with dementia may also reflect a direct effect of hyperglycemia on neuro-degenerative changes as indicated by medial temporal lobe atrophy, or an effect of hyper-insulinemia, or an effect of diabetes-related comorbidities such as hypertension and dyslipidemia (Biessels et al., 2006; Korf et al., 2007).

Hypertension

High blood pressure is a powerful risk factor for CVD, and thus may play a relevant role in vascular dementia and mixed dementia, too. Several studies have provided substantial evidence that midlife uncontrolled high blood pressure is associated with an increased risk of dementia in later life (Qiu et al., 2005). Population-based longitudinal studies of older adults often reported an association of high blood pressure with an increased risk of vascular dementia, but the association with Alzheimer-type dementia was less evident. Instead, among older people very low blood pressure may be associated with an increased risk of dementia.

In support of the association of high blood pressure with dementia, some longitudinal studies show effects of antihypertensive treatment against cognitive decline and dementia (Qiu et al., 2005). The Rotterdam Study found a significant role of use of antihypertensive drugs in reducing the risk of dementia, especially vascular dementia. In the Kungsholmen Project, use of antihypertensive drugs was associated with a slower decline in cognitive function of demented patients and a reduced risk of incident dementia. The beneficial effects of antihypertensive therapy were also reinforced by observations showing that the increased risk of cognitive decline and dementia due to hypertension was less evident among treated individuals with antihypertensive medications (Launer *et al.*, 2000). Some randomized, placebo-controlled clinical trials could partly confirm these observational studies. The Syst-Eur trial showed that among older people with systolic hypertension, active therapy with calcium-channel blockers reduced dementia incidence by more than 50% during a 4-year period. Furthermore, the PROGRESS trial suggested that antihypertensive therapy in older people with a history of stroke or transient ischemic attacks was associated with a reduced risk of dementia and cognitive decline, especially in subjects with recurrent stroke (Tzourio *et al.*, 2003).

Long-standing high blood pressure may cause clinical and silent brain infarcts and induce WMLs; all these lesions are associated with cognitive impairment and vascular dementia. In addition, hypertension has been linked to neurodegenerative markers in the brain, suggesting that high blood pressure may play a causal role in AD by accelerating the neurodegenerative process or causing brain atrophy (Qiu *et al.*, 2005).

Hyperlipidemia

An association of midlife elevated cholesterol and increased risk of late-life dementia has been reported in some studies, but not in the Honolulu–Asia Aging Study. The findings of late-life cholesterol and dementia also have been inconsistent. Some community cohort studies of older people found an elevated risk of vascular dementia and mixed dementia associated with high total cholesterol and low-density lipoprotein cholesterol level, whereas others found no association or even an inverse association of total cholesterol level with the risk of dementia and vascular dementia (Fratiglioni *et al.*, 2008). The long-term follow-up study of Japanese-American men found a decline in total serum cholesterol at least 15 years before

dementia onset. In addition, observational studies suggested a possible role of lowering cholesterol level by use of statins in reducing dementia risk, but this has not yet been confirmed by clinical trials. Thus, high serum cholesterol as a vascular risk factor for dementia remains to be confirmed.

Obesity

Overweight or obesity often occurs in association with high blood pressure and diabetes mellitus. An increased body mass index (BMI) at middle age has been reported in several studies to be associated with an increased risk of dementia in later life, independent of major vascular risk factors (Gorospe and Dave, 2007). In addition, a greater decline in BMI approximately 10 years prior to dementia onset was detected, which is in line with the studies conducted among older adults that suggest an association of accelerated decline in BMI with subsequent development of dementia (Gustafson, 2006). Low BMI in later life may be related to a higher risk of dementia, but low BMI and weight loss can be interpreted as markers of preclinical dementia, especially when measured less than 10 years prior to clinical diagnosis. In summary, these studies imply a lifespan-dependent pattern of the relationship between obesity and the risk of dementia.

Systemic inflammation

Inflammation is known to be involved in the atherosclerotic process as well as in obesity. Thus, serum inflammatory markers may be associated with dementia of vascular origin. In support of this idea, some cohort studies found an association of serum inflammatory markers measured at either midlife or old ages with an increased risk of dementia (Fratiglioni *et al.*, 2008). C-reactive protein seems to be the most promising in predicting the risk of dementia and cognitive impairment. In addition, long-term use (e.g. more than 2 years) of non-steroidal anti-inflammatory drugs was found to be associated with a lower risk of dementia and AD, as concluded in a systematic review (Etminan *et al.*,

2003), further supporting the role of the inflammatory process in dementia. Inflammation may be reduced with pharmacological treatment to prevent cognitive impairment and dementia. However, the major clinical prevention trial with anti-inflammatory drug use has been suspended due to the increased risk of cardiovascular events among the treatment group.

Lifestyles and habits

Cigarette smoking

Cigarette smoking is a well-known risk factor for cardiovascular and cerebrovascular disease. Thus, smoking is expected to play a part in the development of dementia, and of vascular dementia in particular. However, epidemiological studies have been inconclusive. Retrospective studies more often show an inverse association between smoking and risk of dementia, which could be due to survival bias as confirmed by some longitudinal prospective studies (Wang *et al.*, 1999). The cohort study of British doctors found no association between smoking and risk of dementia; however, in this study, the diagnosis of dementia was based on death certificates, and misclassification of dementia might have occurred (Doll *et al.*, 2000). By contrast, several population-based prospective studies have consistently found an increased risk of dementia associated with smoking (Fratiglioni *et al.*, 2008). Thus, cigarette smoking could act as a risk factor for dementia.

Alcohol consumption

Excessive alcohol consumption can cause alcohol-related dementia, and may increase the risk of vascular dementia too. Heavier alcohol intake at middle age was associated with increased risk of late-life dementia, especially among those carrying the APOE ε4 allele (Anttila *et al.*, 2004). By contrast, increasing evidence has emerged that mild-to-moderate alcohol consumption is associated with a reduced risk of dementia and cognitive decline. A

similar effect is reported for cardiovascular disease and all-cause mortality. In the Rotterdam Study, subjects with light-to-moderate alcohol consumption had a lower risk for dementia compared with those who never drank; such an effect was present mainly for vascular dementia and was more prominent in men than in women. Similarly, the Cardiovascular Health Study reported that consumption of one to six drinks weekly was associated with a more than 50% decreased risk of dementia. This study also showed a trend towards greater odds ratios of dementia associated with heavier alcohol consumption in men or in subjects with the APOE ε4 allele. Despite these relatively consistent reports, the inverse association of alcohol consumption with the risk of dementia remains to be confirmed as the confounding effect due to lifestyles, the role of information bias, and differential exposure assessments are not yet well clarified.

Physical exercise

Regular physical activity is known to be associated with a decreased risk of cerebrovascular and cardiovascular events, and thus may confer neuroprotection. A systematic review of longitudinal studies found that physical activity was related to a lower risk of dementia in six of nine studies (Fratiglioni *et al.*, 2004), suggesting that regular physical exercise can act as a protective factor for dementia and cognitive decline. Regular exercise, even low-intensity activity such as walking, was also associated with a reduced risk of dementia and cognitive decline (Larson *et al.*, 2006). A strong protective effect of regular physical activity at middle age against dementia occurring in later life was reported, especially for persons carrying the APOE ε4 allele (Rovio *et al.*, 2005). Some follow-up studies of older adults found that high levels of physical activity might decrease the risk of dementia and cognitive decline independent of initial functional and health status. These studies suggest that maintenance of regular physical activity may protect against cognitive decline and dementia. Intervention studies are warranted to verify its beneficial effects on the maintenance of cognition in older people (Karp *et al.*, 2006).

Dietary and nutritional factors

Epidemiological evidence suggesting an association of dietary factors and nutritional elements with the risk of dementia is still insufficient (Fratiglioni *et al.*, 2008). High intake of fatty acids may affect the development of dementia through various mechanisms, such as atherosclerosis and inflammation. Some studies have shown an association of high intake of saturated fats with an elevated risk of dementia, whereas high intake of fish, shellfish, and n-3 polyunsaturated fatty acid was linked to a decreased risk. Preference for a Western diet (i.e. a diet high in animal fat and protein, but low in complex carbohydrates) as opposed to an Oriental or a mixed diet was found to be protective of vascular dementia among Japanese-American men. Recent studies suggested that higher adherence to a "Mediterranean diet" (i.e. a higher intake of fish, fruits, and vegetables rich in antioxidants) was associated with reduced risk of dementia independent of vascular pathways. In the Rotterdam cohort, the six years' follow-up data found that neither high intake of total and saturated fats nor low intake of polyunsaturated fatty acids was associated with the risk of dementia and its main subtypes.

Some prospective follow-up studies show a decreased risk of dementia related to increasing dietary or supplementary intake of antioxidant vitamins E and C. However, clinical trials of vitamin E supplementation have failed to show any beneficial effect against cognitive impairment. A systematic review of randomized trials found no evidence of any effect of folate, vitamin B_6 or B_{12} supplementation on cognition, although folate plus vitamin B_{12} was effective in reducing serum homocysteine (Balk *et al.*, 2007). High serum homocysteine was associated with an increased risk of dementia in several cohort studies, but randomized clinical trials do not consistently support the possible effect of homocysteine lowering by B vitamins on cognitive performance.

Combination of vascular risk factors

The metabolic syndrome

The metabolic syndrome, characterized by a cluster of several vascular risk factors and disorders, is associated with silent brain infarctions. Studies have reported that the metabolic syndrome contributes to dementia, vascular dementia, and cognitive decline. In the prospective cohort study of Japanese-American men, a higher burden of metabolic risk factors in middle age was associated with an increased risk of dementia detected 25 years later, independent of demographics, smoking, and alcohol consumption (Kalmijn *et al.*, 2000). The metabolic cardiovascular syndrome particularly increased the risk of vascular dementia. The Health, Aging and Body Composition Study found that highly functioning older people with the metabolic syndrome had an increased risk of cognitive impairment, especially for those elders with high levels of serum inflammatory markers (Yaffe *et al.*, 2004). Components of the metabolic syndrome such as obesity, hypertension, and diabetes have each played a role in the pathogenesis of neurodegeneration as well as in the development of vascular dementia. The influence of the metabolic syndrome on cognitive decline and dementia may reflect the joint effect of these vascular risk factors.

Vascular risk factor profile

Vascular risk factors often co-exist in older people and may act interactively to increase the risk of dementia. Several studies have consistently shown that the risk of dementia increases with the increasing number of vascular risk factors (Fratiglioni *et al.*, 2008). Vascular risk scores or vascular indexes have been developed to quantify the risk of dementia associated with clustering of multiple vascular factors. In the population-based CAIDE study in Finland, vascular risk score in midlife could predict the risk of dementia developing 20 years later (Kivipelto *et al.*, 2006). In the Gothenburg H-70 cohort, the vascular risk index could provide robust estimates for the risk of dementia (Mitnitski *et al.*, 2006). The Framingham stroke risk profile, which is based on age, sex, systolic pressure, antihypertensive therapy, diabetes, smoking, history of heart disease, atrial fibrillation, and left ventricular hypertrophy on electrocardiogram, has been associated with lower brain volume and cognitive impairment among stroke and dementia-free subjects (Seshadri *et al.*, 2004). The findings from the middle-aged cohort emphasize the possible greater benefits of implementing intervention measures in midlife to control multiple stroke-related risk factors in preventing cognitive impairment and dementia in later life.

Risk factors in post-stroke dementia

Stroke is related to a two- to ninefold increased risk of dementia, but dementia is not always the ultimate endpoint of a stroke, indicating that other factors may contribute to dementia development. Identifying risk factors for post-stroke dementia may be of considerable relevance in dementia prevention. Table 12.2 summarizes the potential risk factors of post-stroke dementia, including demographic factors, stroke-related features, neuroimaging characteristics, and vascular comorbidities.

Demographic features

The frequency of post-stroke dementia increases with advancing age, which suggests that older age is one of the major risk factors for dementia following stroke (Leys *et al.*, 2005; Qiu *et al.*, 2002). In addition, some studies also suggested that younger old individuals were more likely to develop poststroke dementia compare to the oldest olds. Studies of general community populations often suggest that vascular dementia is more common in males than in females, but no substantial gender difference has been found for the risk of post-stroke dementia

Table 12.2. Putative risk factors in post-stroke dementia.

Demographic features
    Advanced age, male sex, non-whites, and low education
Stroke characteristics
    Stroke types (ischemic vs. hemorrhagic stroke), recurrent stroke, multiple infarcts, strategically located infarcts, more severe clinical features at stroke onset, and left or supratentorial or bilateral lesions
Neuroimaging markers of brain lesions
    Silent brain infarcts, white matter lesions, cerebral atrophy, and cerebral microbleeds (macro- and micro-hemorrhages in the brain)
Vascular disorders and conditions
    Hypertension, atrial fibrillation, diabetes mellitus, myocardial infarction, congestive heart failure, and pre-stroke cognitive status

in most studies. Low education is often reported to be associated with an increased risk of post-stroke dementia. Some studies involving multiple ethnic groups showed that blacks or non-whites were at a higher risk than whites of developing dementia after the occurrence of clinical stroke (Qiu *et al.*, 2002).

Clinical features of stroke

The likelihood of developing dementia for persons having a stroke varies depending on stroke clinical characteristics such as stroke type, volume, numbers, location and severity (Leys *et al.*, 2005; Qiu *et al.*, 2002). Ischemic strokes account for up to 85% of all stroke cases, and patients with ischemic strokes usually have higher survival rates than do people having hemorrhagic strokes, which may explain why ischemic strokes lead to psychiatric morbidity more frequently than do hemorrhagic strokes (Onyike, 2006). Most studies found that more severe clinical deficits at stroke onset were associated with a higher risk of developing post-stroke dementia. Larger volume, multiplicity, strategic locations such as left hemisphere, and bilateral infarcts are the main stroke features associated with an increased risk of post-stroke dementia. In addition, pre-stroke medial–temporal lobe atrophy as well as extensive and more severe WMLs was associated with an increased risk of post-stroke memory dysfunction, a prerequisite for the diagnosis of post-stroke dementia. A history of stroke and recurrent stroke contribute substantially to the increased risk of post-stroke dementia, apparently due to cumulative vascular damage and ischemic injury in the brain. Other clinical features in the acute phase of stroke onset may also predict the occurrence of post-stroke dementia, such as aphasia, dysphasia, low blood pressure, and urinary incontinence (Qiu *et al.*, 2002).

Neuroimaging of brain lesions (see also Chapters 5 and 6)

Some neuroimaging findings, such as WMLs, silent stroke, microbleeds, and cerebral atrophy as detected by computed tomography (CT) or magnetic resonance imaging (MRI), are found to be associated with the occurrence of cognitive decline and dementia among older people with stroke.

White matter lesions

Stroke patients with more severe WMLs usually have an increased risk of recurrent strokes, and among patients with ischemic stroke, WMLs may further increase the risk of developing cognitive impairment. Thus, the presence and severity of WMLs seen on MRI may be predictive of post-stroke dementia (Leys *et al.*, 2005). As other types of brain lesions, such as cerebral atrophy, lacunar infarcts, and silent infarcts are strongly correlated with WMLs, the independent effect of WMLs on cognitive function and dementia among patients with stroke needs to be verified by simultaneously taking into account all other MRI findings.

Silent brain infarcts and microbleeds

Several studies have consistently reported that cerebral silent infarcts detectable with CT or MRI were independently predictive of post-stroke dementia. Silent infarcts may be more important to the delayed onset of dementia in patients with clinical stroke. For example, one study suggested that the presence of silent infarcts was associated with post-stroke dementia detected in the third year, but not in the second year after the clinical stroke (Corea *et al.*, 2001). In addition, microbleeds are radiological hallmarks of CAA that can be detected with the T2*-weighted gradient-echo sequence of MRI. CAA, which is correlated with WMLs and lacunar infarcts, may result in lobar hemorrhages. A recent study in a large cohort of patients attending a memory clinic found a relatively high frequency of microbleeds in patients with vascular dementia (65%), with AD (18%), or with mild cognitive impairment (20%) (Cordonnier *et al.*, 2006). This clinic-based study confirms the neuropathological observations showing that severe CAA in combination with cerebral cortical microinfarcts might represent an underestimated variant of vascular dementia (Haglund *et al.*, 2006).

Cerebral atrophy

Global and medial–temporal lobe atrophy are shown to be associated with post-stroke dementia (Leys *et al.*, 2005). As medial–temporal lobe atrophy is considered a marker of AD, it is likely that the development of post-stroke dementia in subjects with medial–temporal lobe atrophy may be due to the concomitant neurodegenerative process that was ongoing in the preclinical phase at the time of stroke occurrence. In addition, a recent study found that in a group of stroke survivors, medial–temporal lobe atrophy was more strongly associated with subsequent cognitive decline than were WMLs (Firbank *et al.*, 2007), which may suggest a greater role for Alzheimer-type pathology than cerebrovascular lesions in the development of delayed cognitive impairment after the onset of clinical stroke.

In summary, WMLs, silent brain infarcts, global cerebral atrophy, and medial–temporal lobe atrophy are the major neuroimaging predictors of post-stroke dementia. A combination or interaction of different types of brain lesion, including neuro-degenerative markers, may even play a more important role in the development of cognitive decline and dementia after clinical stroke.

Vascular disorders and comorbidities

The APOE ε4 allele has been identified as an independent risk factor for dementia associated with stroke in a population-based study, which implies that stroke-related dementia shares some genetic susceptibility, or that patients were affected by mixed dementia. The attributable risk related to the APOE ε4 allele among demented patients with stroke was estimated to be approximately 41%, and the attributable risk was higher among Alzheimer patients with CVD (44%) than among subjects with vascular dementia (VaD) (33%) (Qiu et al., 2002).

Cognitive impairment has been reported to be a risk factor for clinical stroke, and the association probably reflects the role of silent brain lesions preceding stroke (Zhu et al., 2000). Similarly, pre-stroke cognitive impairment or decline was found to be strongly associated with an increased risk of post-stroke dementia in several studies (Gamaldo et al., 2006). Cognitive impairment occurring prior to stroke is most likely due to either pre-existing Alzheimer-type pathology or asymptomatic CVD or both, suggesting that the underlying neurodegenerative process or cerebrovascular lesions or their interaction may play a relevant role in the development of post-stroke dementia.

Stroke-associated vascular risk factors have not been linked to post-stroke dementia consistently. High blood pressure or hypertension by itself has not yet been firmly linked to dementia among stroke patients. However, uncontrolled high blood pressure, as a powerful risk factor for stroke, also significantly contributes to recurrent stroke, and recurrent strokes significantly increase the risk of post-stroke dementia. Thus, high blood pressure may play an indirect role leading to post-stroke dementia. In addition, clinical trials provide some evidence that high blood pressure might be associated with recurrent stroke-related dementia and cognitive decline (Tzourio et al., 2003).

Among the other stroke-related vascular factors, atrial fibrillation was found to be independently associated with the development of post-stroke dementia in some, but not all, studies (Leys et al., 2005). The role of diabetes mellitus in post-stroke dementia remains to be clarified, although diabetes has been more consistently associated with an increased risk of vascular dementia and of dementia with stroke. A community-based cohort study indicated that high levels of low-density lipoprotein cholesterol were independently related to an increased risk of dementia with stroke (Moroney et al., 1999), but the association between high serum cholesterol and post-stroke dementia has not yet been established. Post-stroke dementia may also be related to myocardial infarction, cardiac arrhythmias, congestive heart failure, daily alcohol consumption, and cigarette smoking, but the association of all these potential factors with post-stroke dementia needs to be confirmed (Leys et al., 2005). In summary, current evidence suggests that although some vascular risk factors or disorders are strongly associated with stroke, their independent contribution to the development of dementia following occurrence of stroke is limited (Gamaldo et al., 2006).

Summary

In the past decade, epidemiological studies have demonstrated that the dementias of both vascular and degenerative types share a number of vascular risk factors. Hypertension and diabetes mellitus are among the most relevant modifiable factors that could explain directly or indirectly a considerable proportion of non-familial dementia cases. The current knowledge of the role of vascular risk factors in the development of dementia provides opportunities for preventing these dementing disorders. As neurodegenerative and vascular dementia, which represent the most common forms of dementia, are currently treatable, but not curable, implementation of primary prevention targeting modifiable or treatable vascular risk factors or disorders seems to be the most promising avenue for reducing the huge burden of dementia.

REFERENCES

Agüero-Torres H, Kivipelto M, von Strauss E. Rethinking the dementia diagnoses in a population-based study: what is Alzheimer's disease and what is vascular dementia? A study from the Kungsholmen Project. *Dementia Geriat Cogn Disord* 2006; **22**: 244–9.

Anttila T, Helkala EL, Viitanen M, *et al.* Alcohol drinking in middle age and subsequent risk of mild cognitive impairment and dementia in old age: a prospective population based study. *Br Med J* 2004; **329**: 539–42.

Balk EM, Raman G, Tatsioni A, Chung M, Lau J, Rosenberg IH. Vitamin B_6, B_{12}, and folic acid supplementation and cognitive function: a systematic review of randomized trials. *Arch Int Med* 2007; **167**: 21–30.

Biessels GJ, Staekenborg S, Brunner E, Brayne C, Scheltens P. Risk of dementia in diabetes mellitus: a systematic review. *Lancet Neurol* 2006; **5**: 64–74.

Cordonnier C, van der Flier WM, Sluimer JD, Leys D, Barkhof F, Scheltens P. Prevalence and severity of microbleeds in a memory clinic setting. *Neurology* 2006; **66**: 1356–60.

Corea F, Henon H, Pasquier F, Leys D. Silent infarcts in stroke patients: patient characteristics and effect on 2-year outcome. *J Neurol* 2001; **248**: 271–8.

Doll R, Peto R, Boreham J, Sutherland I. Smoking and dementia in male British doctors: prospective study. *Br Med J* 2000; **320**: 1097–102.

Etminan M, Gill S, Samii A. Effect of non-steroidal anti-inflammatory drugs on risk of Alzheimer's disease: systematic review and meta-analysis of observational studies. *Br Med J* 2003; **327**: 128–31.

Firbank MJ, Burton EJ, Barber R, *et al.* Medial temporal atrophy rather than white matter hyperintensities predict cognitive decline in stroke survivors. *Neurobiol Aging* 2007; **28**: 1664–9.

Fratiglioni L, Paillard-Borg S, Winblad B. An active and socially integrated lifestyle in late life might protect against dementia. *Lancet Neurol* 2004; **3**: 343–53.

Fratiglioni L, von Strauss E, Qiu CX. Epidemiology of the dementias of old age. In: Dening T, Jacoby R, Oppenheimer C, Thomas A, eds. *The Oxford Textbook of Old Age Psychiatry*, 4th edn., New York: Oxford University Press, 2008; 391–406.

Gamaldo A, Moghekar A, Kilada S, Resnick SM, Zonderman AB, O'Brien R. Effect of a clinical stroke on the risk of dementia in a prospective cohort. *Neurology* 2006; **67**: 1363–9.

Gorospe EC, Dave JK. The risk of dementia with increased body mass index. *Age Ageing* 2007; **36**: 23–9.

Gustafson D. Adiposity indices and dementia. *Lancet Neurol* 2006; **5**: 713–20.

Haglund M, Passant U, Sjobeck M, Ghebremedhin E, Englund E. Cerebral amyloid angiopathy and cortical microinfarcts as putative substrates of vascular dementia. *Int J Geriatr Psychiatry* 2006; **21**: 681–7.

Inzitari D, Simoni M, Pracucci G, *et al.* for the LADIS Study Group. Risk of rapid global functional decline in elderly patients with severe cerebral age-related white matter changes: the LADIS Study. *Arch Int Med* 2007; **167**: 81–8.

Kalmijn S, Foley D, White L, *et al.* Metabolic cardiovascular syndrome and risk of dementia in Japanese-American elderly men: the Honolulu–Asia Aging Study. *Arterioscler Thromb Vasc Biol* 2000; **20**: 2255–60.

Karp A, Paillard-Borg S, Wang H-X, Silverstein M, Winblad B, Fratiglioni L. Mental, physical and social components in leisure activities equally contribute to decrease dementia risk. *Dementia Geriatr Cogn Disord* 2006; **21**: 65–73.

Kivipelto M, Ngandu T, Laatikainen T, Winblad B, Soininen H, Tuomilehto J. Risk score for the prediction of dementia risk in 20 years among middle aged people: a longitudinal, population-based study. *Lancet Neurol* 2006; **5**: 735–41.

Korf ES, van Straaten EC, de Leeuw FE, *et al.* for the LADIS Study Group. Diabetes mellitus, hypertension and medial temporal lobe atrophy: the LADIS Study. *Diabetic Med* 2007; **24**: 166–71.

Kuller LH, Lopez OL, Jagust WJ, *et al.* Determinants of vascular dementia in the Cardiovascular Health Cognition Study. *Neurology* 2005; **64**: 1548–52.

Langa KM, Foster NL, Larson EB. Mixed dementia: emerging concepts and therapeutic implications. *J Am Med Ass* 2004; **292**: 2901–08.

Larson EB, Wang L, Bowen JD, *et al.* Exercise is associated with reduced risk for incident dementia among persons 65 years of age and older. *Ann Int Med* 2006; **144**: 73–81.

Launer LJ, Ross GW, Petrovitch H, *et al.* Midlife blood pressure and dementia: the Honolulu–Asia aging study. *Neurobiol Aging* 2000; **21**: 49–55.

Leys D, Henon H, Mackowiak-Cordoliani MA, Pasquier F. Poststroke dementia. *Lancet Neurol* 2005; **4**: 752–9.

Longstreth WT, Arnold AM, Beauchamp NJ, *et al.* Incidence, manifestations, and predictors of worsening white matter on serial cranial magnetic resonance imaging in the elderly: the Cardiovascular Health Study. *Stroke* 2005; **36**: 56–61.

Mitnitski A, Skoog I, Song X, *et al.* A vascular risk factor index in relation to mortality and incident dementia. *Eur J Neurol* 2006; **13**: 514–21.

Moroney JT, Tang MX, Berglund L, *et al.* Low-density lipoprotein cholesterol and risk of dementia with stroke. *J Am Med Ass* 1999; **282**: 254–60.

Onyike CU. Cerebrovascular disease and dementia. *Int Rev Psychiatry* 2006; **18**: 423–31.

Purandare N, Burns A, Daly KJ, *et al.* Cerebral emboli as a potential cause of Alzheimer's disease and vascular dementia: case-control study. *Br Med J* 2006; **332**: 1119–24.

Qiu C, Winblad B, Fratiglioni L. The age-dependent relation of blood pressure to cognitive function and dementia. *Lancet Neurol* 2005; **4**: 487–99.

Qiu C, Winblad B, Marengoni A, Klarin I, Fastbom J, Fratiglioni L. Heart failure and risk of dementia and Alzheimer disease: a population-based cohort study. *Arch Int Med* 2006; **166**: 1003–08.

Qiu C, Skoog I, Fratiglioni L. Occurrence and determinants of vascular cognitive impairment. In: Erkinjuntti T, Gauthier S, eds. *Vascular Cognitive Impairment.* London: Martin Dunitz Ltd, 2002; 61–83.

Rovio S, Kåreholt I, Helkala EL, *et al.* Leisure-time physical activity at midlife and the risk of dementia and Alzheimer's disease. *Lancet Neurol* 2005; **4**: 705–11.

Selnes OA, Vinters HV. Vascular cognitive impairment. *Nature Clin Pract Neurol* 2006; **2**: 538–47.

Seshadri S, Wolf PA, Beiser A, *et al.* Stroke risk profile, brain volume, and cognitive function: the Framingham Offspring Study. *Neurology* 2004; **63**: 1591–9.

Tzourio C, Anderson C, Chapman N, *et al.* Effects of blood pressure lowering with perindopril and indapamide therapy on dementia and cognitive decline in patients with cerebrovascular disease. *Arch Int Med* 2003; **163**: 1069–75.

van der Flier WM, van Straaten EC, Barkhof F, *et al.* for the LADIS Study Group. Medial temporal lobe atrophy and white matter hyperintensities are associated with mild cognitive deficits in non-disabled elderly people: the LADIS Study. *J Neurol Neurosurg Psychiatry* 2005; **76**: 1497–500.

Vermeer SE, Prins ND, den Heijer T, Hofman A, Koudstaal PJ, Breteler MM. Silent brain infarcts and the risk of dementia and cognitive decline. *N Engl J Med* 2003; **348**: 1215–22.

Viitanen M, Kalimo H. CADASIL: hereditary arteriopathy leading to multiple brain infarcts and dementia. *Ann NY Acad Sci* 2000; **903**: 273–84.

Wang H-X, Fratiglioni L, Frisoni GB, Viitanen M, Winblad B. Smoking and the occurrence of Alzheimer's disease: cross-sectional and longitudinal data in a population-based study. *Am J Epidemiol* 1999; **149**: 640–4.

Xu W, Qiu C, Winblad B, Fratiglioni L. The effect of borderline diabetes on the risk of dementia and Alzheimer's disease. *Diabetes* 2007; **56**: 211–16.

Yaffe K, Kanaya A, Lindquist K, *et al.* The metabolic syndrome, inflammation, and risk of cognitive decline. *J Am Med Ass* 2004; **292**: 2237–42.

Zhu L, Fratiglioni L, Guo Z, Winblad B, Viitanen M. Incidence of stroke in relation to cognitive function and dementia in the Kungsholmen Project. *Neurology* 2000; **54**: 2103–07.

13

Cardiovascular disease, cognitive decline, and dementia

Angela L. Jefferson and Emelia J. Benjamin

Introduction

Over time, vascular risk factors lead to end-organ damage, which includes cardiac and brain injury. The relation between cardiac integrity and brain function is of fundamental importance for the aging population, as the burden of heart disease has shifted to the elderly (Thom *et al.*, 2006). Identifying the risk that cardiovascular disease poses for maladaptive brain aging is critical, because vascular risk factors and cardiovascular disease are amenable to interventions. Such interventions may prevent or delay cognitive decline and dementia, which would have considerable socioeconomic and public health benefits (Brookmeyer *et al.*, 1998), along with implications for the compression of morbidity (Fries, 1980). In this chapter, we review numerous processes involved in the pathogenesis of heart disease and subsequent neurological damage. In particular, we focus on clinically prevalent cardiac disease, including atrial fibrillation, myocardial infarction, coronary artery disease, heart failure, coronary artery bypass grafting, and cardiac arrest.

The diagnosis of vascular dementia (VaD), which is covered in Chapter 1, is challenging because of multiple subtypes and diagnostic schemes. Neuropathological data suggest that VaD and Alzheimer's

disease (AD) share many risk factors (Schmidt *et al.*, 2000) and frequently co-exist (Lim *et al.*, 1999), particularly as adults age (Neuropathology Group of the MRC CFAS, 2001). Because of the overlap between VaD and AD, the present chapter will focus on the risk that clinical heart disease confers for cognitive decline and dementia in general (including AD) and, if data are available, VaD, in particular. Our literature review is drawn from a combination of basic science, animal, post-mortem, subclinical, referral-based, and epidemiological studies. In an effort to better understand the relations between vascular disease and dementia, we discuss shared environmental and genetic risk factors and evidence for common underlying mechanisms of these clinical cardiovascular diseases.

Shared risk factors for cardiovascular disease and cognitive decline

Common risk factors and pathological underpinnings exist between cardiovascular disease and dementia. Such commonalities make it difficult to fully understand the role that vascular disease plays in the etiology and progression of the neurodegenerative process. As an example, animal models suggest that amyloid oligomers, which are similar

Vascular Cognitive Impairment in Clinical Practice, ed. Lars-Olof Wahlund, Timo Erkinjuntti and Serge Gauthier. Published by Cambridge University Press. © Cambridge University Press 2009.

to the amyloid seen post-mortem in Alzheimer's patients, are present in the heart and are associated with cardiac disease (Sanbe *et al.*, 2005). In addition to common pathology, there are numerous shared risk factors between cardiovascular disease and maladaptive cognitive decline, including environmental (Borenstein *et al.*, 2005; Hayden *et al.*, 2006; Hofman *et al.*, 1997; Kivipelto *et al.*, 2005; Luchsinger *et al.*, 2005) and genetic risk factors (Corder *et al.*, 1994; Hébert *et al.*, 2004; Kosunen *et al.*, 1995; Li *et al.*, 2006; Newman *et al.*, 2001b; Slooter *et al.*, 1998). Such shared pathology and risk factors support the theory that there are common mechanisms accounting for the co-morbidity of cardiovascular disease and Alzheimer's disease.

Shared environmental risk factors for cardiovascular disease and dementia include hypertension (Hayden *et al.*, 2006; Kivipelto *et al.*, 2005) and diabetes mellitus (Borenstein *et al.*, 2005; Hayden *et al.*, 2006; Luchsinger *et al.*, 2005). It is difficult to fully account for such shared vascular risks, because multivariable models generally adjust for these factors assessed at a single time point (i.e., contemporaneous measurements). In reality, cardiovascular disease (Wilson *et al.*, 1997) and dementia reflect the lifetime burden of risk factor(s). For instance, investigators from the Framingham Heart Study found that time-integrated estimates of risk factor exposure (i.e. systolic blood pressure, total cholesterol, and cigarette smoking) were related to the presence of carotid stenosis (Wilson *et al.*, 1997).

In addition to well-known shared environmental risk factors, there appear to be shared genetic risk factors between cardiovascular disease and maladaptive cognitive decline and dementia. Several studies, including both animal and clinical models, suggest that heart disease is associated with genetic risk factors for AD. Hébert and colleagues (2004) reported that presenilin 1 and presenilin 2, genetic risk factors associated with familial *early-onset* Alzheimer's, are expressed in the hearts of mice. In clinical models, presenilin 1 and 2 were related to dilated cardiomyopathy, a common cause of heart failure (Li *et al.*, 2006). In

addition to early-onset genetic risk factors, possession of certain polymorphisms of the ApoE gene (i.e. the $\varepsilon 4$ allele) place elders over age 60 years at increased risk for familial *late-onset* AD (Corder *et al.*, 1994). ApoE is involved in the transport of cholesterol in the body, and neuropathological data suggest ApoE $\varepsilon 4$ is associated with the presence of severe coronary atherosclerosis in pathologically confirmed cases of AD (Kosunen *et al.*, 1995). Newman *et al.* (2001b) reported that APOE $\varepsilon 4$-positive patients undergoing coronary artery bypass grafting were significantly younger than APOE $\varepsilon 4$-negative patients undergoing the same surgical procedure. These clinical data from Newman *et al.* (2001b) may be due to increased coronary atherosclerosis severity associated with APOE $\varepsilon 4$, as identified by the former pathological study (Kosunen *et al.*, 1995). Among a clinical referral sample of AD, cardiac ischemia and left ventricular dysfunction were more common among homozygous APOE $\varepsilon 4$ carriers as compared to those patients homozygous for APOE $\varepsilon 3$, a polymorphism that does not confer a significant risk for AD (van der Cammen *et al.*, 1998). A population-based study of non-demented older adults found no significant increased prevalence of atherosclerosis among APOE $\varepsilon 4$ carriers, suggesting that atherosclerosis is not an intermediate factor in the relationship between ApoE and cognitive decline (Slooter *et al.*, 1998). However, adults with both APOE $\varepsilon 4$ and atherosclerosis performed worse on a cognitive screening measure as compared to those adults with either APOE $\varepsilon 4$ or atherosclerosis, suggesting a possible synergistic effect (Slooter *et al.*, 1998).

Collectively, these animal, neuropathological, and clinical data suggest that there may be some shared genetic risk factors between cardiovascular disease and dementia. Though rare mutations with large effects leading to cardiovascular disease and dementia occur (i.e. Mendelian forms), most cases of dementia and cardiovascular disease represent examples of common complex diseases with multiple genetic determinants yet small genetic effects (i.e., so-called *epistatic* effects). Thus, accounting fully for shared burden of genetic variation is difficult.

Atrial fibrillation

Atrial fibrillation is a cardiac arrhythmia characterized by an irregular rhythm and loss of effective atrial contraction. These changes contribute to reduced cardiac efficiency and are thought to impact CNS integrity by reducing cardiac output and cerebral blood flow (Petersen *et al.*, 1989) and increasing thromboembolic risk (Barber *et al.*, 2004), thus contributing to cognitive impairment and dementia.

Atrial fibrillation appears to be related to preclinical and clinical dementia, although research has not supported relationships between atrial fibrillation and cognitive performances among cognitively normal adults. Recent data from Park and colleagues (2005) comparing older adults with atrial fibrillation to those with normal sinus rhythm yielded no cross-sectional relationship between atrial fibrillation and cognitive function. Three-year longitudinal follow-up of this cohort also failed to yield any between-group cognitive differences (Park *et al.*, 2007). In contrast, atrial fibrillation has been linked to risk of conversion to dementia. Ravaglia *et al.* (2006) followed a group of participants with mild cognitive impairment (MCI), a precursor to dementia, and found that atrial fibrillation was more prevalent in those participants that converted to dementia over a mean of 3 years. This research group extended their findings by following a larger sample of participants with MCI (mean follow-up = 2.8 years) and a cognitively normal older adult sample (mean follow-up = 3.8 years) (Forti *et al.*, 2006). Similar to the original work, those MCI participants who developed dementia had a higher prevalence of atrial fibrillation than their MCI peers who did not progress to dementia. However, atrial fibrillation was not associated with conversion to dementia among the cognitively normal sample (Forti *et al.*, 2006). This latter finding that atrial fibrillation is not associated

with cognitive decline among non-demented elderly is consistent with the longitudinal work put forth by Park and colleagues (2007).

Epidemiological data from the Rotterdam Study found that VaD and AD were more than twice as common in older adults with atrial fibrillation than those without, even after adjusting for prevalent cardiovascular disease (Ott *et al.*, 1997). These relations were most prominent for women. However, atrial fibrillation has also been linked to cognitive impairment in community samples of older men (Elias *et al.*, 2006; Kilander *et al.*, 1998). For instance, data from the Framingham Heart Study suggest that men with atrial fibrillation perform worse on cognitive measures assessing verbal reasoning, verbal and visuospatial memory, processing speed, and visual integration (Elias *et al.*, 2006). In an Italian population-based study that included men and women, Di Carlo *et al.* (2000) reported that older adults with "cognitive impairment no dementia" were more likely to have a history of atrial fibrillation as compared to their cognitively normal peers.

Because atrial fibrillation is often a consequence of existing heart disease (including myocardial infarction, heart failure, and valvular heart disease), it is possible that the associations between atrial fibrillation and cognitive impairment are mediated by underlying cardiovascular disease. The co-existence of these cardiovascular conditions complicates the course of each disease process and makes it difficult to tease apart the longitudinal relationships between heart disease and dementia. However, studies examining the longitudinal relations between atrial fibrillation and neurological outcomes may provide important pathophysiological insights regarding the mechanisms for these relations.

Myocardial infarction and coronary artery disease

Myocardial infarctions occur when atherosclerotic plaques rupture and thrombose, leading to acute limitations of coronary artery blood flow. The decrease in coronary artery blood flow may result in myocardial necrosis. The underlying substrate for acute coronary events is progressive coronary artery atherosclerosis. Myocardial infarction is thought to contribute to low cardiac output, reduction in cerebral blood flow, and micro-embolism. Although limited, recent animal model data suggest neurobiological changes occur following acute myocardial infarction, including apoptotic events in the prefrontal cortex and hypothalamus (Wann et al., 2007). The presence of atherosclerosis prior to myocardial infarction may also affect the brain through shared genetic factors (Slooter et al., 2004), lipid peroxidation, and oxidative stress (Napoli and Palinski, 2005). Collectively, these mechanisms for CNS injury are the theoretical basis for empirical studies relating myocardial infarction or coronary artery disease to cognitive decline and dementia.

Pathological data suggest relationships between atherosclerosis, or plaques, and maladaptive cognitive decline. For instance, post-mortem measures of intracranial atherosclerosis (i.e. atheromatous involvement in the circle of Willis) were significantly more severe in individuals diagnosed in vivo with dementia, including VaD and AD, as compared to dementia-free subjects (Beach et al., 2007). As mentioned above, neuropathological data have linked a genetic risk factor for AD (APOE ε4) to severe coronary atherosclerosis in pathologically confirmed AD cases (Kosunen et al., 1995). These latter findings suggest that shared genetic factors may underlie the aforementioned clinical and neuropathological observations relating atherosclerosis to dementia. Additional neuropathological data based on a large data set suggest that, independent of stroke, AD (i.e. neuritic plaques) was associated with atherosclerosis (i.e. large-vessel CVD) but not arteriosclerosis (i.e. small-vessel CVD) (Honig et al., 2005).

Findings from small clinical referral samples have related myocardial infarction to risk of vascular-based dementias. Tresch and colleagues

(1985) reported that patients with multi-infarct dementia (MID) were more likely to have a history of myocardial infarction compared to patients with AD. In a case-control study of Japanese men, Watanabe et al. (2004) demonstrated that those with VaD had significantly more frequent atherosclerotic plaque deposition and increased carotid intima-media thickness compared to those with AD. These authors recently extended their prior findings by reporting that the presence of atherosclerosis was significantly increased in Japanese men and women with VaD relative to their dementia-free peers (Ban et al., 2006). In both studies, the groups were statistically comparable for vascular risk factors, such as age, systolic and diastolic blood pressure, fasting glucose, and triglycerides, yet these variables were not included as covariates in the between-group comparisons. Although increased atherosclerosis is likely involved in the pathogenesis and progression of dementia, future research is needed to assess these relations while adjusting for vascular risk factors.

Epidemiological studies in this area have supported the pathological and clinical findings linking myocardial infarction and atherosclerosis to CNS variables. Data from the Bronx Aging Study suggest that women with a history of myocardial infarction are five times more likely to have dementia than their peers without a previous myocardial infarction (Aronson et al., 1990). Among Japanese-American men in the Honolulu–Asia Aging Study, coronary heart disease was associated with an increased risk for VaD (Ross et al., 1999). In a large, Italian population-based study, Di Carlo and colleagues (2000) found that older adults with "cognitive impairment no dementia" had a greater prevalence of myocardial infarction as compared to cognitively normal older adults. Cross-sectional epidemiological data from the Rotterdam Study has linked increased atherosclerosis of the carotids and large vessels of the leg to the presence of dementia (Hofman et al., 1997). Odds ratios for both AD and VaD increased as the burden of atherosclerosis increased (Hofman et al., 1997). More recent longitudinal data from the Cardiovascular Health Study extend the Rotterdam findings, such that common carotid artery wall thickness was related to incident dementia over a mean follow-up period of 5.4 years (Newman *et al.*, 2005).

Taken together, these findings suggest that a history of myocardial infarction and increased atherosclerosis are associated with increased risk for dementia. Relations between prior myocardial infarction and dementia may be due to amplified systemic burden of atherosclerosis that led to the initial myocardial infarction or reduced cardiac function as a result of damage caused by the myocardial infarction. Alternatively, as suggested by recent animal data, apoptotic events in the brain may follow acute myocardial infarction (Wann *et al.*, 2007).

Heart failure

Heart failure occurs if the left or right ventricle is not contracting (systolic heart failure) or relaxing (diastolic heart failure) normally and is unable to pump blood efficiently to the body. Heart failure purportedly contributes to neurological impairment by reducing blood flow to the brain. This theoretical model is supported by data documenting that restoration of heart function results in cerebral blood flow increases (Gruhn *et al.*, 2001). However, additional mechanistic pathways between heart failure and CNS injury may include neurohumoral factors (Felder *et al.*, 2003), thromboemboli (Freudenberger and Massie, 2005), and oxidative stress (Mariani *et al.*, 2005).

Clinical data from referral-based samples of heart failure patients have shown that markers of disease severity are associated with cognitive functioning. Zuccala *et al.* (1997) showed that very poor left ventricular systolic function (i.e. assessed by ejection fraction) was related to global cognitive impairment. More recent work from this group suggests that patients with heart failure who have arterial hypotension are at greatest risk for cognitive impairment (Zuccala *et al.*, 2001). Trojano and

colleagues (2003) compared patients with heart failure to a "control" sample of cardiovascular patients without heart failure. Findings suggest that the heart failure patients performed significantly worse on neuropsychological measures assessing global cognition, attention, verbal fluency, and memory (Trojano *et al.*, 2003). Although left ventricular dysfunction and reduced cardiac efficiency may contribute to CNS damage, another mechanism for such damage is cardiac output, or blood flow exiting the heart's left ventricle. Among heart failure patients awaiting transplantation, cardiac output was inversely associated with sequencing performance, an element of executive functioning (Putzke *et al.*, 1998). More recent work has extended this finding to older cardiovascular patients free of end-stage heart failure (Jefferson *et al.*, 2007). Specifically, those cardiovascular patients with reduced cardiac output performed significantly worse on cognitive measures assessing planning and sequencing as compared to patients with normal cardiac output values (Jefferson *et al.*, 2007). These findings collectively suggest that proxy measures of systemic blood flow may be related to the integrity of executive functioning.

Epidemiological data have extended the research between heart failure and maladaptive cognitive decline from small, referral-based samples into larger cohorts. In a large Italian cohort, a history of heart failure was more frequently found in adults with "cognitive impairment no dementia" as compared to cognitively normal older adults (Di Carlo *et al.*, 2000). More recent epidemiological data extend these findings by linking heart failure to dementia. In a population-based Swedish cohort, Qiu *et al.* (2006) found that heart failure was associated with an 80% increased risk of dementia and AD over a nine-year follow-up period. Results were modestly attenuated if antihypertensive medication usage was considered in the multivariable analyses.

These clinical and epidemiological data suggest that heart failure is associated with both cognitive impairment and an increased risk for dementia. In the absence of heart failure, markers of subclinical cardiac dysfunction are also related to cognitive impairments, specifically elements of executive functioning (Jefferson *et al.*, 2007). Epidemiological data suggest that antihypertensive drug use attenuates the risk that heart failure confers for dementia (Qiu *et al.*, 2006). Therefore, future studies may wish to examine the benefit of antihypertensive therapeutic intervention on dementia conversion among patients with heart failure, as prior clinical trials in this area have yielded promising results (Forette *et al.*, 1998).

Coronary artery bypass grafting

The most common cardiac surgery in the USA is coronary artery bypass grafting (CABG), which is used to treat coronary artery disease. Coronary artery disease consists of narrowing of the arteries supplying blood to the myocardium, and such narrowing is usually caused by atherosclerosis. By grafting arteries or veins, CABG provides a conduit for blood to pass around arterial blockages.

The neurological and psychological correlates of cardiac surgery have been of interest to investigators for more than 50 years (Samuels, 2006). In particular, cognitive complications following CABG have generated considerable interest with most studies focusing on perioperative factors. Initially, alterations in cerebral blood flow were proposed as the underlying mechanism for the cognitive decline seen in CABG (Patel *et al.*, 1993), particularly because of intraoperative hypotension associated with use of the cardiopulmonary bypass machine (Sendelbach *et al.*, 2006). However, studies comparing off-pump and on-pump CABG patients yield comparable longitudinal cognitive decline, regardless of intervention methodology (van Dijk *et al.*, 2007). Alternatively, diffusion-weighted and perfusion MRI data suggest that cerebral microembolism is common with heart surgery and contributes to cognitive decline (Wityk *et al.*, 2001), perhaps because of perioperative manipulation of the vessels. Basic science models have suggested that the use of general anesthetics

may be one possible underlying mechanism accounting for the increased risk of cognitive impairment and dementia following surgery (Eckenhoff *et al.*, 2004; Xie *et al.*, 2006). As an example, isoflurane is a commonly applied general inhalation anesthetic. Using a clinically appropriate concentration of isoflurane in human cell cultures, Xie and colleagues (2006) reported that isoflurane alters amyloid precursor protein processing and increases β-amyloid protein, both pathogenic features of AD.

In addition to perioperative variables, research has suggested that post-operative factors may account for the cognitive decline seen in CABG. For instance, the incidence of atrial fibrillation is increased following cardiac surgery and its presence is associated with worse cognitive outcome post-CABG (Stanley *et al.*, 2002). This association may be due to the aforementioned association between atrial fibrillation, increased thromboembolic risk, and reduced cardiac output. Inflammation and oxidative stress may also account for relations between CABG and CNS injury. Circulating markers of inflammation and oxidative stress increase following CABG, and these markers are more elevated in those patients who present post-CABG with cognitive decline compared to those patients without such cognitive decline (Ramlawi *et al.*, 2006).

Although immediate neurological complications following cardiac surgery are well known, it was previously thought that these complications resolved over time. For instance, earlier work suggested that the majority of immediate cognitive complications following CABG resolved within the first 6 months post-surgery (Savageau *et al.*, 1982). More extended follow-up periods of cardiac surgical patients have revealed that late cognitive impairments may manifest several years after surgery. Newman *et al.* (2001a) reported that cognitive difficulties following CABG dissipated over a six-month follow-up period following discharge. However, nearly half of all study patients experienced significant cognitive impairment 5 years post-surgery. Significant predictors of late cognitive impairment included older age, lower education attainment, and cognitive impairment at discharge. Such late-onset cognitive decline following CABG, however, is an inconsistent finding in the literature. Müllges and others (2002), for example, followed a small cohort of patients over a median follow-up of 55 months. Of the original 91 patients examined, 52 were re-examined, and none of these patients exhibited long-term cognitive impairment compared to baseline performance (Müllges *et al.*, 2002). In fact, cognitive test performances were stronger at the follow-up examination as compared to baseline, particularly for verbal intellectual functioning. Such dramatic improvement in stable cognitive functions may suggest a possible survival bias for this small cohort of patients or, as the authors purport, these improvements may reflect a reduction of cognitive deterioration because of well-controlled vascular risk factors (Müllges *et al.*, 2002).

A criticism of the longitudinal work examining the cognitive correlates of CABG is that CABG patients are rarely compared to "control" groups with comparable coronary artery disease. Such atherosclerotic disease may worsen with age and account for cognitive decline seen several years later. In an effort to address this methodological problem, McKhann *et al.* (2005) compared CABG patients with three groups, including off-pump cardiac surgery patients, medically treated cardiac patients, and healthy adults free of cardiovascular disease. Baseline data yielded significant cognitive performance differences between the coronary heart disease groups as compared to the heart-healthy group. However, one-year follow-up data revealed that the slope of change in cognitive performance was comparable among all four groups.

In light of the mixed findings linking CABG to cognitive difficulties, there has been increased interest in whether CABG increases risk for dementia. Using a case-control design that included dementia and age-matched control participants, Knopman and others (2005) did not find differences between the groups with respect to a history of CABG. In contrast, a very large study by Lee and colleagues (2005) followed CABG patients ($n = 5216$) for 6 years, and findings suggest CABG is

indeed a risk factor for dementia. The discrepancy between these studies may be the relatively few number of dementia and control participants with a history of CABG in the study of Knopman *et al.* (2005), yielding insufficient power to detect an association.

These clinical and epidemiological data suggest CABG is related to cognitive decline and dementia. Underlying substrates accounting for these relations are likely multi-factorial and include the aforementioned peri-operative factors, such as microembolism (Wityk *et al.*, 2007) and anesthesia (Xie *et al.*, 2006), and post-operative factors, such as changes in cardiac function (Stanley *et al.*, 2002) and inflammation (Ramlawi *et al.*, 2006). One needed research direction is long-term follow-up studies using "control" groups to clarify discrepancies in the late cognitive decline–CABG literature.

Cardiac arrest

Cardiac arrest occurs if there is an abrupt cessation of the heart beat, often due to ventricular fibrillation or asystole. Although resuscitation immediately restores heart function and blood flow, animal models of cardiac arrest suggest that following reperfusion, cardiac function is altered and oxygen delivery to the brain is reduced (Oku *et al.*, 1994). Thus, cardiac arrest's adverse impact on the brain commences with an acute reduction in cerebral blood flow, followed by resuscitation and subsequent cerebral reperfusion that results in abnormal cerebral hemodynamics.

Research directed at understanding the neuropathological consequences of cardiac arrest has capitalized on animal models. These studies suggest that neuropathological features associated with AD are present following cardiac arrest. For instance, Pluta (2000) examined neuropathological features of rats subjected to 10 min cardiac arrest. Diffuse increases in beta-amyloid peptide and amyloid precursor protein expression were observed in regions such as the hippocampus and entorhinal cortex. These data suggest that the molecular events following the ischemic–reperfusion process are similar to those seen in the pathogenesis of AD. Human models, although subject to less experimental control, have supported the neuropathological findings from the animal models. Wisniewski and Maslinska (1996) examined neuropathological correlates among 12 non-demented adults age 44–78. Patients were resuscitated within a few minutes following cardiac arrest but came to autopsy within 36 days. All cases exhibited overexpression of beta protein precursor, suggesting that cardiac arrest is associated with Aβ-amyloidosis, a pathological process associated with AD.

Clinical data based on longitudinal follow-up of cardiac arrest patients has yielded mixed findings regarding the risk cardiac arrest confers for dementia. One of the first patient series was conducted by Nielsen and colleagues (1983), which followed 13 cardiac arrest patients and 13 myocardial infarction "control" patients for approximately 3 years. Findings revealed that a greater proportion of patients with cardiac arrest had dementia at the end of follow-up. In contrast, a study by Horsted and others (2007) followed 33 patients over a 2-year period without a reference group and found global cognition was in the normal range for 94% of the sample.

Treatment advances suggest that the devastating neurological outcome following cardiac arrest can be improved using hypothermia, a technique that was initially introduced in the 1950s but abandoned secondary to difficulties associated with its use (Marion et al., 1996). Animal data have consistently shown that systemic hypothermia may diminish CNS injury following cardiac arrest (Horn et al., 1991; Leonev et al., 1990). Subsequent clinical trial data have more recently supported the animal studies' findings, such that therapeutic hypothermia is associated with a more positive neurological outcome following cardiac arrest as compared to normothermia (Bernard et al., 2002; Hypothermia After Cardiac Arrest Study Group, 2002). One plausible mechanism accounting for the therapeutic benefit of hypothermia includes suppression of biochemical

reactions that contribute to mitochondrial damage and cell death (Busto et al., 1989).

Collectively, data suggest that cardiac arrest is associated with neuropathological features associated with AD as well as an increased risk of clinical dementia. Although animal studies in this area are experimentally well-controlled, clinical data are limited and subject to less experimental control regarding the etiology and duration of cardiac arrest. Future, larger-scale longitudinal studies are warranted to better understand the long-term clinical significance of cardiac arrest on dementia. Treatment advances that reduce the severity of neurological symptoms post-cardiac arrest (Bernard et al., 2002; Hypothermia After Cardiac Arrest Study Group, 2002) may contribute to increased survival rates and greater opportunities to explore the long-term CNS outcomes for cardiac arrest.

Future directions

Understanding the complex relations between cardiac integrity and brain function requires a number of future research directions, including the diversity of samples investigated, methodological considerations, prevention advances, and genetic discoveries. One major need is to expand the racial and ethnic populations of interest and increase the diversity of samples studied. For instance, the majority of literature in this area has been conducted in North American and Western European samples, with focus on whites of European descent. It is well-known that cardiovascular disease disproportionately impacts minorities (Mensah et al., 2005). Thus, it is critical that future research in this area expands to include more ethnically and racially diverse groups.

There are many shared risk factors associated with cardiovascular disease, cognitive impairment, and dementia (Borenstein et al., 2005; Hayden et al., 2006; Kivipelto et al., 2005; Luchsinger et al., 2005). Such shared factors make it difficult to discern if relationships observed between cardiovascular disease and cognitive decline are secondary to common underlying risks or reflect a unique relation between cardiac integrity and dementia. Future studies should implement methodology that accounts for important shared vascular and subclinical risk factors, as existing research linking clinical events and cardiac conditions to dementia risk may reflect shared underlying disease processes rather than a unique relation.

Identification of subclinical risk factors and early intervention is another important area of future research focus because of implications for cardiovascular risk factor management and cardiac disease prevention. Such early identification and management of subclinical vascular risk factors is a critical next step to dementia prevention. Past research suggests that interventions targeted at managing cardiovascular risk factors can result in a substantial reduction in dementia cases. For example, management of hypertension (an important vascular risk factor) appears to reduce the incidence of dementia. Observational work from the Cache County Study suggests that antihypertensive medication usage is associated with a reduced incidence of AD (Khachaturian *et al.*, 2006). A clinical trial targeted at managing hypertension yielded a 50% reduction in the incidence of dementia over a five-year follow-up period (Forette *et al.*, 1998). Taken together, these data emphasize that identifying and managing vascular risk factors for dementia has strong potential for improving health and reducing functional disability through dementia prevention.

Finally, identifying genetic risk factors associated with AD and understanding how these factors simultaneously confer risk for heart disease is a future area of research emphasis. Multiple studies are underway to provide opportunities for studying genetic risk factors for complex diseases (like dementia and heart disease), such as the Genetic Association Information Network (GAIN). Such large, collaborative projects will shed light on shared genetic risk factors and their interaction with environmental factors in understanding relations between heart disease and dementia.

ACKNOWLEDGMENTS

Preparation of this chapter was supported, in part, by AG022773, AG027480, and HD043444 (ALJ); HL70100; N01-HC25195; R01-NS17950; HL076784, and AG028321 (EJB); P30-AG13846 (Boston University Alzheimer's Disease Core Center). The authors wish to thank Ms. Susan Vanderhill and Laura Byerly for their administrative assistance in preparing this chapter.

REFERENCES

Aronson MK, Ooi WL, Morgenstern H, *et al.* Women, myocardial infarction, and dementia in the very old. *Neurology* 1990; **40**: 1102–06.

Ban Y, Watanabe T, Miyazaki A, *et al.* Impact of increased plasma serotonin levels and carotid atherosclerosis on vascular dementia. *Atherosclerosis* 2006; **195**(1): 153–9.

Barber M, Tait RC, Scott J, Rumley A, Lowe GD, Stott DJ. Dementia in subjects with atrial fibrillation: hemostatic function and the role of anticoagulation. *J Thromb Haemost* 2004; **2**: 1873–8.

Beach TG, Wilson JR, Sue LI, *et al.* Circle of Willis atherosclerosis: association with Alzheimer's disease, neuritic plaques and neurofibrillary tangles. *Acta Neuropathol (Berl)* 2007; **113**: 13–21.

Bernard SA, Gray TW, Buist MD, *et al.* Treatment of comatose survivors of out-of-hospital cardiac arrest with induced hypothermia. *N Engl J Med* 2002; **346**: 557–63.

Borenstein AR, Wu Y, Mortimer JA, *et al.* Developmental and vascular risk factors for Alzheimer's disease. *Neurobiol Aging* 2005; **26**: 325–34.

Brookmeyer R, Gray S, Kawas C. Projections of Alzheimer's disease in the United States and the public health impact of delaying disease onset. *Am J Pub Hlth* 1998; **88**: 1337–42.

Busto R, Globus MY, Dietrich WD, Martinez E, Valdes I, Ginsberg MD. Effect of mild hypothermia on ischemia-induced release of neurotransmitters and free fatty acids in rat brain. *Stroke* 1989; **20**: 904–10.

Corder EH, Saunders AM, Risch NJ, *et al.* Protective effect of apolipoprotein E type 2 allele for late onset Alzheimer disease. *Nature Genet* 1994; **7**: 180–4.

Di Carlo A, Baldereschi M, Amaducci L, *et al.* Cognitive impairment without dementia in older people: prevalence, vascular risk factors, impact on disability. The Italian Longitudinal Study on Aging. *J Am Geriatr Soc* 2000; **48**: 775–82.

Eckenhoff RG, Johansson JS, Wei H, *et al.* Inhaled anesthetic enhancement of amyloid-beta oligomerization and cytotoxicity. *Anesthesiology* 2004; **101**: 703–09.

Elias MF, Sullivan LM, Elias PK, *et al.* Atrial fibrillation and cognitive performance in the Framingham offspring men. *Int J Stroke Cardiovasc Dis* 2006; **15**: 214–22.

Felder RB, Francis J, Zhang ZH, Wei SG, Weiss RM, Johnson AK. Heart failure and the brain: new perspectives. *Am J Physiol Regul Integr Comp Physiol* 2003; **284**: R259–76.

Forette F, Seux ML, Staessen JA, *et al.* Prevention of dementia in randomised double-blind placebo-controlled Systolic Hypertension in Europe (Syst-Eur) trial. *Lancet* 1998; **352**: 1347–51.

Forti P, Maioli F, Pisacane N, Rietti E, Montesi F, Ravaglia G. Atrial fibrillation and risk of dementia in non-demented elderly subjects with and without mild cognitive impairment. *Neurol Res* 2006; **28**: 625–9.

Freudenberger RS, Massie BM. Silent cerebral infarction in heart failure: vascular or thromboembolic? *J Cardiac Fail* 2005; **11**: 490–1.

Fries JF. Aging, natural death, and the compression of morbidity. *N Engl J Med* 1980; **303**: 130–5.

Gruhn N, Larsen FS, Boesgaard S, *et al.* Cerebral blood flow in patients with chronic heart failure before and after heart transplantation. *Stroke* 2001; **32**: 2530–3.

Hayden KM, Zandi PP, Lyketsos CG, *et al.* Vascular risk factors for incident Alzheimer disease and vascular dementia: the Cache County study. *Alzheimer Dis Assoc Disord* 2006; **20**: 93–100.

Hébert SS, Serneels L, Dejaegere T, *et al.* Coordinated and widespread expression of gamma-secretase in vivo: evidence for size and molecular heterogeneity. *Neurobiol Dis* 2004; **17**: 260–72.

Hofman A, Ott A, Breteler MM, *et al.* Atherosclerosis, apolipoprotein E, and prevalence of dementia and Alzheimer's disease in the Rotterdam Study. *Lancet* 1997; **349**: 151–4.

Honig LS, Kukull W, Mayeux R. Atherosclerosis and AD: analysis of data from the US National Alzheimer's Coordinating Center. *Neurology* 2005; **64**: 494–500.

Horn M, Schlote W, Henrich HA. Global cerebral ischemia and subsequent selective hypothermia. A neuro-pathological and morphometrical study on ischemic neuronal damage in cat. *Acta Neuropathol (Berl)* 1991; **81**: 443–9.

Horsted TI, Rasmussen LS, Meyhoff CS, Nielsen SL. Long-term prognosis after out-of-hospital cardiac arrest. *Resuscitation* 2007; **72**: 214–18.

Hypothermia After Cardiac Arrest Study Group. Mild therapeutic hypothermia to improve the neurologic outcome after cardiac arrest. *N Engl J Med* 2002; **346**: 549–56.

Jefferson AL, Poppas A, Paul RH, Cohen RA. Systemic hypoperfusion is associated with executive dysfunction in geriatric cardiac patients. *Neurobiol Aging* 2007; **28**: 477–83.

Khachaturian AS, Zandi PP, Lyketsos CG, *et al.* Anti-hypertensive medication use and incident Alzheimer disease: the Cache County Study. *Arch Neurol* 2006; **63**: 686–92.

Kilander L, Andren B, Nyman H, Lind L, Boberg M, Lithell H. Atrial fibrillation is an independent determinant of low cognitive function: a cross-sectional study in elderly men. *Stroke* 1998; **29**: 1816–20.

Kivipelto M, Ngandu T, Fratiglioni L, *et al.* Obesity and vascular risk factors at midlife and the risk of dementia and Alzheimer disease. *Arch Neurol* 2005; **62**: 1556–60.

Knopman DS, Petersen RC, Cha RH, Edland SD, Rocca WA. Coronary artery bypass grafting is not a risk factor for dementia or Alzheimer disease. *Neurology* 2005; **65**: 986–90.

Kosunen O, Talasniemi S, Lehtovirta M, *et al.* Relation of coronary atherosclerosis and apolipoprotein E genotypes in Alzheimer patients. *Stroke* 1995; **26**: 743–8.

Lee TA, Wolozin B, Weiss KB, Bednar MM. Assessment of the emergence of Alzheimer's disease following coronary artery bypass graft surgery or percutaneous transluminal coronary angioplasty. *J Alzheim Dis* 2005; **7**: 319–24.

Leonov Y, Sterz F, Safar P, *et al.* Mild cerebral hypothermia during and after cardiac arrest improves neurologic outcome in dogs. *J Cerebr Blood Flow Metab* 1990; **10**: 57–70.

Li D, Parks SB, Kushner JD, *et al.* Mutations of presenilin genes in dilated cardiomyopathy and heart failure. *Am J Hum Genet* 2006; **79**: 1030–9.

Lim A, Tsuang D, Kukull W, *et al.* Clinico-neuropathological correlation of Alzheimer's disease in a community-based case series. *J Am Geriatr Soc* 1999; **47**: 564–9.

Luchsinger JA, Reitz C, Honig LS, Tang MX, Shea S, Mayeux R. Aggregation of vascular risk factors and risk of incident Alzheimer disease. *Neurology* 2005; **65**: 545–51.

Mariani E, Polidori MC, Cherubini A, Mecocci P. Oxidative stress in brain aging, neurodegenerative and vascular diseases: an overview. *J Chromatogr B, Analyt Technol Biomed Life Sci* 2005; **827**: 65–75.

Marion DW, Leonov Y, Ginsberg M, *et al.* Resuscitative hypothermia. *Crit Care Med* 1996; **24**: S81–9.

McKhann GM, Grega MA, Borowicz LM Jr, *et al.* Is there cognitive decline 1 year after CABG? Comparison with surgical and nonsurgical controls. *Neurology* 2005; **65**: 991–9.

Mensah GA, Mokdad AH, Ford ES, Greenlund KJ, Croft JB. State of disparities in cardiovascular health in the United States. *Circulation* 2005; **111**: 1233–41.

Müllges W, Babin-Ebell J, Reents W, Toyka KV. Cognitive performance after coronary artery bypass grafting: a follow-up study. *Neurology* 2002; **59**: 741–3.

Napoli C, Palinski W. Neurodegenerative diseases: insights into pathogenic mechanisms from atherosclerosis. *Neurobiol Aging* 2005; **26**: 293–302.

Neuropathology Group of the Medical Research Council Cognitive Function and Ageing Study (MRC CFAS). Pathological correlates of late-onset dementia in a multicentre, community-based population in England and Wales. *Lancet* 2001; **357**: 169–75.

Newman AB, Fitzpatrick AL, Lopez O, *et al.* Dementia and Alzheimer's disease incidence in relationship to cardiovascular disease in the Cardiovascular Health Study cohort. *J Am Geriatr Soc* 2005; **53**: 1101–07.

Newman MF, Kirchner JL, Phillips-Bute B, *et al.* Longitudinal assessment of neurocognitive function after coronary-artery bypass surgery. *N Eng J Med* 2001a; **344**: 395–402.

Newman MF, Laskowitz DT, White WD, *et al.* Apolipoprotein E polymorphisms and age at first coronary artery bypass graft. *Anesth Analg* 2001b; **92**: 824–9.

Nielsen JR, Gram L, Rasmussen LP, *et al.* Intellectual and social function of patients surviving cardiac arrest outside the hospital. *Acta Med Scand* 1983; **213**: 37–9.

Oku K, Kuboyama K, Safar P, *et al.* Cerebral and systemic arteriovenous oxygen monitoring after cardiac arrest. Inadequate cerebral oxygen delivery. *Resuscitation* 1994; **27**: 141–52.

Ott A, Breteler MM, de Bruyne MC, van Harskamp F, Grobbee DE, Hofman A. Atrial fibrillation and dementia in a population-based study. The Rotterdam Study. *Stroke* 1997; **28**: 316–21.

Park HL, Hildreth AJ, Thomson RG, O'Connell J. Non-valvular atrial fibrillation and cognitive function – baseline results of a longitudinal cohort study. *Age Ageing* 2005; **34**: 392–5.

Park H, Hildreth A, Thomson R, O'Connell J. Non-valvular atrial fibrillation and cognitive decline: a longitudinal cohort study. *Age Ageing* 2007; **36**: 157–63.

Patel RL, Turtle MR, Chambers DJ, Newman S, Venn GE. Hyperperfusion and cerebral dysfunction. Effect of differing acid–base management during cardiopulmonary bypass. *Eur J Cardiothor Surg* 1993; **7**: 457–63; discussion, 464.

Petersen P, Kastrup J, Videbaek R, Boysen G. Cerebral blood flow before and after cardioversion of atrial fibrillation. *J Cerebr Blood Flow Metab* 1989; **9**: 422–5.

Pluta R. The role of apolipoprotein E in the deposition of beta-amyloid peptide during ischemia–reperfusion brain injury. A model of early Alzheimer's disease. *Ann NY Acad Sci* 2000; **903**: 324–34.

Putzke JD, Williams MA, Rayburn BK, Kirklin JK, Boll TJ. The relationship between cardiac function and neuropsychological status among heart transplant candidates. *J Cardiac Fail* 1998; **4**: 295–303.

Qiu C, Winblad B, Marengoni A, Klarin I, Fastbom J, Fratiglioni L. Heart failure and risk of dementia and Alzheimer disease: a population-based cohort study. *Arch Int Med* 2006; **166**: 1003–08.

Ramlawi B, Rudolph JL, Mieno S, *et al.* Serologic markers of brain injury and cognitive function after cardiopulmonary bypass. *Ann Surg* 2006; **244**: 593–601.

Ravaglia G, Forti P, Maioli F, *et al.* Conversion of mild cognitive impairment to dementia: predictive role of mild cognitive impairment subtypes and vascular risk factors. *Dementia Geriatr Cogn Disord* 2006; **21**: 51–8.

Ross GW, Petrovitch H, White LR, *et al.* Characterization of risk factors for vascular dementia: the Honolulu–Asia Aging Study. *Neurology* 1999; **53**: 337–43.

Samuels MA. Can cognition survive heart surgery? *Circulation* 2006; **113**: 2784–6.

Sanbe A, Osinska H, Villa C, *et al.* Reversal of amyloid-induced heart disease in desmin-related cardiomyopathy. *Proc Natl Acad Sci USA* 2005; **102**: 13592–7.

Savageau JA, Stanton BA, Jenkins CD, Frater RW. Neuropsychological dysfunction following elective cardiac operation. II. A six-month reassessment. *J Thorac Cardiovasc Surg* 1982; **84**: 595–600.

Schmidt R, Schmidt H, Fazekas F. Vascular risk factors in dementia. *J Neurol* 2000; **247**: 81–7.

Sendelbach S, Lindquist R, Watanuki S, Savik K. Correlates of neurocognitive function of patients after off-pump coronary artery bypass surgery. *Am J Crit Care* 2006; **15**: 290–8.

Slooter AJ, van Duijn CM, Bots ML, *et al.* Apolipoprotein E genotype, atherosclerosis, and cognitive decline: the Rotterdam Study. *J Neural Transm Supplem* 1998; **53**: 17–29.

Slooter AJ, Cruts M, Hofman A, *et al.* The impact of APOE on myocardial infarction, stroke, and dementia: the Rotterdam Study. *Neurology* 2004; **62**: 1196–8.

Stanley TO, Mackensen GB, Grocott HP, *et al.* The impact of postoperative atrial fibrillation on neurocognitive outcome after coronary artery bypass graft surgery. *Anesth Analg* 2002; **94**: 290–5.

Thom T, Haase N, Rosamond W, *et al.* Heart disease and stroke statistics – 2006 update: a report from the American Heart Association Statistics Committee and Stroke Statistics Subcommittee. *Circulation* 2006; **113**: e85–151.

Tresch DD, Folstein MF, Rabins PV, Hazzard WR. Prevalence and significance of cardiovascular disease and hypertension in elderly patients with dementia and depression. *J Am Geriatr Soc* 1985; **33**: 530–7.

Trojano L, Antonelli Incalzi R, Acanfora D, Picone C, Mecocci P, Rengo F. Cognitive impairment: a key feature of congestive heart failure in the elderly. *J Neurol* 2003; **250**: 1456–63.

van der Cammen TJ, Verschoor CJ, van Loon CP, *et al.* Risk of left ventricular dysfunction in patients with probable Alzheimer's disease with APOE*4 allele. *J Am Geriatr Soc* 1998; **46**: 962–7.

van Dijk D, Spoor M, Hijman R, *et al.* Cognitive and cardiac outcomes 5 years after off-pump vs. on-pump coronary artery bypass graft surgery. *J Am Med Assoc* 2007; **297**: 701–08.

Wann BP, Bah TM, Boucher M, *et al.* Vulnerability for apoptosis in the limbic system after myocardial infarction in rats: a possible model for human postinfarct major depression. *J Psychiatry Neurosci* 2007; **32**: 11–16.

Watanabe T, Koba S, Kawamura M, *et al.* Small dense low-density lipoprotein and carotid atherosclerosis in relation to vascular dementia. *Metabolism* 2004; **53**: 476–82.

Wilson PW, Hoeg JM, D'Agostino RB, *et al.* Cumulative effects of high cholesterol levels, high blood pressure, and cigarette smoking on carotid stenosis. *N Engl J Med* 1997; **337**: 516–22.

Wisniewski HM, Maslinska D. Beta-protein immunoreactivity in the human brain after cardiac arrest. *Folia Neuropathol* 1996; **34**: 65–71.

Wityk RJ, Goldsborough MA, Hillis A, *et al.* Diffusion- and perfusion-weighted brain magnetic resonance imaging in patients with neurologic complications after cardiac surgery. *Arch Neurol* 2001; **58**: 571–6.

Xie Z, Dong Y, Maeda U, *et al.* The common inhalation anesthetic isoflurane induces apoptosis and increases amyloid beta protein levels. *Anesthesiology* 2006; **104**: 988–94.

Zuccala G, Cattel C, Manes-Gravina E, Di Niro MG, Cocchi A, Bernabei R. Left ventricular dysfunction: a clue to cognitive impairment in older patients with heart failure. *J Neurol Neurosurg Psychiatry* 1997; **63**: 509–12.

Zuccala G, Onder G, Pedone C, *et al.* Hypotension and cognitive impairment: selective association in patients with heart failure. *Neurology* 2001; **57**: 1986–92.

14

Vascular factors in Alzheimer's disease: from diagnostic dichotomy to integrative etiology

Miia Kivipelto, Alina Solomon and Tiia Ngandu

Introduction

Alzheimer's disease (AD) and vascular dementia (VaD) are nowadays widely accepted as the most common dementia forms. Just as widely accepted and applied in clinical practice is the traditional rule of diagnostic parsimony, urging physicians to look for the fewest possible causes which can account for all the patient's symptoms. It is thus no wonder that AD and VaD have been approached separately so far, and most studies have focused on identifying means for sharply differentiating neurodegenerative from vascular dementia types.

A century of research and discovery since Alois Alzheimer's first description of the AD pathological hallmarks (amyloid plaques and neurofibrillary tangles) was celebrated in 2006. However, the fact that Alzheimer has written many more papers on vascular dementia is less cited (Libon *et al.*, 2006). Although at the beginning of the twentieth century both Alzheimer and Kraepelin had accurately recognized the complexity of the group of vascular dementias, in clinical practice the term "arteriosclerotic dementia" was synonymous with "senile dementia". According to the general view of that time, brain atrophy in the elderly resulted from ischemic–hypoxic neuronal death due to progressive narrowing of cerebral blood vessels, and the

eponym *Alzheimer's disease* (as introduced by Kraepelin in the 1910 edition of his *Psychiatry* textbook), designated a presenile rarity. The shift towards an opposite view – unification of AD and senile dementia and simultaneous separation from vascular dementia – began to occur in the 1960s, when the neuropathologic changes described by Alzheimer were found to be very common in elderly demented patients. And so it has been during the past 30 years: AD dominating the field of dementia research, closely followed by its diagnostic competitor, vascular dementia.

The "Alzheimerization" of the dementia field, apart from assigning an inferior, second-place status to vascular dementia, had another characteristic with important consequences. The intense focus on amyloid and tau proteins and on the genes involved in their processing has somehow shadowed the fact that "AD" is not a single nosological entity. The majority of AD cases are sporadic, but the image of the disease has been strongly influenced by research on the familial AD type (which accounts for only 1–2% of all cases). The inherited form is mainly the result of an interaction between genes and proteins, but the sporadic form differs from the familial type and presents considerable heterogeneity in terms of risk factor profiles, pathogenesis, and neuropathological findings. The

Vascular Cognitive Impairment in Clinical Practice, ed. Lars-Olof Wahlund, Timo Erkinjuntti and Serge Gauthier. Published by Cambridge University Press. © Cambridge University Press 2009.

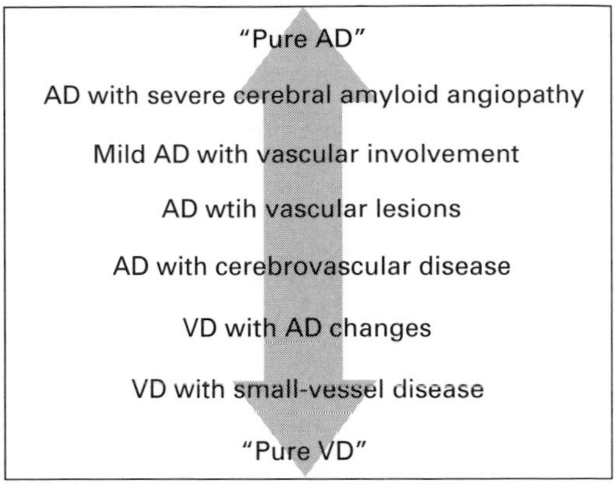

Figure 14.1 Alzheimer's disease and vascular dementia continuum. (Adapted from Kalaria and Ballard (1999), with permission.)

fact that the brain is entirely dependent on a properly functioning vascular system can no longer be disregarded when it comes to the markedly multifactorial sporadic AD.

AD-type and cerebrovascular changes are both so common that they inevitably occur together in many cases. However, the association seems to be more complex than a mere coincidence, as there is now evidence for a significant AD–VaD overlapping in terms of risk factors, clinical features, and pathology. "Pure" AD and "pure" VaD can be considered the opposite ends of a dementia etiology continuum, where most cases are "in between" and have combinations of AD type and vascular changes in different degrees (Figure 14.1). This chapter focuses on the overlap of the two dementia groups, discussing risk factors, symptoms, pathologies and some possible mechanisms of interaction.

Risk factors for AD

Until quite recently, the only established risk factors for AD were advanced age, familial aggregation and the presence of the apolipoprotein E (APOE) ε4 allele. As the available treatments are still symptomatic, the step to a fatalistic view of the disease was easily taken. However, during the past years, evidence has accumulated from long-term population based studies that modifiable risk factors (vascular- and lifestyle-related) are important not only for VaD but also for AD. AD is now considered to be a multi-factorial disease resulting from an interaction between genetic susceptibility and environmental factors, which opens opportunities for prevention.

Dementia of Alzheimer type is, in most cases, a syndrome occurring late in life. There is, however, a long preclinical stage characterized by progressive neuropathological changes, which at a certain point become clinically detectable in the form of cognitive impairment. Therefore this window of opportunity for preventive interventions covers a wide time span, turning the classical "late-life" view of AD into a more appropriate "life-long" view.

Hypertension

Hypertension has received a lot of attention because it may represent a common and potentially modifiable risk factor not only for cardiovascular and cerebrovascular disorders but also for AD. Long-term population-based follow-up studies have shown that high blood pressure (BP) especially at mid-life is associated with an increased AD risk later in life (Kivipelto *et al.*, 2002; Launer *et al.*, 2000). High BP even later in life (Skoog *et al.*, 1996) and closer to dementia onset has also been linked with a higher AD risk, but results have been more inconsistent.

In the few autopsy studies conducted, hypertension has been associated with amyloid plaques and neurofibrillary tangles (e.g. Honolulu–Asia Ageing Study (HAAS)). Hypertension has also been related to increased brain atrophy. These findings suggest that hypertension may be linked with neurodegenerative changes besides its known contributions as a risk factor for cerebrovascular lesions.

BP values often fall during aging, before the manifestation of dementia, and during the course of AD. AD is a catabolic disorder and, besides BP, cholesterol values and body weight often decline during the disease course. Decline in BP may be at least partly related to neurodegenerative processes and brain lesions (e.g. several brain regions affected in AD are involved in BP regulation), and thus be secondary to the AD process, but other factors may also be involved. Whether low BP accelerates the AD process is still a matter of debate. Longstanding hypertension may lead to various changes in cerebral arteries and alter autoregulation of blood flow to the brain. Under these conditions, episodes of hypotension may lead to hypoperfusion and ischemia in vulnerable brain areas (e.g. deep white matter). These brain changes may further impair cognition and interact with AD changes as discussed below.

Some observational studies indicated that anti-hypertensive medication, especially long-term treatment, may reduce the risk of dementia, including AD (Peila et al., 2006). In the Systolic Hypertension in Europe (Syst-Eur) trial, active treatment of isolated systolic hypertension with nitrendipine, a calcium-channel blocker, was found to halve the incidence of AD. The Study on Cognition and Prognosis in the Elderly (SCOPE) showed that lowering BP among elderly (70–89 years) with mild hypertension is beneficial and safe. Cognitive functions were well maintained both in the candesartan (an angiotensin receptor blocker) group and in the control group, which besides placebo often received other BP medications to control BP levels. In the sub-group analyses, it was shown that among the subjects with lower baseline cognition (MMSE 24–28), MMSE score declined less in the candesartan than in the control group. It is no longer ethical to leave persons with high BP without treatment because of the risk of cardiovascular and cerebrovascular disorders, and, thus, true placebo-controlled trials in this issue may no longer be possible to conduct as the SCOPE study indicated.

Hypercholesterolemia

It has been reported that high serum total cholesterol (TC) values at mid-life increase the risk of late-life AD (Kivipelto et al., 2002; Whitmer et al. 2005). Mid-life TC has also been related to AD-type brain changes in autopsy studies (Launer et al., 2001; Pappolla et al., 2003). The role of high cholesterol later in life and closer to dementia onset is less clear, as some studies indicate either no association or an inverse association of hypercholesterolemia with subsequent AD development. Recent data from the Cardiovascular Risk Factors, Aging and Dementia (CAIDE) study suggest a bidirectional relationship between TC and dementia; high TC is a risk factor for subsequent AD 20 years later, but decreasing TC after midlife may reflect ongoing disease processes and may represent a risk marker for late-life dementia (Solomon et al., 2007). The hypothesis that a decline in TC may be associated with early stages in dementia development is also supported by results from the HAAS. A decrease over time in BP and BMI has also been described, but with somewhat different patterns. Dementia-associated additional decline in these other factors becomes detectable about 3–6 years before the clinical expression of the disease, while the decline in TC seems to start much earlier, with little subsequent acceleration prior to the onset of dementia (Stewart et al., 2007). These changes may explain at least partly the inconsistent/negative results from the cross-sectional and short-term follow-up studies and studies having the baseline measurement of cholesterol at late-life.

Little information is currently available regarding other cholesterol types (LDL, HDL, triglycerides). Serum HDL-C would be of specific interest because HDL is the major carrier of cholesterol in the brain, and serum HDL-C levels, but not LDL-C or TC, were found to be correlated with CSF cholesterol in elderly human subjects.

As serum and brain cholesterol are two separate pools, studies measuring serum cholesterol can only observe the tip of the iceberg. The brain is the most cholesterol-rich organ in the body, and disturbances in brain cholesterol metabolism have been linked with all the main neuropathological changes in AD. The links between serum and brain cholesterol are not fully known, but one link is represented by oxysterols, mono-oxygenated derivates of cholesterol with a unique ability to pass the blood–brain barrier (BBB). 24S-hydroxycholesterol (24OHC) and 27-hydroxycholesterol (27OHC) are increased in the CSF of patients with established AD. Recently, an uptake of 27OHC into the brain from the periphery was described; this may be important for neurodegeneration, and may be one of the links between hypercholesterolemia and AD (Björkhem, 2006).

There is strong biological evidence linking cholesterol to AD. Sparks et al. (1994) reported already more than a decade ago that rabbits, which normally do not develop β-amyloid deposits, rapidly accumulate β-amyloid in the brain after being fed with cholesterol. Experimental studies later revealed that cholesterol may directly affect amyloid precursor protein (APP) metabolism, and that cholesterol reduction with statins may modulate the major APP secretases in such a way that they switch from the amyloidogenic to the non-amyloidogenic pathway. Supporting this hypothesis, some experimental studies have shown that statins may reduce β-amyloid production in vitro and in vivo. It is also important to notice that statins have a variety of actions which may also be beneficial for central nervous system and be associated with reduced risk of AD, including endothelial protection via actions on the nitric oxide synthase system, antioxidant, anti-inflammatory, anti-platelet effects, and immunomodulatory effects.

The currently available epidemiological and clinical data on statins and AD give a rather mixed picture (Rockwood, 2006). Cross-sectional studies consistently showed a reduced occurrence of dementia among statin users. Two-wave epidemiological studies investigated the effects of statins on AD incidence, but without showing any statistical benefit related to statin use. The number of treated persons who developed AD was, however, small, questioning whether these studies were sufficiently powered to detect any putative statin effects. A few clinical trials have also addressed the statins–dementia issue. Cognitive arms were added to ongoing cardiology studies (Heart Protection Study and PROSPER), but no significant influence of statins on cognition or dementia incidence was found. However, the add-on design and the possible lack of power question again the results. Two small studies indicated that statins might be effective in delaying the progression of cognitive decline in persons with AD (Simons et al., 2002; Sparks et al., 2005). Two much larger studies (LEADe and CLASP) are now ongoing. In these trails of patients with mild to moderate AD with normal cholesterol values and receiving background AchE treatment, statins had no additional benefits on cognition and global function over 18 months (sub-analyses ongoing).

Obesity

Obesity is increasing across the world, with severe consequences on cardiovascular health, but its association with the risk of AD has so far been less extensively studied. Weight loss seems to occur during the pre-clinical phases of dementia, and recent follow-up studies (e.g. PAQUID and HAAS) have suggested that low body mass index (BMI) could actually be an early sign of dementia. There is increasing evidence from long-term population-based studies (e.g. CAIDE study, Kaiser Permanente Study) that high BMI at mid-life, or at late-life 9–18 years prior to dementia (Gothenburg study), is associated with an increased AD risk (Gustafson et al., 2003; Kivipelto et al., 2005).

Obesity is related to vascular disorders, which could be the link to AD. For example, obesity is an essential feature in metabolic syndrome, which is also characterized by dyslipidemia, hypertension, glucose intolerance and insulin resistance. Higher BMI and waist-to-hip ratio were related to white matter lesions (WML) in some studies, and higher BMI was associated with greater temporal lobe atrophy and greater brain atrophy rate. These associations were independent of several vascular risk factors, suggesting a more direct role of obesity in neurodegeneration. Insulin resistance is one possible factor related to AD pathogenesis, as discussed below. Furthermore, adipose tissue is the largest endocrine organ in the human body and secretes hormones and several other bioactive compounds, and thus other adipose-associated (e.g. sex hormones) and adipose-derived factors (e.g. leptin, interleukins, growth factors) may also be involved.

Vascular diseases

Until recently, clinical vascular diseases (which can be considered consequences of elevated BP, cholesterol and obesity) have quite seldom been studied in relation to AD. Because of the diagnostic criteria for AD, patients with clinical vascular diseases are less likely to be diagnosed with AD. However, recent studies have reported an association between various vascular disorders such as myocardial infarction, atrial fibrillation, heart failure, and AD. In addition, coronary artery disease at autopsy has been linked with an increase in cortical senile plaques. In the Rotterdam study, generalized atherosclerosis was also associated with AD.

Diabetes and metabolic syndrome

Diabetes has been associated with an increased risk of AD in several cohort studies, while others have found no association (Martins *et al.*, 2006). However, the definition of diabetes varies between studies. In the elderly, the true prevalence of DM is over 30%, and more than half are asymptomatic and undiagnosed. In addition, more than 30% have impaired glucose tolerance, which makes more than half of elderly people affected with hyperglycemia. The potential biological mechanisms underlying the diabetes–AD association are many. These associations may reflect the direct effects on the brain of hyperglycemia and advanced glycation end products, or the effects of diabetes-associated co-morbidities (hypertension, dyslipidemia, or

hyperinsulinemia). Diabetes is associated with changes in cerebral microvessels and the BBB. Some studies have indicated that higher insulin levels are associated with the risk of dementia–AD. Insulin resistance may be important in AD pathogenesis by influencing APP and β-amyloid regulation, cerebral glucose metabolism, and inflammatory processes. Insulin-degrading enzyme (IDE) has received a lot of interest recently as a potential link between hyperinsulinemia and AD; the enzyme degrades insulin, amylin, and β-amyloid, and hyperinsulinemia may elevate β-amyloid through insulin's competition with β-amyloid for IDE (Qiu and Folstein, 2006).

Besides indicators of diabetes and metabolic syndrome, inflammatory markers (e.g. high CRP levels in the HAAS study), have also been suggested as risk factors for cognitive decline and AD.

Dietary factors

Diet is an important lifestyle factor affecting vascular health. It has been reported that a diet rich in saturated fat and cholesterol may increase the risk of AD, whereas polyunsaturated fatty acids and fish may be protective. However, contradictory findings exist as well (Luchsinger and Mayeux, 2004). The studies conducted so far had a relatively short follow-up, and are therefore prone to bias due to sub-clinical dementia (i.e. poor diet could be a consequence rather than a cause of disease), and long-term prospective studies are still needed to clarify the issue. Recent data from the CAIDE study indicate that moderate intake of unsaturated fats at mid-life is protective, whereas a moderate intake of saturated fats may increase the risk of AD, especially among APOE ε4 carriers (Laitinen *et al.*, 2006).

There are several putative pathways through which fat intake may be related to AD. The effect could be through vascular factors and oxidative stress caused by a high saturated fat intake. Unsaturated fatty acids may confer protection through their anti-inflammatory properties. Fatty acids may play important roles in the synthesis and fluidity of nerve cell membranes and for synaptic plasticity and neuronal degeneration. Experimental studies using transgenic mouse models of AD have shown that essential omega-3 fatty acids protect against neuronal deficits, decrease β-amyloid levels, and decrease the number of activated microglia in the brain (Calon *et al.*, 2004; Oksman *et al.*, 2006).

In a recent randomized controlled trial, omega-3 fatty acid supplementation did not influence cognitive functioning during a follow-up of 6 months. However, positive effects were observed in a small group of patients with very mild AD (MMSE >27) (Freund-Levi *et al.*, 2006). These data together with epidemiological evidence support the idea that omega-3 may have a role in the primary and maybe secondary prevention of the disease, but not when the disease process has already taken over.

Oxidative stress is one central feature in the AD brain, and some studies have suggested that a diet rich in antioxidants might protect against AD, while others did not find such an association (Luchsinger and Mayeux, 2004). A recent study indicated that a "Mediterranean diet" might protect against AD. As the association remained even after controlling for several vascular factors, other mechanisms (e.g. oxidative or inflammatory) may also be involved (Scarmeas *et al.*, 2006). In addition, low B12 and folate levels and their marker high homocysteine have been linked with an increased AD risk in some studies.

Physical exercise and active lifestyle

Another lifestyle-related factor that has been connected with AD is physical activity. Some shorter-term longitudinal studies indicated an inverse association between regular and high-intensity leisure time physical activity, or some specific form of physical activity (e.g. dancing, walking) and dementia/AD risk, whereas others found no association (Fratiglioni *et al.*, 2004). The CAIDE study showed that regular leisure time physical activity at mid-life may protect against dementia and AD later

in life. The risk reduction was 50% for dementia and 60% for AD, even after controlling for several vascular and lifestyle related factors (Rovio *et al.*, 2005). This association was more pronounced among APOE4 ε4 carriers.

Physical activity is important in promoting general and vascular health, but it may confer its effects against AD through other mechanisms as well. It may promote brain plasticity (Colcombe *et al.*, 2004) and affect several gene transcripts and neurotrophic factors that are relevant for maintenance of cognitive functions (Berchtold *et al.*, 2002; Tong *et al.*, 2001). Social and mental activities have also been suggested to protect against AD (Fratiglioni *et al.*, 2004). Generally active lifestyle may increase cognitive reserve (Kramer *et al.*, 1999), reduce stress and protect against development or expression of dementia also through these mechanisms.

Smoking and alcohol drinking

It is important to notice that the possible effects of other proposed risk factors for AD such as smoking and alcohol drinking may also be mediated through vascular mechanisms. Smoking (which is a strong risk factor for vascular diseases and is also associated with oxidative stress) may result in modestly increased risk for AD. Heavy drinking may increase dementia risk, and a J- or U-shaped relation between alcohol drinking and dementia/AD has also been described, suggesting that light-to-moderate alcohol use might have a protective effect, but in some studies alcohol consumption was not related to AD.

Several possible mechanisms lay behind these associations. Alcohol may have beneficial effects on several cardiovascular risk factors, including hypertension, lipid and lipoprotein levels, inflammatory and hemostatic factors, and moderate alcohol drinking has been related to a reduced risk of cardiovascular diseases. Moderate alcohol drinking has also been associated with fewer brain infarcts, and a U-shape relationship with WMLs has been described (Mukamal *et al.*, 2001). On the other hand, excessive alcohol drinking has clear detrimental effects on brain, and even light drink-ing levels have been related to increased brain atrophy (Ding *et al.*, 2004).

The protective effect of alcohol may also be due to the effect of specific antioxidant substances in wine. Further, moderate amounts of alcohol could act directly by releasing acetylcholine in the hippo-campus. Apart from the effect of alcohol per se, other social and lifestyle-related factors associated with certain drinking habits may be the reasons behind the favorable association between moderate alcohol drinking and cognitive functioning.

Apolipoprotein E and other genetic factors

To date, the apolipoprotein E (apoE) ε4 allele is the only genetic risk factor for AD of established general significance. The association has been confirmed in several studies world-wide, in both sporadic and late-onset familial AD cases. APOE ε4 is a suscepti-bility gene for AD, being neither necessary nor suf-ficient for AD development. The risk of AD increases, and the age of onset decreases with the number of the ε4 alleles, in a dose-dependent manner. The very mechanisms relating ApoE ε4 allele to AD are not completely understood. APOE has a central role in lipid metabolism, and the APOE ε4 allele is associated with increased serum total and LDL cholesterol levels, atherosclerosis, and coronary heart disease, but the effect for AD seems to be at least partly independent of these peripheral vascular factors (Kivipelto *et al.*, 2002).

Interestingly, APOE has been linked to all the major features in AD pathogenesis, including β-amyloid generation and clearance, neurofibrillary tangle formation, oxidative stress, apoptosis, dys-function in lipid transport and homeostasis, modulation of intracellular signalling, and synaptic plasticity (Cedazo-Mínguez and Cowburn, 2001). In all cases, the presence of the APOE ε4 allele has been shown to exacerbate these disturbances, in contrast to the protection seen with other ApoE isoforms. Further, ApoE plays a key role in the maintenance and repair of neurons, and the APOE ε4 allele carriers show a poor compensation

of neuronal loss in different brain regions. Consequently, the lack of function observed in the apoE4, compared with other isoforms, could act in concert with environmental deleterious factors and lead to neuropathological processes. Recent epidemiological studies have suggested that ApoE ε4 carriers would be more vulnerable to a variety of environmental factors (e.g. physical inactivity, sat-urated fat intake, alcohol drinking, diabetes, high BP, low B12/folate), and thus give support to this hypothesis. Further investigation of gene–environ-ment interactions both in epidemiologic and experimental settings are needed to increase our understanding of the disease process.

Interestingly, many of the other suggested can-didate genes for AD are vascular related, e.g. CYP46 (cholesterol 24-hydroxylase), IDE, ACE (angio-tensin-converting enzyme), PPARγ (peroxisome proliferator-activated receptor gamma), and IL-1 (interleukin 1).

Vascular factors in AD: suggested mechanisms

The exact role of vascular factors in the develop-ment of AD and manifest dementia syndrome is still unknown, but several possible pathways have been proposed. Vascular risk factors may directly induce AD neuropathology, or lead to arteriosclerosis, impaired brain blood flow and metabolism, and neuronal dysfunction. Vascular risk factors may also induce small- and large-vessel cerebrovascular dis-ease and infarcts. Accumulation of various lesions might lead to an increased risk of development of clinically manifest AD (Figure 14.2).

There is a discrepancy between AD-type neu-ropathologic changes in the brain and the clinical manifestation of dementia. There have been attempts to explain this, for example by the cog-nitive reserve hypothesis: the individuals that do not have manifest dementia in spite of abundant neuropathologic changes in their brains may have a greater reserve capacity, and thus greater pathological changes are needed to reach the threshold for clinically manifest dementia than in individuals with a lower reserve capacity. The

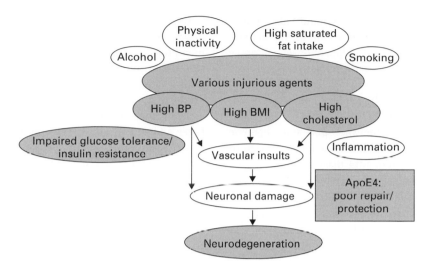

Figure 14.2 Possible processes for the development of AD and dementia.

variability in the amount of cognitive reserve between persons could be both genetic and due to early life factors and/or a result of lifelong mental stimulation due to education, occupation, leisure time and other activities.

Methodological considerations

The commonly accepted diagnostic criteria for AD have their limitations, as they refuse the pathogenic participation of vascular factors a priori. This has an important influence on the analysis of risk factors involved in AD. For example, stroke is one of the diagnostic criteria for VaD and generally excludes a diagnosis of AD, which may result in a negative association between the risk factors for stroke and AD. In addition, as the current diagnostic criteria for dementia focus on the later stages of cognitive impairment and are heavily biased toward the diagnosis of AD, the accuracy of clinical AD diagnosis in epidemiological studies has often been questioned. However, in many of the recent epidemiological studies, participants underwent detailed and structured clinical and differential diagnostic procedures, and many such studies also included neuroimaging methods. It is important to notice that, while neuroimaging can detect vascular lesions, the significance of these lesions may be difficult to determine, i.e., if they are a cause, a contributing factor, or just a coincidental finding in the dementia syndrome. Neuropathological examination, the golden diagnostic standard, is rarely available in epidemiological studies. Even when neuropathological information is available, interpretation of findings concerning the cause(s) of dementia is not totally free of problems (see below).

Clinical features: rethinking dementia diagnoses

The textbook clinical picture of AD includes a long preclinical phase and an insidious onset of dementia, while the classical description of cognitive decline due to vascular causes comprises a step-wise onset and course. There are indeed cases matching this traditional representation. However, vascular dementias constitute a pathologically and clinically heterogeneous group of disorders, and AD seems to be less homogenous than previously thought, which often makes the clinical distinction between AD and VaD a theoretical exercise with limited benefit for the patient. For example, identifying a date of onset will prove impossible in many cases; ministrokes affecting small subcortical vessels will probably lead to symptoms with gradual onset and slower progression, mimicking AD.

To acknowledge the fact that the cognitive effects of cerebrovascular disease can be significant even when dementia diagnostic criteria are not met, the term "vascular cognitive impairment" (VCI) was recommended instead of VaD. The transitional period between normal aging and dementia is also described as "mild cognitive impairment" (MCI). MCI was initially meant to represent prodromal AD, but it is now clear that persons with MCI constitute a highly heterogeneous group in terms of underlying pathology and clinical course. MCI is a state with high dementia risk, but not all MCI cases develop dementia, and those who do can progress to AD, VaD or other dementia types. The problems related to defining VCI and MCI therefore reflect the separation between the "vascular field" and the "Alzheimer field", from which the two concepts originated.

The association of AD and VaD has been recognized since the beginning of the last century and categorized as "mixed dementia". However, until recently, admitting the co-existence of AD and VaD in the same patient did not necessarily imply recognition of their interactions. The controversy in "mixed dementia" conceptualization is clearly reflected by the current lack of validated clinical criteria, generally accepted and validated neuropathologic guidelines and exact epidemiologic data. "Mixed dementia" seems to imply that the patient has both "AD symptoms" and "VaD symptoms", when in reality there is a high variability in the form and degree to which the degenerative and vascular components express themselves clinically. To make things even more confusing, the term "mixed dementia" is not reserved for the AD/VaD combination, and can be used to describe dementia resulting from any combination of pathologies (AD, VaD, vitamin B12 deficiency, hypothyroidism, etc.).

The issue of co-occurring AD and cerebrovascular disease was recently investigated in the Kungsholmen Project by retrospectively reclassifying dementias based on information concerning vascular disorders, and dementia onset and course (Aguero-Torres et al., 2006). Only 47% of the AD cases were reclassified as "pure" AD without any vascular disorder, and only 25% of VaD cases were reclassified as "pure" VaD. Furthermore, 26% of the "pure" AD cases developed a vascular disorder in the following three years. The study confirmed that vascular involvement is frequent in AD, and "pure" dementia types occur in a minority of very old subjects.

Pathology

Diagnostic issues

Besides the classical neuritic plaques and neurofibrillary tangles, Alzheimer's initial case (Auguste D) showed cerebral infarcts and endothelial changes, as well as atherosclerosis of the basal artery. However, the role of vascular lesions when neurodegenerative disorders and vascular changes coincide was discounted for a long time.

That the two types of pathologies can interact with each other was first clearly shown by findings from the Nun Study (Snowdon et al., 1997). Elderly nuns could carry a heavy load of typical AD changes without having cognitive impairment as long as they did not have, in addition, cerebrovascular lesions (CVLs). CVLs thus have the potential to tip the balance so that persons with AD pathology express a dementia syndrome. For the same degree of dementia severity, AD patients with CVLs can present a lower burden of degenerative lesions than "pure" AD cases. Also, in many individuals, a combination of minor AD-type and vascular pathologies may cause dementia, when these minor pathologies would not have done so individually, which indicates their synergistic effect.

Several clinical–pathologic studies have pointed out a low correspondence between clinical and neuropathologic diagnosis. Currently available clinical diagnostic criteria can detect pathology, but not "pure" pathology, and thus may fail to reflect the complexity of the underlying lesions. A high proportion of individuals fulfilling the neuropathological criteria for AD also have significant CVLs lesions, just like VaD cases diagnosed by current criteria can have considerable AD pathology at autopsy.

Two main issues concerning the diagnosis of "pure" AD or VaD are identifying the actual pathological burden and relating it to cognitive impairment. Although pathology protocols for AD-type changes have been renewed recently, no generally accepted criteria for VaD/VCI have been established to date. VaD can be related to variable types, sizes and locations of lesions (e.g. larger or smaller vessels) determined by a large variety of causes (e.g. emboli, thrombosis, amyloidosis, vasculitis). There are no available criteria for synthesizing a global "vascular pathology score" in cases with multiple pathologies (Jellinger, 2007). Also, relating structural changes to cognitive findings can be problematic, as CVLs and AD-type lesions can be present even in cognitively intact elderly.

Under these circumstances, diagnosing dementia of mixed etiology is unsurprisingly complicated. The main conceptual difficulty is considering concomitantly the type, location, and number of AD and vascular lesions, when the interactions and clinical significance of these lesions are still controversial. For example, some neuropathologists diagnose "mixed dementia" when there are enough vascular and degenerative lesions for AD and VaD diagnosis to be made independently, whereas others require only the presence of any ischemic lesion associated with severe AD pathology. Although there is a general consensus regarding the negative impact of large macrovascular lesions on cognition, the role of lacunes and microvascular lesions, such as microscopic infarcts and demyelination is controversial. Minor cerebrovascular lesions appear not essential for cognitive decline in full-blown AD, while both mild AD pathology and small-vessel disease may interact synergistically. Although infarct location, size and numbers are important, other factors, such as age, systemic disease, other brain lesions, and level of education, are involved in determining intellectual decline (Jellinger, 2007).

Nowadays, neuroimaging methods allow the easy detection of CVLs long before autopsy, but they do not necessarily make the identification of causal relationships with cognition easier. However, it has to be kept in mind that the causality requirement for CVLs usually starts from the assumption that cognitive deficits rely on the focal impact of the lesion, when this may not always be the case. An alternative viewpoint is that CVLs merely signal a "brain at risk". For example, it has been shown that cortical metabolic dysfunction can be seen in relation to neuroimaged subcortical infarction, even in the absence of cortical infarction demonstrable by MRI (Rockwood, 2006). Neuropathological parameters other than lesions may thus determine cognitive performance. Mean microvessel diameters (e.g. in entorhinal cortex and CA1 region of hippocampus) have been suggested as independent predictors of cognitive status in old individuals. Moving away from the classical link between lesion development and loss of function, these new data suggest that *microvascular integrity*, which is closely related to the adaptive capacities of the brain, may be an important determinant of cognition (Giannakopoulos *et al.*, 2007).

Behind AD and vascular lesions: some interaction mechanisms

Cerebrovascular structure is profoundly altered in AD. AD patients can have atherosclerosis in large cerebral arteries at the base of the brain (circle of Willis) and in extracranial vessels supplying the brain. It is increasingly recognized that several pathogenic mechanisms promoting atherosclerosis (e.g. oxidative stress, inflammation, immune responses) may also contribute to neurodegenerative diseases. Moreover, atherosclerosis has been associated with increased frequency of neuritic plaques (Honig *et al.*, 2005). One possible mechanism is through cerebral infarcts which influence β-amyloid processing (see below), although additional mechanisms may exist.

Cerebral amyloid angiopathy (CAA) is also present in vessels of persons with AD, and has been associated with microbleeds. In addition, the number of cerebral microvessels is reduced, endothelial cells are flattened, smooth muscle cells are modified, and there is basement membrane pathology, with β-amyloid deposits in the microvascular wall (Girouard and Iadecola, 2006).

Cerebrovascular dysfunction is also present in persons with AD. Resting cerebral blood flow (CBF) is reduced, and the increase in CBF produced by activation is attenuated, and β-amyloid seems to be one of the factors involved in CBF dysregulation. Most of the deleterious effects of β-amyloid were initially attributed to the form deposited in plaques, but more recent data indicate that soluble β-amyloid oligomers may actually be the culprit. β-Amyloid has long been known to have neurotoxic and pro-inflammatory properties. However, a growing body of evidence indicates that it also has profound effects on blood vessels, causing vasoconstriction and attenuating acetylcholine-induced vasodilatation. Neurons, glia and vascular cells act as an integrated unit which maintains the homeostasis of the brain's microenvironment, and β-amyloid-induced dysfunction of this unit can result in vascular dysregulation. In turn, ischemia may upregulate APP and β-amyloid cleavage. Vascular dysfunction can affect β-amyloid trafficking across the BBB, reducing the rate of β-amyloid clearance from the brain (Girouard and Iadecola, 2006). These two processes reinforce each other, and vascular dysregulation becomes more pronounced as the disease progresses. This connection between ischaemia and Aβ is a possible explanation for the fact that co-occurrence of ischemic lesions and AD pathology aggravates dementia. It remains to be established whether neurofibrillary tangles also contribute to vascular dysregulation and, if so, the mechanism through which they exert their effect.

Resting CBF reductions observed in AD may not be sufficient to produce acute ischemic injury. However, cerebral protein synthesis (which is crucial for learning, memory, and for normal cognitive functioning) is susceptible to reductions in CBF (Girouard and Iadecola, 2006). Also, due to an altered cerebrovascular autoregulation, reduced arterial pressure (for example, during sleep, induced by drugs, or cardiac failure) might result in reductions in CBF severe enough to cause ischemic cell injury. Recurrent ischemia in susceptible territories such as deep white matter could explain the frequent occurrence of WML in patients with AD.

Cholinergic mechanisms also play a role in the modulation of regional blood flow in the brain. The cholinergic system and CBF appear to be linked in a reciprocal manner: CBF changes may affect central cholinergic neurons, and unimpaired cholinergic function is necessary to regulate regional CBF. Cholinergic deficits have been shown in both AD and VaD, and the ChAT activity deficit is more pronounced in patients diagnosed with mixed dementia, AD and VaD, (Roman and Kalaria, 2006).

Although research has moved ahead considerably since the days of Alois Alzheimer, the question of the very essence of AD still remains to be answered. Ironically, the view that AD is actually a vascular disorder has (re)emerged in recent years (de la Torre, 2002). It is also interesting that soluble β-amyloid and tau proteins (usually associated with AD) have been identified by immunocytochemical methods in a high proportion of VaD cases, even when conventional histopathological analysis did not reveal classical AD pathology (Kalaria, 2002). Thus, it can be hypothesized that the β-amyloid-driven neurodegenerative process may predominate in some cases, while in others ischemia may be the main pathogenic process. However, the more the disease progresses and the pathological changes interact and accumulate, the harder it becomes to disentangle the degenerative and vascular components and to identify the "true cause".

Practical implications for treatment and prevention

Attempting to sharply distinguish between AD and VaD may lead to an oversimplification of reality.

Instead of trying to decide whether to apply the "AD" or "VaD" tag on a patient, more efforts should be made to try to identify all etiopathogenic factors involved. As many studies have shown, mixed pathology is the rule, rather than the exception, in dementia. It is not yet known to what extent AD-type and vascular changes are coincidental, contributory or causal, but the concept of a dementia spectrum (from purely degenerative to combinations of AD type and vascular changes in different degrees to purely vascular) seems now more adequate than the previous dichotomy. Clearly, diagnostic criteria will have to be adjusted accordingly.

The classical view "vascular versus degenerative diseases" has strongly influenced dementia therapy, making it difficult to tailor treatments to the patients' various needs. If the diagnosis is VaD, there is a chance that cognition-directed treatment is overlooked, while if the diagnosis is AD, vascular changes may be overlooked. Therefore, therapeutic interventions aimed at a single dementia etiology might have only a limited efficacy.

At the moment there is no curative treatment for dementia and AD, and they already represent a major public health challenge. As life expectancy increases and more and more people live to a very old age, dementia prevalence is expected to increase dramatically. To influence the future occurrence of dementia diseases, effective preventive measures are required. During the past years, research has shown that modifiable risk factors do exist, as well as the means to deal with them on an individual level and in the general population. What is now necessary are practical tools for assessing dementia risk by taking into account the set of risk factors present in each individual, and for identifying individuals who can benefit from intensive lifestyle consultations and pharmacological interventions. Such tools are already available for predicting the risk of cardiovascular outcomes (e.g. the Framingham score) and diabetes, but they have only started to be formulated for dementia. Based on the data from the CAIDE study, we have recently developed the Dementia Risk Score, which includes easily measurable variables that are associated with the risk of dementia later in life (Kivipelto et al., 2006; Table 14.1). The risk score should be validated and further improved (e.g. by adding new variables) to increase its predictive value, but it can already be used as an educational tool to demonstrate the role of modifiable vascular factors in dementia syndrome.

Most dementias are and will remain late-life syndromes managed within geriatric specialties. However, AD has a long preclinical phase and the pathological changes begin quite early in adulthood, outside the classical age borders of geriatrics. Thus, as for many other chronic diseases, efficient prevention can only be achieved by taking a lifelong view of the disease.

Table 14.1 CAIDE dementia risk score. Probability of dementia in late life according to the risk score categories in middle age.

Risk factor		Points
Age	< 47 years	0
	47–53 years	3
	> 53 years	4
Education	> 10 years	0
	7–9 years	2
	< 9 years	3
Sex	Female	0
	Male	1
Blood pressure	< 140 mmHg	0
	> 140 mmHg	2
Body mass index	< 30 kg m^{-2}	0
	> 30 kg m^{-2}	2
Total cholesterol	< 6.5 mmol l^{-1}	0
	> 6.5 mmol l^{-1}	2
Physical activity	Yes	0
	No	1
Total score	Dementia risk (%)	
0–5	1.0	
6–7	1.9	
8–9	4.2	
10–11	7.4	
12–5	16.4	

REFERENCES

Aguero-Torres H, Kivipelto M, von Strauss E. Rethinking the dementia diagnoses in a population-based study: what is Alzheimer's disease and what is vascular dementia? A study from the Kungsholmen Project. *Dementia Geriatr Cogn Disord* 2006; **22**: 244–9.

Berchtold NC, Kesslak JP, Cotman CW. Hippocampal brain-derived neurotrophic factor gene regulation by exercise and the medial septum. *J Neurosci Res* 2002; **68**: 511–21.

Björkhem I. Crossing the barrier: oxysterols as cholesterol transporters and metabolic modulators in the brain. *J Int Med* 2006; **260**: 493–508.

Calon F, Lim GP, Yang F, *et al*. Docosahexaenoic acid protects from dendritic pathology in an Alzheimer's disease mouse model. *Neuron* 2004; **43**(5): 633–45.

Cedazo-Minguez A, Cowburn RF. Apolipoprotein E: a major piece in the Alzheimer's disease puzzle. *J Cell Mol Med* 2001; **5**: 254–66.

Colcombe, SJ, Kramer, AF, Erickson, KI, *et al*. Cardiovascular fitness, cortical plasticity, and aging. *Proc Natl Acad Sci USA* 2004; **101**(9): 3316–21.

de la Torre JC. Alzheimer disease as a vascular disorder: nosological evidence. *Stroke* 2002; **33**: 1152–62.

Ding J, Eigenbrodt ML, Mosley TH Jr, *et al*. Alcohol intake and cerebral abnormalities on magnetic resonance imaging in a community-based population of middle-aged adults: the Atherosclerosis Risk in Communities (ARIC) study. *Stroke* 2004; **35**(1): 16–21.

Fratiglioni L, Paillard-Borg S, Winblad B. An active and socially integrated lifestyle in late life might protect against dementia. *Lancet Neurol* 2004; **3**(6): 343–53.

Freund-Levi Y, Eriksdotter-Jonhagen M, Cederholm T, *et al*. Omega-3 fatty acid treatment in 174 patients with mild to moderate Alzheimer disease: OmegAD study: a randomized double-blind trial. *Arch Neurol* 2006; **63**(10): 1402–08.

Giannakopoulos P, Gold G, Kovari E, *et al*. Assessing the cognitive impact of Alzheimer disease pathology and vascular burden in the aging brain: the Geneva experience. *Acta Neuropathol (Berl)* 2007; **113**(1): 1–12.

Girouard H, Iadecola C. Neurovascular coupling in the normal brain and in hypertension, stroke, and Alzheimer disease. *J Appl Physiol* 2006; **100**(1): 328–35.

Gustafson D, Rothenberg E, Blennow K, Steen B, Skoog I. An 18-year follow-up of overweight and risk of Alzheimer disease. *Arch Intern Med* 2003; **163**: 1524–8.

Honig LS, Kukull W, Mayeux R. Atherosclerosis and AD. Analysis of data from the US National Alzheimer's Coordinating Center. *Neurology* 2005; **64**: 494–500.

Jellinger KA. The enigma of vascular cognitive disorder and vascular dementia. *Acta Neuropathol* 2007; **113** (4): 349–88.

Kalaria RN. Overlap with Alzheimer's disease. In: Erkinjuntti T, Gauthiers, eds. *Vascular Cognitive Impairment*. London: Martin Dunitz Ltd, 2002.

Kalaria RN, Ballard C. Overlap between pathology of Alzheimer disease and vascular dementia. *Alzheimer Dis Assoc Disord* 1999; Oct–Dec; **13** Suppl 3: S115–23.

Kivipelto M, Helkala E-L, Laakso MP, *et al*. Apolipoprotein E ε4 allele, elevated midlife total cholesterol level and high midlife systolic blood pressure are independent risk factors for late-life Alzheimer's disease. *Ann Intern Med* 2002; **137**: 149–55.

Kivipelto M, Ngandu T, Fratiglioni L, *et al*. Obesity and vascular risk factors at midlife and the risk of dementia and Alzheimer's disease. *Arch Neurol* 2005; **62**: 1556–60.

Kivipelto M, Ngandu T, Laatikainen T, Winblad B, Soininen H, Tuomilehto J. Risk score for prediction of dementia risk in 20 years among middle aged people: a longitudinal population based study. *Lancet Neurol* 2006; **9**: 735–41.

Kramer A, Hahn S, Cohen NJ, *et al*. Ageing, fitness and neurocognitive function. *Nature* 1999; **400**: 418–19.

Laitinen M, Ngandu T, Rovio S, *et al*. Fat intake at midlife and risk of dementia and Alzheimer's disease: a population-based study. *Dement Geriatr Cogn Disord* 2006; **22**: 99–107.

Launer LJ, Ross GW, Petrovitch H, *et al*. Midlife blood pressure and dementia: the Honolulu–Asia aging study. *Neurobiol Aging* 2000; **21**: 49–55.

Launer LJ, White LR, Petrovitch H, Ross GW, Curb JD. Cholesterol and neuropathologic markers of AD: a population-based autopsy study. *Neurology* 2001; **57**: 1447–52.

Libon DJ, Price CC, Heilman KM, Grossman M. Alzheimer's 'other dementia'. *Cognit Behav Neurol* 2006; **19**: 112–16.

Luchsinger JA, Mayeux R. Dietary factors and AD. *Lancet Neurol*, 2004; **3**: 579–87.

Martins IJ, Hone E, Foster JK, *et al*. Apolipoprotein E, cholesterol metabolism, diabetes, and the convergence of risk factors for Alzheimer's disease and cardiovascular disease. *Molec Psychiatry* 2006; **11**: 721–36.

Mukamal KJ, Longstreth WT Jr, Mittleman MA, Crum RM, Siscovick DS. Alcohol consumption and subclinical findings on magnetic resonance imaging of the brain in older adults: the cardiovascular health study. *Stroke* 2001; **32**(9): 1939–46.

Oksman M, Iivonen H, Hogyes E, *et al.* Impact of different saturated fatty acid, polyunsaturated fatty acid and cholesterol containing diets on beta-amyloid accumulation in APP/PS1 transgenic mice. *Neurobiol Dis* 2006; **23**(3): 563–72.

Pappolla MA, Bryant-Thomas TK, Herbert D, *et al.* Mild hypercholesterolemia is an early risk factor for the development of Alzheimer amyloid pathology. *Neurology* 2003; **61**(2): 199–205.

Peila R, White LR, Masaki K, Petrovitch H, Launer LJ. Reducing the risk of dementia: efficacy of long-term treatment of hypertension. *Stroke* 2006; **37**(5): 1165–70.

Qiu WQ, Folstein MF. Insulin, insulin-degrading enzyme and amyloid-β peptide in Alzheimer's disease: review and hypothesis. *Neurobiol Aging* 2006; **27**: 190–8.

Roman GC, Kalaria RN. Vascular determinants of cholinergic deficits in Alzheimer disease and vascular dementia. *Neurobiol Aging* 2006; **27**: 1769–85.

Rockwood K. The mixed dementias. In: Erkinjuntti T, Gauthiers, eds. *Vascular Cognitive Impairment*. London: Martin Dunitz Ltd, 2002.

Rockwood K. Epidemiological and clinical trials evidence about a preventive role for statins in Alzheimer's disease. *Acta Neurol Scand Suppl* 2006; **185**: 71–7.

Rovio S, Ka?reholt I, Helkala E-L, *et al.* Leisure time physical activity at midlife and the risk of dementia and Alzheimer's disease. *Lancet Neurol* 2005; **4**: 705–10.

Scarmeas N, Stern Y, Mayeux R, Luchsinger JA. Mediterranean diet, Alzheimer disease, and vascular mediation. *Arch Neurol* 2006; **63**(12): 1709–17.

Skoog I, Lernfelt B, Landahl S, *et al.* 15-year longitudinal study of blood pressure and dementia. *Lancet* 1996; **347**: 1141–5.

Simons M, Schwarzler F, Lutjohann D, *et al.* Treatment with simvastatin in normocholesterolemic patients with Alzheimer's disease: a 26-week randomized, placebo-controlled, double-blind trial. *Ann Neurol* 2002; **52**: 346–50.

Snowdon DA, Greiner LH, Mortimer JA, *et al.* Brain infarction and the clinical expression of Alzheimer disease. *JAMA* 1997; **277**: 813–17.

Solomon A, Ka?reholt I, Ngandu T, *et al.* Serum cholesterol changes after midlife and late-life cognition: 21-year follow-up study. *Neurology* 2007; **68**(10): 751–6.

Sparks DL, Scheff SW, Hunsaker JC 3rd, Liu H, Landers T, Gross DR. Induction of Alzheimer-like beta-amyloid immunoreactivity in the brains of rabbits with dietary cholesterol. *Exp Neurol* 1994; **126**(1): 88–94.

Sparks DL, Sabbagh MN, Connor DJ, *et al.* Atorvastatin for the treatment of mild to moderate Alzheimer disease: preliminary results. *Arch Neurol* 2005; **62**: 753–7.

Stewart R, White LR, Xue QL, Launer LJ. Twenty-six-year change in total cholesterol levels and incident dementia: the Honolulu–Asia Aging Study. *Arch Neurol* 2007; **64**(1): 103–07.

Tong L, Shen H, Perreau VM, Balazs R, Cotman CW. Effects of exercise on gene-expression profile in the rat hippocampus. *Neurobiol Dis* 2001; **8**: 1046–56.

Whitmer RA, Sidney S, Selby J, Johnston SC, Yaffe K. Midlife cardiovascular risk factors and risk of dementia in late life. *Neurology* 2005; **64**(2): 277–81.

Treatment

15

Treatment of cognitive changes

Serge Gauthier and Timo Erkinjuntti

Introduction

Cerebrovascular disease (CVD) frequently contributes to cognitive loss in patients with Alzheimer's disease (AD). Progress in understanding the pathogenesis of vascular dementia (VaD) has resulted in promising symptomatic and preventive treatments of these conditions. Cholinergic deficits associated with VaD are due to ischemia of cholinergic pathways and can be treated with the use of the cholinesterase inhibitors (ChEI): controlled clinical trials with donepezil, galantamine, and rivastigmine in VaD, as well as galantamine in patients with AD with CVD, have demonstrated improvement in cognition and other symptomatic domains discussed in the next two chapters of this book. The use of the NMDA receptor antagonist, memantine, has also demonstrated symptomatic benefit in VaD in comparison to placebo. This chapter will review available evidence for a cognitive improvement associated with ChEI and memantine in VaD and AD with CVD. Although there is much interest in the pre-dementia or prodromal stage of VaD (also referred to in the literature as Vascular Mild Cognitive Impairment), there is as yet no standard treatment other than secondary prevention of stokes. Thus only cognitive changes associated with the dementia stage of VaD are discussed in this chapter.

Issues in the measurement of cognition in VaD

Randomized clinical trials in VaD have closely used the instruments from AD trials as recommended by the United States Food and Drug Administration (FDA) regulatory specifications (Sawada and Whitehouse, 2002). The instruments adopted as primary outcome measures for the current generation of clinical trials include the cognitive portion of the Alzheimer's Disease Assessment Scale (ADAS-Cog; Rosen et al., 1984). The European Commission for Medicinal and Pharmaceutical Compounds (CPMC) mostly requires positive impact on cognition and ADL and a responder analysis. To the extent that ADAS-cog and global measures such as the CIBIC-plus have proved to be sensitive in cholinergic AD trials, and since the cholinergic hypothesis is being endorsed in VaD (Roman and Kalaria, 2006), it is not unreasonable to use the same measures in both patient populations (Ferris and Gauthier, 2002). Furthermore, the VADAS-cog has been proposed by Ferris as an ADAS-cog with additional items sensitive to executive dysfunction. The heterogeneity of pathology in VaD will impact on the nature and severity of cognitive changes, and a higher variance in the measurement of cognitive changes should be expected compared to AD, whatever instrument is used to measure these changes.

Vascular Cognitive Impairment in Clinical Practice, ed. Lars-Olof Wahlund, Timo Erkinjuntti and Serge Gauthier. Published by Cambridge University Press. © Cambridge University Press 2009.

Cholinergic dysfunction in vascular dementia

A cholinergic deficit has been demonstrated in VaD, independently of any concomitant AD pathology (Roman and Kalaria, 2006). Cholinergic structures are vulnerable to ischemic damage. For instance, hippocampal CA1 neurons are particularly susceptible to experimental ischemia, and hippocampal atrophy is common in patients with VaD in the absence of AD (Gottfries *et al.*, 1994; Vinters *et al.*, 2000). Selden *et al.* (1998) described two highly organized and discrete bundles of cholinergic fibers in human brains that extend from the nucleus basalis to the cerebral cortex and amygdala. Both pathways travel in the white matter, and together carry widespread cholinergic input to the neocortex. Localized strokes may interrupt these cholinergic bundles (Swartz *et al.*, 2003). Mesulam *et al.* (2003) demonstrated cholinergic denervation from pathway lesions, in the absence of AD, in a young patient with CADASIL, a pure genetic form of VaD, and Keverne *et al.* have described similar findings in nine additional CADASIL cases (Keverne *et al.*, 2007).

In experimental rodent models, such as the spontaneously hypertensive stroke-prone rat, there is a significant reduction in cholinergic markers including acetylcholine (ACh) in the neocortex, hippocampus and cerebrospinal fluid (CSF) (Togashi *et al.*, 1994). In human disease, there is a reported loss of cholinergic neurons in 70% of AD cases and in 40% of VaD patients examined neuropathologically, and reduced ACh activity in the cortex, hippocampus, striatum, and CSF (Court *et al.*, 2002).

Evidence for the efficacy of cholinesterase inhibitors in VaD and AD with CVD

Donepezil and rivastigmine have been studied using randomized clinical trials in VaD and galantamine in a mixed population of VaD and AD with CVD.

The safety and efficacy of *donepezil* has been studied in three large, 24-weeks randomized placebo-controlled clinical trials of VaD, two fully reported (Black *et al.*, 2003; Wilkinson *et al.*, 2003) and 1 concluded last year. The first 2 studies had a pooled analysis reported by Roman *et al.* (2005), for a total of 1219 subjects. The patients were randomized to one of three groups: placebo, donepezil at a dosage of 5 mg per day or donepezil, 10 mg per day. The group receiving 10 mg per day initially received 5 mg per day for 4 weeks; the dosage was then titrated up to 10 mg per day. Patients with a diagnosis of either possible or probable VaD according to the NINDS-AIREN criteria were eligible for inclusion in the study. All patients had brain imaging prior to the study (CT or MRI) with demonstration of relevant cerebrovascular lesions. Patients with pre-existing AD were excluded, as were AD with CVD patients. Although patients with concomitant AD may not be totally excluded, the NINDS-AIREN criteria are able to classify patients into probable or possible VaD categories.

Probable VaD was present in 73% of the patients in the two studies. Probable VaD was diagnosed by the presence of mild to moderate dementia, clinical and brain imaging evidence of relevant CVD, and a clear temporal relationship between stroke and cognitive decline, with onset of dementia within three months of a clinically eloquent stroke or a step-wise course. Possible VaD was diagnosed in cases with indolent onset of the cognitive decline, and accounted for 27% of the cases. Possible VaD included patients with silent stroke, extensive white matter disease, or an atypical clinical course. There were no differences in trial results between these two subgroups.

The endpoints included cognition measured with the ADAS-cog and the MMSE, global function as measured with the CIBIC-plus and the Sum of Boxes of the Clinical Dementia Rating (CDR-SB) and ADL as measured with Alzheimer's Disease Functional Assessment and Change Scale (ADFACS). The results of changes in cognitive measures will be summarized in this chapter: in one trial, the donepezil treatment group showed statistically significant improvement in cognitive functioning measured with the ADAS-cog; the mean changes from baseline score were: donepezil 5 mg per day, -1.90 ($p = 0.001$); donepezil 10 mg per day, -2.33 ($p < 0.001$). The MMSE also showed statistically significant improvement vs. placebo. In the second trial, the donepezil treatment group showed statistically significant improvement in cognitive functioning measured with the ADAS-cog; the mean changes from baseline score were: donepezil 5 mg per day, -1.65 ($p = 0.003$); donepezil 10 mg per day, -2.09 ($p = 0.0002$). The MMSE also showed statistically significant improvement vs. placebo.

Of interest, cognitive decline in untreated patients with VaD in these trials was less severe than in placebo-treated patients with AD during 24 weeks of study, using similar instruments. These differences were also notable for their global impact, measured by the CIBIC-plus version; and, in contrast with AD, patients with VaD showed improvements in global function. In contrast with AD trials, these VaD studies enrolled more men than women (58% vs. 38%), their mean age was older (74.5±0.2 vs. 72±0.2 yrs), their Hachinski score more elevated (6.6±0.2 vs. < 4), with higher percentages of subjects with hypertension, cardiovascular disease, diabetes, smoking, hypercholesterolemia, previous stroke and transient ischemic attacks, suggesting that the two populations are clearly different.

Donepezil was generally well tolerated, although more adverse effects were reported in the 10 mg group than in the 5 mg or placebo groups. The adverse effects were assessed as mild to moderate and transient, and were typically diarrhea, nausea, arthralgia, leg cramps, anorexia, and headache. The incidence of bradycardia and syncope was not significantly different from the placebo group. The discontinuation rates for the groups were 15% for placebo, 18% for 5 mg, and 28% for the 10 mg group. There was no significant interaction with the numerous cardiovascular medications and antithrombotic agents used by this patient population. In the partially reported third study, there

was an imbalance for deaths of any case in favor of placebo; no obvious explanation has been found, and a pooled analysis of mortality in AD and in VaD showed no imbalance for any of the ChEI (Lon Schneider, unpublished data).

Galantamine is a cholinesterase inhibitor that also modulates central nicotinic receptors to increase cholinergic neurotransmission. A randomized, double-blind, controlled clinical trial studied patients diagnosed with probable VaD, or with AD combined with CVD, who received galantamine 24 mg per day ($n = 396$) or placebo ($n = 196$) over 6 months (Erkinjuntti *et al.*, 2002). Eligible patients met the clinical criteria of probable VaD by NINDS-AIREN criteria, or of possible AD according to the NINCDS-ADRDA criteria. They also showed significant radiological (CT/MRI) evidence of CVD (i.e., AD *plus* CVD). Evidence of CVD on a recent (within 12 months) scan included multiple large-vessel infarcts or a single, strategically placed infarct (angular gyrus, thalamus, basal forebrain, territory of the posterior or anterior cerebral artery), or at least two basal ganglia and white matter lacunae, or white matter changes involving at least 25% of the total white matter. The MMSE score was 10–25 and 12 or more in the ADAS-cog/11; age ranged from 40 to 90 years.

Primary endpoints were cognition, as measured using the ADAS-cog/11, and global functioning as measured using the CIBIC-plus. Secondary endpoints included assessments of ADL, using the Disability Assessment in Dementia, and behavioral symptoms, using the Neuropsychiatric Inventory. The analyses of both groups as a whole showed that galantamine demonstrated efficacy on all outcome measures. In terms of cognition, galantamine showed greater efficacy than placebo on ADAS-cog (2.7 points, $p \leq 0.001$). In an open-label extension, the original galantamine group with probable VaD or AD with CVD showed similar sustained benefits in terms of maintenance of or improvement in cognition (Erkinjuntti *et al.*, 2003).

Probable VaD was diagnosed in 81 (41%) of the placebo patients and in 171 (43%) of those on galantamine. In the probable VaD group, ADAS-cog scores improved significantly (mean change from baseline, 2.4 points, $p < 0.0001$) in patients treated with galantamine for 6 months, but not with placebo (mean change from baseline, 0.4; treatment difference vs. galantamine 1.9, $p = 0.06$); this difference appeared to be maintained at least up to 12 months, demonstrating a mean change of -2.1 in the ADAS-cog score compared to baseline, and the active group was still close to baseline at 24 months.

Rivastigmine is an acetylcholinesterase and butyrylcholinesterase inhibitor. The effects of rivastigmine in the treatment of cognitive impairment associated with VaD remain to be established. In a small open-label study of patients with subcortical VaD, rivastigmine improved cognition (clock-drawing test), reduced caregiver stress and improved behavior (Moretti *et al.*, 2001, 2002; Erkinjuntti *et al.*, 2002). AD patients with vascular risk factors showed a relatively larger effect size in cognitive response (ADAS-cog) than those without vascular risk factors.

Evidence for the efficacy of memantine in VaD

Memantine is a moderate-affinity, voltage-dependent, uncompetitive NMDA receptor antagonist with fast receptor kinetics. Initial data from a double-blind, placebo-controlled nursing home trial in severe dementia of mixed etiology (51% of patients had VaD) showed that memantine (10 mg per day) was well-tolerated, improved function, and reduced care dependency in treated patients with severe dementia, compared to patients on placebo (Winblad and Porotis, 1999). Based on the hypothesis of glutamate-induced neurotoxicity in cerebral ischemia, two randomized, placebo-controlled 6-month trials have studied memantine (20 mg per day) in patients with mild to moderate probable VaD by NINDS-AIREN criteria.

In the MMM 300 study 147 patients were randomized to memantine and 141 to placebo (Orgogozo *et al.*, 2002). After 28 weeks, the mean ADAS-cog scores were significantly improved relative to placebo: the memantine group mean score had gained an average of 0.4 points, whereas the placebo group mean score declined by 1.6, i.e., a difference of 2.0 points ($p = 0.0016$).

In the MMM 500 study, 277 patients were randomized to memantine and 271 to placebo (Wilcock *et al.*, 2002). At 28 weeks the active group had gained 0.53 points and the placebo declined by 2.28 points in ADAS-cog, a significant difference of 1.75 ADAS-cog points between the groups ($p < 0.05$). The MMSE did not reveal differences between the groups. Memantine was well-tolerated in the two studies. In a post-hoc pooled subgroup analysis of these two studies by baseline severity as assessed by MMSE, the more advanced patients obtained a larger cognitive benefit than did mildly affected patients. The subgroup with an MMSE score <15 at baseline showed an ADAS-cog improvement of 3.2 points over placebo (Möbius *et al.*, 2002). Sub-group analyses by radiological findings at baseline showed that the cognitive treatment effect for memantine was more pronounced in the small-vessel type group without cortical infarctions by CT or MRI. In addition, the placebo decline in this group was clearly more pronounced than in patients with (cortical) large-vessel type VaD.

Practical recommendations for use of ChEI and memantine for cognitive changes in VaD

Although there is as yet no regulatory approval for the specific indication of ChEI and memantine in VaD, these classes of drugs remain a therapeutic option to consider in patients where there is a suspicion of or evidence for a degenerative component to the dementia, which is likely the case for most patients over age 75 where the prevalence of "mixed AD–CVD" may very well be higher than AD and certainly of "pure VaD". Cognitive tests should be performed before treatment, preferable using those with an executive component, to be repeated at set intervals in the order of six months. These tests should be supplemented by questions on activities of daily living and behavior appropriate for the stage of dementia.

REFERENCE

Black S, Roman GC, Geldmacher DS, *et al.* Efficacy and tolerability of Donepezil in vascular dementia. Positive results of a 24-week, multicenter, international, randomized, placebo-controlled clinical trial. *Stroke* 2003; **34**: 2323–32.

Court JA, Perry EK, Kalaria RN. Neurotransmitter control of the cerebral vasculature and abnormalities in vascular dementia. In: Erkinjuntti T, Gauthier S, eds. *Vascular Cognitive Impairment.* London: Martin Duniz Ltd, 2002; 167–85.

Erkinjuntti T, Skoog I, Lane R, Andrews C. Rivastigmine in patients with Alzheimer's disease and concurrent hypertension. *Int J Clin Pract* 2002; **56**: 791–6.

Erkinjuntti T, Kurz A, Small GW, *et al.* An open-label extension trial of galantamine in patients with probable vascular dementia and mixed dementia. *Clin Therap* 2003; **25**: 1765–82.

Ferris S, Gauthier S. Cognitive outcome measures in vascular dementia. In: Erkinjuntii T, Gauthier S, eds. *Vascular Cognitive Impairment.* London: Martin Duniz Ltd, 2002; 395–400.

Gottfries CG, Blennow K, Karlsson I, Wallin A. The neurochemistry of vascular dementia. *Dementia* 1994; **5**: 163–7.

Keverne JS, Low WCR, Ziabreva I, Court JA, Oakley AE, Kalaria RN. Cholinergic neuronal deficits in CADASIL. *Stroke* 2007; **38**: 188–91.

Mesulam M, Siddique T, Cohen B. Cholinergic denervation in a pure multi-infarct state: observations on CADASIL. *Neurology* 2003; **60**: 1183–5.

Möbius HJ, Stöffler A. New approaches to clinical trials in vascular dementia: Memantine in small vessel disease. *Cerebrovasc Dis* 2002; **13**(S2): 61–6.

Moretti R, Torre P, Antonello RM, Cazzato G. Rivastigmine in subcortical vascular dementia: a comparison trial on efficacy and tolerability for 12 months follow-up. *Eur J Neurol* 2001; **8**: 361–2.

Moretti R, Torre P, Antonello RM, Cazzato G, Bava A. Rivastigmine in subcortical vascular dementia: an open 22-month study. *J Neurol Sci* 2002; **203**: 141–6.

Roman GC, Wilkinson DG, Doody RS, *et al.* Donepezil in vascular dementia: combined analysis of two large-scale clinical trials. *Dement Geriatr Cogn Disord* 2005; **20**: 338–44.

Roman GC, Kalaria RJ. Vascular determinants of cholinergic deficits in Alzheimer disease and vascular dementia. *Neurobiol Aging* 2006; **27**: 1769–85.

Rosen WG, Mohs RC, Davis KL. A new rating scale for Alzheimer's disease. *Am J Psychiatry* 1984; **141**: 1356–64.

Orgogozo J-M, Rigaud A-S, Stöffler A, Möbius H-J, Forette F. Efficacy and safety of Memantine in patients with mild to moderate vascular dementia. A randomized, placebo-controlled trial (MMM 300). *Stroke* 2002; **33**: 1834–9.

Sawada T, Whitehouse PJ. Regulatory guidelines for anti-dementia drugs. In: Erkinjuntti T, Gauthier S, eds. *Vascular Cognitive Impairment.* London: Martin Duniz Ltd, 2002; 619–27.

Selden NR, Gitelman DR, Salamon-Murayama N, Parrsh TB, Mesulam MM. Trajectories of cholinergic pathways within the cerebral hemispheres of the human brain. *Brain* 1998; **121**: 2249 57.

Swartz RH, Sahlas DJ, Black SE, *et al.* Strategic involvement of cholinergic pathways and executive dysfunction: does location of white matter signal hyperdensities matter? *J Stroke Cerebrovasc Dis* 2003; **12**: 29–36.

Togashi H, Matsumoto K, Yoshida M. Neurochemical profiles in cerebrospinal fluid of stroke-prone spontaneously hypertensive rat. *Neurosci Lett* 1994; **166**: 117 20.

Vinters HV, Ellis WG, Zarow C, *et al.* Neuropathologic substrates of ischemic vascular dementia. *J Neuropathol Exp Neurol* 2000; **60**: 658–9.

Wilkinson D, Doody R, Helme R, *et al.* Donepezil in vascular dementia. A randomized, placebo-controlled study. *Neurology* 2003; **61**: 479–86.

Wilcock G, Möbius HJ, Stöffler A, on behalf of the MMM 500 group. A double-blind, placebo-controlled multicentre study of memantine in mild to moderate vascular dementia (MMM500). *Int Clin Psychopharmacol* 2002; **17**: 297–305.

Winblad B, Porotis N. Memantine in severe dementia: results of the 9M-Best Study. *Int J Geriatr Psychiatry* 1999; **14**: 135–46.

16

Treatment of functional decline

Lena Borell

Functional decline is most often referred to as the impaired ability to perform activities of daily living (ADL) including instrumental activities of daily living (IADL), motor and sensory status. Limited ability to perform ADL in vascular dementia should be seen as a result of several interacting circumstances, such as comorbid medical and psychiatric illness, barriers in the environment, and also from other family members (Nygård, 2006; Wimo *et al.*, 1999).

The well-defined concept of *disability* can be appropriate to apply in clinical work when we want to better understand functional decline in vascular dementia (Gauthier *et al.*, 1999). The ICF (*International Classification of Functioning, Disability and Health*; WHO, 2001) offers a model for classification of illness and disability. Figure 16.1 illustrates how disability phenomena are outcomes of interactions between the environment, the person and the health condition.

The World Health Organization (WHO) identified kinds of human functioning and developed a classification of Impairments, Disabilities and Handicaps (ICIDH; WHO, 1990) followed by a second generation, the ICF (WHO, 2001) for use in international research and clinical work world-wide. The ICF identifies three dimensions of human functioning.

(1) *Body function* or *structure*, physiological and psychological functions of body systems, and anatomical parts of the body, organs, limbs and their components.
(2) *Activity*, the execution of a task or action by an individual.
(3) *Participation*, involvement in a life situation.

The IFC provides a coding structure that identifies specific categories of functioning related to the three dimensions: (1) *impairments* of body function, (2) activity *limitations*, and (3) participation *restrictions*; all three can be observed and/or measured. The model also identifies environmental factors, features of the physical, the human built, the social and attitudinal world that may have an impact on activity limitations and participation restrictions. The choice of the ICF as a model in clinic work also has implications for the choice of assessment and measurements to identify limitations to the ability to perform ADL and other activity limitations.

It is interesting to note that in the case of vascular dementia the *body function/organ* in terms of subcortical neuropathology does not predict IADL impairment in the *activity and performance dimension* (Boyle *et al.*, 2004). These findings also demonstrate how *activity limitations* measured in ADL is a different construct compared to *functional impairments* in the body organs, and that there is

Vascular Cognitive Impairment in Clinical Practice, ed. Lars-Olof Wahlund, Timo Erkinjuntti and Serge Gauthier. Published by Cambridge University Press. © Cambridge University Press 2009.

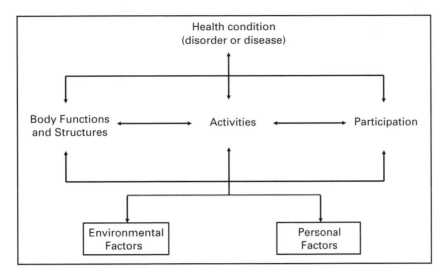

Figure 16.1 Interactions between the components of ICF.

no apparent causal relationship between the two. Therefore, measuring activity limitations is of great importance for treatment planning.

Activity limitations and participation restrictions in vascular dementia

A diagnosis of vascular dementia implies activity limitations and participation restrictions. Assessment and measurement of disability, functional abilities and decline is of importance for diagnosis, treatment planning, and the analysis of treatment outcomes in vascular dementia (Gauthier *et al.*, 1999).

Pohjasvaara *et al.* (2003) found the most significant clinical features in vascular dementia to be: apraxlic–atactic gait, impaired ADL functions, and depression. Several studies have demonstrated how cognitively complex activities included in IADL are affected by cognitive limitations, and how more basic and physical ADL activities are affected by cognitive and physical impairments together, for example, limitations in walking (Bennet, 2002).

It is common to find impaired function in memory functions among persons with vascular dementia. These impairments will clearly affect the individual's ability to independently manage activities in daily life (Wimo *et al.*, 1999). Research also suggests a difference between vascular dementia and dementia of Alzheimer's type when it comes to carrying out specific steps in some daily tasks (Giovannetti *et al.*, 2006). The cognitive impairment also affects the executive functioning of the individual; for example, initiation, planning and self-monitoring in daily living. These are all functions that enable the person to engage independently in complex everyday tasks.

Obviously, limitations will not only affect performance in daily living. The whole living situation for the individual and the family and friends will change dramatically after the onset of dementia.

The measure of ADL/IADL

Assessments of ADL/IADL are conducted through various techniques, most commonly through formal assessments, but also through observations and informal interviews (Miller and Butin, 2000; Tuokko and Morris, 1999).

It has been discussed whether the person with dementia performs better in a familiar environment such as the home, and if there is a difference compared to a clinical setting. Research examining the impact of different environments on outcome in assessment and intervention has demonstrated mixed findings (Nygård, 1998; Ward et al., 1990). Nygård (1998) suggests that assessment should take place in the environment where the person is actually living (home vs. clinic).

Research suggests that persons in the early stages of dementia can report in interviews on what they find most important in daily living, but find it harder to reflect on the consequences of the disease in daily life (Nygård, 2006). Findings from research suggest that conducting interviews with, and observations of, the person with dementia is recommended in order to get the best type of knowledge about activity limitations and participation restrictions. To invite a client to report about his/her interest could also be a way of getting to know the client better.

Cotter et al. (2002) investigated whether caregivers of persons with dementia give valid reports of the level of patients' ADL and the amount of time they spend providing ADL assistance. Findings from these studies suggest that caregiver reports of ADL assistance should be used with caution, since caregivers could overestimate the time they provide assistance.

The importance of using standardized measures should be stressed, although measures in terms of naturalistic descriptions of ADL/IADL abilities are common in practice. When standardized measures are applied in the clinic, included key concepts are most often well-defined, and it is possible to repeat and measure an individual over time. Another great advantage in standardized measures is that the results are easy to transfer and interpret. When applying an ADL measure, it is also of importance to pay attention to floor and ceiling effects in the measure. An ADL measure used in the early

detection of disability might not be relevant for use later or when the individual is more severely off in the disease (Nygård, 2004). It is also a well-known problem in the rehabilitation of persons with dementia that ADL/IADL scales can be more sensitive to physical disabilities than to the cognitive dimension of performance, which causes a problem for clinicians in choosing relevant measures of ADL. Consultations with occupational therapists are recommended on the choice of approach to measure ADL (Borell, 1992).

ADL/IADL assessments are developed with different purposes. For example, the Katz ADL index was developed to measure burden of care and to identify needs of assistance. In research including persons with vascular dementia, the Lawton (1971) scale for measurement of IADL is one of the most common measures of limitations in activities of daily living (Bennett et al., 2002; Pohjasvaara et al., 2003). Gitlin et al. (2002) developed a measure focusing on the interaction between a person with dementia and the environment, including, for example, safety issues in the home environment, overall ability, and ability to orient and overall well-being in the environment.

The choice of measure for ADL outcomes in therapeutic drug studies has been discussed by Gauthier et al. (1999), who recommended the use of ADL scales developed for therapeutic research in Alzheimers' disease in the care and research of patients with vascular dementia.

Rehabilitation interventions

Rehabilitation with the aim to maintain an optimum level of physical, psychological and social functioning will facilitate participation in preferred activities and social roles (WHO, 2007). Rehabilitation goals for persons suffering from vascular dementia necessarily need to change over time, due to the severity of the problem. At one point in time, it will not be possible to regain function, just to make efforts to maintain function and to compensate for the loss of function.

The underpinning idea in rehabilitation is that practice of daily activities has the potential to improve and/or maintain functioning. Dependency upon other people is often the result of activity limitations, and dependency is often seen as the main factor affecting health-related quality of life (Wimo *et al.*, 1999). Support for compensating and, if possible, overcoming memory problems can be important in the early stages of dementia.

Even though the consequences of vascular dementia lead to long-term care in institutions in many cases, it is of great importance for the general level of health to stay physically and socially active. Studies have demonstrated how it is possible in vascular dementia to increase the general level of functional fitness and reduce disability through, for example, taking daily walks (Singh, 2002; Yaffe *et al.*, 2001). To make use of physical and cognitive capacity will enable the person to keep his/her abilities for a longer time. The actual doing of a number of taken-for-granted things when living at home, such as taking care of one's hygiene, dressing and preparing food, are then to be carried out by the individual himself/herself as long as possible in order to postpone hospitalization (Corcoran and Gitlin, 1992; Gitlin *et al.*, 2001).

The most important aspect for planning a successful intervention to support a person with dementia to maintain functions needed in independent daily living, is knowledge about the person's own motivation (Kielhofner *et al.*, 2002). Rehabilitation efforts should support the individual to keep his/her roles and habits. This includes the identification of realistic goals for the maintenance of memory skills and cognitive abilities in daily life.

Cognitive rehabilitation intends to help people with cognitive impairments to identify personally relevant goals and devices (Wilson *et al.*, 2001). The emphasis is not on enhancing performance on cognitive tasks; instead, the function in an everyday context is the focus for therapy. To be unable to handle and use the telephone or understand how to make use of a remote control for the TV are common consequences of impaired memory. At this point, the individual can be helped by developing a few simple strategies for reminding one's self (Nygård, 2003).

Treatment for family members

Family members are always involved in caregiving for people with dementia living at home. Still, there a few descriptions of good support programs directed to family members who are taking care of, for example, a spouse.

Hence, formal caregivers can provide support for the primary caregivers in several ways. One option for the professionals is to provide home environmental skill-building programs (Gitlin *et al.*, 2005) and coaching for family members in everyday tasks (Josephsson *et al.*, 1993; Vikström *et al.*, 2005). Especially in the early phases of dementia, educational efforts might be beneficial for spouses or for family caregivers (Clare *et al.*, 2003; Gitlin *et al.*, 2001). These educational efforts could include guidance in problematic everyday activities, and would typically include environmental modifications.

Besides home-based interventions, there is also a need to provide other types of care and support for people with a dementing disease. For example, there is the need for daycare and or a short-term stay in a nursing home, so the spouse or family gets a chance to rest for some time.

The National (American) Alzheimer's Association (1997) proposed an approach to support family caregivers which includes efforts on (1) the environmental design; to be simple and easy to understand, (2) policies and procedures; for example, reduced expectation of perfection, and (3) individual staff action; for example, prompt and assist when needed.

Technology developments to support function

Environmental modifications are in general recommended by professionals so that people with disabilities can choose to remain in their homes for a longer time. Still, with a huge population of older adults and persons suffering from cognitive problems such as dementia, the designers of new products need to pay attention to persons with cognitive impairments.

Until recently, home modifications have focused just on the physical environment with the goal, for example, to ease transfer in the home and increase mobility. Assistive technology, such as digital calendars, adaptable watches, and locators (finds lost objects) for people with cognitive deficits has rapidly developed, although their usability has been little researched. Recently, technology for people with dementia has been successfully designed in an EU project (www.enableproject.org), and examples of clinical cases have been published (Nygård, 2006). These studies demonstrated that aspects such as the user's motivation, the adaptability of the technology and the support from the environment are crucial for successful use in people with dementia.

New technology needs to be adaptable to the individual's needs, and introduced early after the onset of cognitive decline. In order to be useful, technology needs to be incorporated in the user's everyday life, and this process involves learning and adaptation.

However, of special interest for the future is the provision of cognitive support through "built-in-the-home ICT". There is still a lack of evidence to support provision of IT-based support in the home in terms of modifications in the environment. Still, the time is ripe to learn more about the new possibilities provided by technology developments to support persons with vascular dementia.

Summary

Functional decline is often referred to as the impaired ability to perform activities of daily living. Vascular dementia is associated both with activity limitations and with participation restrictions. The limitations will affect the individual's ability to independently manage activities in daily life. The *International Classification of Functioning, Disability and Health* (ICF) introduced in this chapter offers a model for classification of disability related to vascular dementia. Rehabilitation with the aim of maintaining an optimum level of physical, psychological and social functioning will facilitate participation in preferred activities and social roles among persons who suffer from vascular dementia.

REFERENCES

Bennet HP, Corbett A, Gaden S, Grayson D, Kril J, Broe GA. Subcortical vascular disease and functional decline, a 6 year predictor study. *J Am Geriatr Soc* 2002; **50**: 1969–77.

Borell L. The activity life of people with dementia. Dissertation, Karolinska Institutet, 1992.

Boyle P, Paul RH, Mose DJ and Cohen RA. Executive impairments predict functional declines in vascular dementia. *Clin Neuropsychol* 2004; **18**: 75–82.

Clare L, Woods RT, Moniz Cook ED, Orell M, Spector A. Cognitive rehabilitation and cognitive training for early stage Alzheimer's disease and vascular dementia. *The Cochrane Database of Systematic Reviews* 2003, issue 4. Art no. CD003260.DOI:10.1002/14651858 .CD003260.

Corcoran M, Gitlin L. Dementia management – an occupational therapy home based intervention for caregivers. *Am J Occup Ther* 1992; **46**(9): 801–08.

Cotter E, Burgio L, Stevens A, Gitlin L. Correspondence of the functional independence measure (FIM) self care subscale with real-time observations of dementia patients' ADL performance in the home. *Clin Rehab* 2002; **16**: 36–45.

Gauthier S, Rockwood K, Gelinas I, *et al.* Outcome measures for the study of activities of daily living in vascular dementia. *Alzheimers Dis Assoc Disord* 1999; **13** (Supp. 3): S143–7.

Giovannetti T, Schmidt K, Gallo J, Sestito N, Libon D. Everyday action in dementia: Evidence for differential deficits in Alzheimers disease versus subcortical vascular dementia. *J Int Neuropsychol Soc* 2006; **12**: 45–53.

Gitlin LN, Corcoran M, Winter L, Boyce A, Hauck W. A randomized controlled trial of a home environmental intervention; effect on efficacy and upset in caregivers and on daily function of persons with dementia. *The Gerontol* 2001; **41**(1): 4–14.

Gitlin LN, Schinfeld S, Winter L, Corcoran M, Boyce A, Hauck W. Evaluating home environments of persons with dementia: interrater reliability ad validity of the Home Environment Assessment Protocol (HEAP). *Disability Rehab* 2002; **24**(1/2/3): 59–71.

Gitlin, LN, Hauch W, Dennis MP, Winter L. Maintenance of effects of the home environmental skill-building program for family caregivers and individuals with Alzheimers disease and related disorders. *J Gerontol* 2005; **60A**(3): 368–74.

Josephsson S, Bäckman L, Borell L, Bernspång B, Nygård L, Rönnberg L. Supporting everyday activities in dementia; an intervention study. *Int J Geriatr Psychiatry* 1993; **8**: 395–400.

Kielhofner G, Borell L, Freidheim L, *et al.* Crafting occupational life. In: Kielhofner G, ed. *Model of human occupation*. Baltimore, MD: Lippincott Williams & Wilkins, 2002.

Lawton M. The functional assessment of elderly people. *J Am Geriatr Soc* 1971; **19**(6): 465–81.

Miller P, Butin D. The role of occupational therapy in dementia – C.O.P.E. (Caregiver Options for Practical Experiences). *Int J Geriatr Psychiatry*, 2000; **15**: 86–9.

National (American) Alzheimers Association, The. Key elements of dementia care. 1997. www.alz.org.

Nygård L. Assessing ADL/IADL in persons with dementia. In. Winblad B, Wimo A, Jönsson B, Karlsson G, eds. *The health economics of dementia*. Chichester: John Wiley & Sons Ltd, 1998.

Nygård L. Instrumental activities of daily living: A stepping stone towards Alzheimer's disease diagnosis in subjects with mild cognitive impairment? *Acta Neurol Scand* 2003; **107**(Suppl. 179): 42–6.

Nygård L. The responses of persons with dementia to challenges in daily activities: A synthesis of findings from empirical studies. *Am J Occup Therapy* 2004; **58**: 435–45.

Nygård L. How can we get access to the experiences of people with dementia? Suggestions and reflections. *Scand J Occup Therapy* 2006; **13**: 101–12.

Pohjasvaara T, Mäntylä R, Ylikoski R, Kaste M, Erikjuntti T. Clinical features of MRI defined subcortical vascular disease. *Alzheimers Dis Assoc Disord* 2003; **17**: 236–42.

Singh MA. Exercise come of age: Rationale and recommendations for a geriatric exercise prescription. *J Gerontol A Biol Med Sci* 2002; **57**: M262–82.

Tuokko H, Morris C, Ebert P. Mild cognitive impairment and everyday functioning in older adults. *Neurocase* 2005; **11**: 40–7.

Vikström S, Stigdotter-Neely A, Borell L, Josephsson S. Caregivers' self-initiated support towards their partners with dementia when performing an everday occupation together at home. *Occupation, Participation & Health* 2005; **25**(4): 149–59.

World Health Organisation (WHO). *International classification of impairments, disabilities, and handicaps*. Geneva: WHO, 1990.

World Health Organisation, WHO. ICF, *International classification of functioning, disability and health*. Geneva: WHO, 2001.

Wilson BA, Emslie HC, Quirk K, Evans JJ. Reducing everyday memory and planning problems by means of a paging system: A randomised control and crossover study. *J Neurol Neurosurg Psychiatry* 2001; **70**: 477–82.

Wimo A, Winblad B, Grafström M. The social consequences for families with Alzheimer's disease patients. Potential impact of new drug treatment. *Int J Geriatr Psychiatr* 1999; **14**: 338–47.

Yaffe K, Barnes D, Nevitt M, Lui LY, Covinsky K. A prospective study of physical activity and cognitive decline in elderly women: Women who walk. *Arch Intern Med* 2001; **161**: 1703–08.

Treatment of behavioral symptoms in vascular dementia

Catherine Cole and Alistair Burns

Introduction

Behavioral and psychological symptoms in vascular dementia (VaD) are common, and are now recognized as an integral part of the condition. These symptoms may constitute the greatest burden in dementia, being associated with diminished quality of life for both patient and carer (Finkel, 2000), referral to specialist services (Lawlor, 2002) and transfer to residential care (O'Donnell *et al.*, 1992). They also make a significant contribution to the financial cost of dementia (Finkel, 2000).

Defining and categorizing behavioral and psychological symptoms in dementia (BPSD)

BPSD are defined as "symptoms of disturbed perception, thought content, mood or behavior that frequently occur in patients with dementia" (Finkel *et al.*, 1997). The symptoms are divided into those usually assessed at the patient/carer interview (anxiety, depressed mood, hallucinations and delusions) and symptoms usually assessed by behavioral observation of the patient/relative (aggression, screaming, restlessness, agitation, wandering, culturally inappropriate behaviors, sexual disinhibition, hoarding, cursing and shadowing).

Epidemiology

BPSD are common in all types of dementia, and it has been estimated that up to 80% of patients will exhibit them at some point (Overshott and Burns, 2005). BPSD generally become more frequent as the severity of dementia increases (Swearer *et al.*, 1988), and tend to be observed most frequently among those patients in residential care settings (Kozman *et al.*, 2006).

Symptom profile may differ between types of dementia, suggesting a role for different etiological pathways in the emergence of symptoms, and indicating the possible need for alternative management strategies for different diagnoses (Chiu, 2003). One of the difficulties in establishing prevalence figures is that VaD represents a heterogeneous group of conditions, and BPSD may be more prevalent in some types of vascular dementia, e.g. small-vessel disease affecting the prefrontal–subcortical circuit (Cummings, 1994; Erkinjuntti *et al.*, 2000). Whereas particular symptoms seem to emerge and decline at predictable points during the clinical course of Alzheimer's disease (AD), there may be a less predictable symptom pattern in VaD (Purandare *et al.*, 2000), and symptoms may emerge abruptly (Rockwood and Shea, 2003). Some authors have found no significant differences in symptom profile between AD and VaD (Cohen *et al.*, 1993; Kunik *et al.*, 2000; Swearer *et al.*, 1988),

Vascular Cognitive Impairment in Clinical Practice, ed. Lars-Olof Wahlund, Timo Erkinjuntti and Serge Gauthier. Published by Cambridge University Press. © Cambridge University Press 2009.

and one study found the highest level of psychiatric disturbance in patients with mixed AD and VaD (Cohen *et al.*, 1993; Kozman *et al.*, 2006).

Mood disorders

There is a well-documented association between vascular disease and depressive symptoms (O'Brien, 2003a): 30–40% of stroke patients develop a major depressive episode. The prevalence of depression in VaD is around 13.1% in community settings, and 21.4% in clinical samples (Ballard, 1996a). It is associated with a past history of depression, a family history of depression, a lower level of education, longer hospital stay and delay in rehabilitation, social isolation and a larger volume of infarction (Ballard 1996a; O'Brien 2003a).

Various authors have found an increased prevalence or incidence of depressive symptoms in VaD compared with AD (Ballard *et al.*, 1996; Ballard *et al.*, 2000a; Cooper and Mungas, 1993; Groves *et al.*, 2000; Kozman *et al.*, 2006; Li *et al.*, 2001; Lyketsos *et al.*, 2000; Newman, 1999; Sultzer *et al.*, 1993). In patients with VaD, the prevalence of depressive symptoms is around 8–66% (mean 32%), compared to 20% in AD (Ballard and O'Brien, 2002; Ballard *et al.*, 1996).

Other mood disorders

Estimates for the prevalence of anxiety in VaD may depend on study setting, and range from 19% (Lyketsos *et al.*, 2000) to over 50% (O'Brien, 2003a). Most authors report similar levels of anxiety in AD and VaD (Erkinjuntti, 2000), but Ballard and colleagues (2000a) found a greater prevalence (71%) in VaD than in AD.

There are no prevalence studies for hypomania in VaD, but the prevalence is probably similar to that in AD, around 1% (Hope *et al.*, 1997; Lyketsos *et al.*, 2000; O'Brien, 2003a). Clinically, the patient may present with irritability, elation, restlessness, poor sleep, and sometimes inappropriate sexual behavior (Ballard and O'Brien, 2002).

Psychotic symptoms

Delusions occur in around a third of patients with dementia (Ballard and O'Brien, 2002) and may be more common in AD than VaD (Lyketsos *et al.*, 2000; O'Brien, 2003a; Pinto and Seethalakshmi, 2006) although some studies found no difference in prevalence between AD and VaD (Leroi *et al.*, 2003). Visual hallucinations are more common than auditory hallucinations in organic mental disorders, and may be more common in multi-infarct dementia (MID) than AD (Cohen *et al.*, 1993; Cummings, 1993; Purandare *et al.*, 2000). Visual hallucinations in AD may be related to the cholinergic deficit; there is also a cholinergic deficit in VaD, but it is not clear whether the same etiological pathways apply (O'Brien, 2003a). Patients with Lewy body dementia have a high prevalence of visual hallucinations which occur early and tend to persist (McKeith, 2006) (see Table 17.1).

Agitation and aggression

Agitation has been defined as "inappropriate verbal, vocal, or motor activity that is not explained by needs or confusion per se" (Cohen-Mansfield and Billig, 1986), and has been reported to occur in around 50% of patients with dementia (Tariot, 1999). Aggression occurs in 25–33% of patients with dementia (Tariot, 1999). It is the commonest cause of referral to specialist services, and the commonest cause of admission to residential care (Ballard and O'Brien, 2002; O'Brien, 2003a). The prevalence is probably similar in VaD and AD (Ballard and O'Brien, 2002).

Emotional lability

This has been described in patients following stroke, and may occur in over a quarter of patients with VaD (Lavretsky and Chui, 2006). It manifests as sudden episodes of crying or laughing, which

Table 17.1 Adapted from Ballard *et al.,* (2000a). Prevalence rates of psychosis in VaD and AD in 92 patients with VaD and 92 with AD. With permission from Elsevier.

	VaD%	AD%
1 month prevalence of psychotic symptoms	46	38
Delusions	36	28
Visual hallucinations	22	16
Auditory hallucinations	8	3
Delusional misidentification	23	17

In the above study, there were no significant differences in prevalence rates for psychotic symptoms between VaD and AD.

may occur in response to minor triggers, and are not under normal social control (O'Brien, 2003a). The patient does not exhibit other signs of depression.

Etiology

The precise mechanisms for development of BPSD in vascular dementia are unclear (Erkinjuntti, 2000). It has been postulated that different factors may operate in AD and VaD, suggesting that different treatment strategies may be appropriate for BPSD in different types of dementia (Chiu, 2003). Debate continues about to what degree BPSD may arise from focal lesions in specific areas, or be due to a more generalized effect of subcortical changes (Erkinjuntti *et al.*, 2000).

Patients with subcortical VaD often present with a syndrome of depressed mood, lability, dysexecutive syndrome and personality changes (Lind, 2002; Moretti *et al.*, 2006; Rockwood and Shea, 2003) and have evidence of lesions in the prefrontal–subcortical circuits, including the prefrontal cortex (Moretti *et al.*, 2006). Post-stroke depression may be more likely if there is involvement of the prefrontosubcortical circuits, espe-

cially on the left side (O'Brien *et al.*, 2003; Vataja *et al.*, 2001).

At an individual level, careful history-taking and assessment may reveal the etiology of the patient's behavior. For example, it is not uncommon for female patients in residential or daycare settings to become agitated mid-afternoon when they believe they must leave "to pick up the children from school". Pacing may be a response to lack of physical exercise, or boredom (Tariot, 1999). Disorientation in time and a need to make sense of an unpredictable world may lead to repetitive questioning of the carer. Too much stimulation, or too little, may increase agitation, as may pain, excess noise, or extremes of temperature (Tariot *et al.*, 1997). Agitation may also arise from depression, anxiety or psychosis (Howard *et al.*, 2001) and may be an appropriate response to a distressing environment (e.g. a very unsettled nursing home).

Assessment

1. Define the problem.
2. Review of patient's history.
3. Observation and mental state examination.
4. Physical examination.
5. Differential diagnosis.
6. Rating scales.
7. Investigations.
8. Carer response.

1. Define the problem

The first task for the clinician is to ascertain whether there is a problem, and who it is affecting. Some behavioral problems may be distressing for carers, but have little impact on the patient (Lawlor, 2002); indeed, some may even be comforting for the patient (Cohen-Mansfield, 2003), and reassurance for the carer may be all that is required. Carers cite aggression, sleep disturbance and paranoia as being among the most upsetting symptoms (O'Donnell *et al.*, 1992).

The process of defining and describing the problem may in itself be therapeutic (Tariot *et al.*, 1997), and apparently random behavior may, in fact, follow a predictable pattern. Is the behavior associated with any particular time of day, particular tasks, or the gender of the carer? Have there been recent important life events or changes of carer which might have coincided with the onset of the problem? Are there any clues to physical discomfort or changes in sensory impairment? Have there been any recent changes in medication? Some patients may respond better with lower levels of stimulation, and some may require more.

It is often helpful to know why the patient is presenting now; has there been a recent change of symptoms, or, for example, has the carer reached a point where they are unable to cope? An "ABC" approach (Antecedents – Behavior – Consequences) will provide some basic information, which may be expanded on by interviewing the patient and carers.

For psychotic symptoms, it is important to gain a precise description of the experiences, as this will have a bearing on treatment choices. What may appear to be delusions may, in fact, be the disorientated patient's attempts to make sense of his surroundings, rather than having the characteristics of persistent and unshakeable beliefs. Forgetful patients may accuse others of stealing the objects they have mislaid, and relatives and friends may be misidentified as impostors.

2. Review of patient's past medical history, current medication, physical history

It may be possible to gain some understanding of the symptoms in the context of the patient's personal history or narrative, and their pre-morbid personality. Many psychotropic drugs and medications for physical illnesses may contribute to BPSD, and polypharmacy associated with patients in residential care has been well-described. Is there any chronic or acute medical condition which could be contributing to the symptoms? Undiagnosed pain in patients with severe dementia may

be a factor in BPSD, and in some cases behavioral symptoms have been shown to respond to small doses of opioid analgesia.

3. Mental state examination

The clinician should observe the patient in their usual residential setting, and conduct an interview with the patient, making an assessment of appearance and behavior, speech, thoughts, mood, perceptions, cognition, and insight in the usual manner.

4. Physical examination

A brief physical examination will give information about general health, pulse, blood pressure, temperature, hydration, nutritional state, sensory impairments and mobility.

5. Differential diagnosis

Delirium is common in patients in residential care and in medical inpatients, and dementia is a risk factor for delirium. It must be excluded as a possible cause for the development of new BPSD, and treated accordingly. The clinician should keep in mind the common causes of delirium (infection, side effects of medication, metabolic disturbances, alcohol, etc., Tariot, 1999) and attempt to find a cause where possible. Symptoms and signs suggestive of delirium would include an acute onset, disorientation, disruption of the sleep–wake cycle, fluctuating course and change in psychomotor behavior (increased or decreased).

6. Rating scales

Standardized scales may be used to provide a baseline measure and to assess response to treatment. In choosing a scale, the clinician must be clear about what exactly is to be measured. Some scales may be useful for pragmatic, day-to-day use, and others may be better reserved for research. The time taken to administer the scale, whether it is carer-completed or observed by the clinician or nursing staff, its reported sensitivity to change and its applicability to various groups (e.g. different ethnic groups, patients with learning disability) will all inform the choice of scale (Teri *et al.*, 2002). Many of the commonly used scales were initially validated in AD, but appear to be valid in VaD (O'Brien *et al.*, 2003).

BPSD may be assessed using uni-dimensional scales such as the Cornell Scale for Depression in Dementia (Alexopoulos *et al.*, 1988), which measure a particular symptom, or a multi-dimensional scale such as the Behavioural Pathology in Alzheimer's Disease (BEHAVE-AD) (Reisberg *et al.*, 1987). Given that patients with vascular dementia often present with a variety of symptoms, a multi-dimensional scale may be more appropriate (Rosler, 2002). The Neuropsychiatric Inventory is a widely used, carer-completed, multi-dimensional scale which examines the frequency and severity of symptoms in the following domains: delusions, hallucinations, agitation, depression/dysphoria, anxiety, euphoria/elation, apathy/indifference, disinhibition, irritability/lability, and aberrant motor behavior (Cummings *et al.*, 1994; Rosler, 2002). Agitation may be measured separately on the Cohen-Mansfield Agitation Inventory (CMAI) (Cohen-Mansfield and Billig, 1986).

7. Investigations

These will follow on from the history and examination, but may include full blood count, erythrocyte sedimentation rate, urea and electrolytes, thyroid function tests, bone profile, liver function tests, vitamin B12 and folate, midstream urine specimen, chest X-ray, electrocardiogram, electroencephalogram, and CT brain scan.

8. Carer response

Informal carers of people with dementia show high levels of psychological disturbance and physical health problems (Donaldson *et al.*, 1997). A carer

assessment should form part of the interview, and the clinician must be aware of the possibility of elder abuse, both in the family home and in institutional settings.

General principles of treatment

1. Setting treatment goals.
2. Non-pharmacological treatment.
3. Pharmacological treatment.

1. Setting treatment goals

Defining specific treatment goals for particular symptoms will assist the clinician in tailoring an individualized treatment plan, and monitoring response. Ideally, carers will be involved in this process, and it may provide an opportunity to discuss risks and benefits and to explain that not all behaviors may be amenable to treatment.

2. Non-pharmacological interventions

The first line of treatment should usually be non-pharmacological. There is evidence for the effectiveness of various treatments for BPSD in dementia, although not specifically in VaD. Non-pharmacological interventions have the advantage of having little in the way of adverse effects and no unwanted interactions with the patient's medication (Teri *et al.*, 2002). However, they may be more time-consuming to implement and require more carer input than pharmacological interventions, so the clinician may be under some pressure to prescribe medication prematurely. On the positive side, the greater involvement of the carer may enable the carer to access additional support (Teri *et al.*, 2002). A range of therapies are available, but the most effective interventions appear to be those which are tailored to the needs of the individual patient (Livingston *et al.*, 2005; Rockwood and Shea, 2003).

Once an "ABC" formulation of the patient's symptoms has been described, it may be possible to identify a non-pharmacological intervention for the particular symptom. Once again, there is a paucity of rigorous research, and no studies addressing non-pharmacological management of BPSD in VaD specifically. Non-pharmacological therapies for BPSD may be broadly divided into:

- *Environmental strategies*: manipulating aspects of the patient's environment to modify the symptoms.
- *Creative therapies, exercise and social interaction*: music therapy, art therapy and increasing social interaction may be cost-effective ways to address agitation and mood symptoms.
- *Behavioral techniques*: although patients with dementia have a limited capacity for new learning, it may be possible to implement simple behavioral strategies for specific behaviors.
- *Psychological therapies*: these include therapies specific to dementia (reality orientation therapy, cognitive stimulation therapy, reminiscence therapy, validation therapy) and brief psychotherapies (CBT, interpersonal therapy).
- *Alternative therapies*: bright light therapy, aromatherapy, multi-sensory stimulation (Snoezelen).

Recent guidelines published by the National Institute for Health and Clinical Excellence in the UK (2006) have encouraged the use of creative and alternative therapies in the management of BPSD.

Environmental strategies

These techniques may be employed if, for example, the patient is wandering. Various measures have been tried in residential settings, including disguising door handles, visual barriers on exits, mirrors on doors (Mayer and Darby, 1991) and pleasant areas within the ward to encourage patients to linger there (Cohen-Mansfield and Werner, 1989; Opie *et al.*, 1999). Most of these interventions are inexpensive and easy to implement. Clearly labeling lavatories, dining areas, etc., may also be beneficial. If patients do wander, then electronic tagging systems and identity bracelets may assist with the patient's safe return

(Teri, 2002). Whall and colleagues (1997) used enhanced bathing rooms to make bathing a more pleasant sensory experience, and observed reduced levels of agitation and aggression. Removing sources of inappropriate visual stimulation such as mirrors or television screens may be helpful in the management of visual hallucinations.

Exercise

Providing patients with regular, gentle exercise has beneficial effects on sleep, agitation and aggression (Alessi *et al.*, 1999; Holmberg, 1997; King *et al.*, 1997; Namazi *et al.*, 1994). Dance therapy has also had encouraging results, and may provide patients with therapeutic physical contact (Ballard *et al.*, 2001; Perrin, 1998).

Bright light therapy

Disturbances in diurnal rhythms may lead to an altered sleep–wake cycle and the syndrome of "sundowning" in dementia. Bright light therapy improves sleep and agitation in dementia (Allen *et al.*, 2003; Douglas *et al.*, 2004; Lyketsos *et al.*, 1999). Most studies have used a light box daily over several weeks, for 1–2 h at a time.

Aromatherapy

Aromatherapy is gaining popularity as an extremely well-tolerated intervention which is usually delivered either by inhalation or topically as a cream or massage oil. The most common essential oils used in BPSD are lavender and *Melissa* (lemon) balm. A number of studies have reported improvements in agitation and well-being (Burns *et al.*, 2002).

Management of sleep disorders

Disturbed nights may make a large contribution to carer burden. The first approach is "sleep hygiene", incorporating consistent bedtimes and rising times, encouraging exercise, limiting daytime sleep and restricting caffeine and alcohol in the evenings (Teri, 2002). Environmental approaches to limiting night-time noise and maximizing comfort may also be of benefit (Teri, 2002).

Carer education

Carers may be educated in how to approach the agitated patient, and use techniques to refocus them and de-escalate aggression. However, if physical aggression continues to be a problem, the clinical team may also have a role in helping the carer find alternative provision for the patient's care.

3. Pharmacological interventions

Important considerations when prescribing in vascular dementia include:
- General considerations for prescribing in the elderly (pharmacokinetics and pharmacodynamics): "start low, go slow".
- Interactions with other medications.
- Cardiovascular side effects in a population already known to have vascular risk factors; it is essential to avoid causing further cerebrovascular damage where possible (Chiu, 2002).
- Avoid anticholinergic side effects (Chiu, 2002).
- Adequate supervision of medication in the cognitively impaired patient.
- Aim for evidence-based treatment of specific symptoms where possible (Lawlor, 2002).
- Individual patient factors (e.g. if sleep is a problem, avoid alerting drugs).
- Need for frequent medication review.

Antidepressants

Treatment with an antidepressant may be indicated for patients with VaD who present with moderate to severe depressive symptoms, or in whom mild depressive symptoms or emotionality have not responded to non-pharmacological measures.

Selective serotonin reuptake inhibitors (SSRIs)

The SSRIs are often used as a first-line treatment for depression in dementia, due to their lower propensity for causing adverse effects, particularly cardiotoxic and anticholinergic effects (BNF, 2006). They also have the advantage of once-daily administration. The most common side-effects associated with the SSRIs are gastrointestinal effects, anorexia and weight loss, and they must be used with caution in those patients at higher risk of gastric bleeding. SSRIs have also been shown to be effective in stroke-associated lability of mood (Burns *et al.*, 1999).

Other antidepressants

Venlafaxine, trazodone and mirtazapine appear to be well-tolerated alternatives to SSRIs. Tricyclic antidepressants must be used with caution in this group of patients, in view of their cardiotoxicity and propensity to cause anticholinergic side effects.

Anticonvulsants

If the patient is presenting with apparent manic symptoms, agitation or aggressive behavior, it may be appropriate to treat with an anticonvulsant. Carbamazepine has been shown to reduce agitation in patients with AD (Lawlor, 2002; Tariot *et al.*, 1998), but does have side effects of sedation, ataxia and skin rash, as well as interacting with many other medications (Rockwood and Shea, 2003). Sodium valproate may have a role in the treatment of agitation in dementia (Porsteinsson *et al.*, 2001; Kozman *et al.*, 2006; Sandborn, 1995; Herrmann, 1998), although Sival and colleagues (2002) found no beneficial effect of valproate in aggressive behavior in dementia in a three-week trial. There is some evidence from case series that gabapentin may be well-tolerated and effective in BPSD, including aggressive symptoms (Hawkins *et al.*, 2000; Herrmann, 2001; Miller, 2001).

Anxiolytics

The benzodiazepines have often been used to treat agitation, aggression and anxiety in patients with VaD, but have the drawbacks of dependence, sedation and ataxia. Agitation may increase paradoxically with the use of benzodiazepines (Rockwood and Shea, 2003). If a benzodiazepine is used, it is recommended that the lowest possible dose of a short-acting medication is prescribed, and the prescription is reviewed regularly. There is little evidence for their use in agitation in dementia from randomized controlled trials (Howard *et al.*, 2001). A randomized, double-blind study of haloperidol, oxazepam and diphenhydramine (no placebo) in BPSD resulted in improvements in all three groups, although most improvement was seen in the antipsychotic group (Coccaro *et al.*, 1990).

Buspirone 30 mg per day was found to be no more effective than placebo in a 4-week trial (Lawlor *et al.*, 1994), but showed some positive effects on anxiety in a trial versus haloperidol (Cantillon *et al.*, 1996; Rockwood and Shea, 2003).

Antipsychotics

Typical antipsychotics

If the patient presents with delusions or hallucinations, it is reasonable to begin treatment with antipsychotic medication. The conventional antipsychotics have been used widely in the treatment of BPSD. Unfortunately, many of the clinical trials have involved only patients with AD, or patients with dementia unselected by diagnosis.

The conventional antipsychotics have modest efficacy in agitation, aggression, psychosis and sleep disturbance (DeDeyn *et al.*, 1999; Devanand, 2000; Lawlor, 2002; Rosler, 2002; Street *et al.*, 2000) but have the disadvantage of causing side effects including extrapyramidal effects (EPSE), sedation, anticholinergic effects, cardiac conduction disturbances and postural hypotension (Rockwood and Shea, 2003). Older patients are at a higher risk of tardive dyskinesia than younger patients (Jeste *et al.*, 1995), and antipsychotics may also exacerbate cognitive decline (McShane *et al.*, 1997). In terms of efficacy, there is little difference between the various classes of conventional antipsychotics (Devanand, 2000; Howard *et al.*, 2001).

Antipsychotics have been used, often over-used, in the treatment of agitation and non-specific behavioral disturbance in dementia as well as psychotic symptoms. A Cochrane review of haloperidol for the treatment of agitation in dementia (Lonergan *et al.*, 2002) examined five randomized controlled trials. The authors concluded that although haloperidol was effective in reducing aggression in agitated patients, overall there was no improvement in other aspects of agitation compared with controls, and there were adverse effects associated with treatment. This study did not specifically examine treatment of patients with VaD.

Atypical antipsychotics

The atypical antipsychotic drugs, risperidone and olanzapine in particular, have been used widely as a well-tolerated alternative to the typical antipsychotics in the treatment of BPSD (Schneider *et al.*, 2006). Although they may be similar to the conventional neuroleptics in terms of efficacy (Devanand, 2000), they carry a lower risk of EPSE and tardive dyskinesia. Risperidone is effective in controlling agitation, psychosis and aggression in dementia (Brodaty *et al.*, 2003b; DeDeyn *et al.*, 1999; Katz *et al.*, 1999). DeDeyn and colleagues and Brodaty and colleagues found no significant increase in EPSE in the risperidone group over placebo, and Katz and colleagues found increased somnolence and EPSE at higher doses. All three trials included patients with VaD, although results were not broken down by diagnosis. Risperidone also resulted in improvements on the BEHAVE-AD and CMAI, and was associated with a lower rate of EPSE than haloperidol in a double-blind randomized controlled trial which included patients with VaD (Chan *et al.*, 2001). Olanzapine produced comparable reductions in NPI scores when compared to conventional antipsychotics in an open-label, controlled study in 346 patients with subcortical VaD or MID, and was well tolerated. No increased incidence of cerebrovascular events was found (Moretti *et al.*, 2005). Olanzapine produced reductions in agitation/aggression, hallucinations and delusions on the NPI modified for nursing homes in patients with Alzheimer's disease (Street *et al.*, 2000).

Risperidone and olanzapine have been associated with a threefold rise in the risk of stroke, and a twofold rise in mortality in patients with BPSD, leading to a recommendation from the US Food and Drug Administration that they should not routinely be used in this group of patients (Schneider *et al.*, 2005). Various authors have questioned this advice, especially as the alternatives to risperidone and olanzapine may have similar or even less desirable side effects. If it is necessary to consider prescribing these drugs in a patient with VaD, the clinician is advised to weigh up the risks and benefits of the proposed medication for the individual patient.

Quetiapine has not thus far been associated with concerns about stroke, and is gaining in popularity as a treatment for psychotic symptoms and agitation in BPSD. It has been found to be helpful in psychosis in dementia in a small, open-label trial (McManus *et al.*, 1999), and has been associated with improvements in delusions, activity disturbances, diurnal rhythm disturbance, and aggressiveness (McManus *et al.*, 1999), and decreased scores on the CMAI and BEHAVE-AD (Fujikawa *et al.*, 2004). Side effects include dizziness, sedation and postural hypotension (Chiu *et al.*, 2002). However, Ballard and colleagues (2005) found that quetiapine may have no benefit for agitation, and may worsen cognitive performance.

Cholinesterase inhibitors

The cholinergic deficit in AD has been well documented. There is emerging evidence of a cholinergic deficit in VaD also, independent of any co-existing AD pathology (Roman, 2004, 2005), and this may be implicated in the etiology of BPSD (Robert, 2002; Rosler, 2002). Inhibition of cholinesterase enzymes partially corrects the cholinergic deficit (Robert, 2002). The cholinesterase inhibitors (donepezil, galantamine and rivastigmine) have been studied mainly for their effects on the cognitive deficits in AD, but some studies have also included measures of BPSD, and there is evidence that the cholinesterase inhibitors may improve or stabilize existing BPSD, and delay the emergence of new symptoms (Cummings, 2000; Robert, 2002). Depression, anxiety, and apathy in AD improve with cholinesterase inhibitors, and rivastigmine also appears to improve psychotic symptoms (Rosler, 2002). Although much of the literature relates to AD, there have been a number of studies involving patients with VaD. Decline in cholinergic function affects cerebral blood flow, and treatment with cholinesterase inhibitors may have beneficial effects on regional cerebral blood flow, particularly in frontal brain areas (Roman, 2005). The commonest side effects of the cholinesterase inhibitors are nausea and vomiting, anorexia and diarrhea; these often settle within the first few weeks of treatment (Roman, 2005). Caution is advised in patients with a history of gastric bleeding or chronic obstructive pulmonary disease.

Conclusion

Behavioral and psychological symptoms are common in vascular dementia, and carry a significant burden for patients and carers. The symptom profile of BPSD in VaD may differ from that in AD. It is essential to gain a clear description of symptoms as the most beneficial management strategies appear to be those tailored closely for the

Table 17.2 Drug treatment of behavioral and psychological symptoms of vascular dementia.

Class of drug	Indications	Comments
Antidepressants	Moderate to severe depressive symptoms, mild symptoms unresponsive to non-pharmacological methods	SSRI first line (gastrointestinal side effects, gastric bleeding), venlafaxine, mirtazepine. Avoid tricyclics
Anticonvulsants	Manic symptoms, aggression, agitation	Carbamazepine reduces agitation but may cause sedation, ataxia and skin rash, and interacts with other medications. Some evidence for sodium valproate, gabapentin
Anxiolytics	Sometimes used to treat agitation, aggression, although little evidence of benefit	Benzodiazepines may cause dependence, sedation, ataxia, paradoxical increase in agitation
Conventional antipsychotics	Agitation, psychosis, aggression, sleep disturbance	May cause extrapyramidal effects (EPSE), sedation, anticholinergic effects, cardiac conduction disturbances, postural hypotension, tardive dyskinesia, exacerbation of cognitive decline
Atypical antipsychotics	Agitation, psychosis, aggression	Less EPSE, but risperidone and olanzapine have been linked to an increased risk of cerebrovascular events
Cholinesterase inhibitors	Depression, anxiety, apathy, psychotic symptoms	Gastrointestinal side effects, cardiac conduction problems. Caution in patients with a history of chronic obstructive pulmonary disease or gastric bleeding

individual patient. Non-pharmacological treatments should be the first line of management.

REFERENCES

Alessi CA, Yoon EJ, Schnelle JF, Al Samarrai NR, Cruise PA. A randomized trial of a combined physical activity and environment intervention in nursing home residents: do sleep and agitation improve? *J Am Geriatr Soc* 1999; **47**: 784–91.

Alexopoulos G, Abrams R, Young R, Shamoian C. Cornell scale for depression in dementia. *Biol Psychiatry* 1988; **23**: 271–84.

Allen H, Byrne EJ, Sutherland D, Tomenson B, Butter B, Burns A. Bright light therapy, diurnal rhythm and sleep in dementia. *Int Psychogeriatrics* 2003; **15**(S12): 97–8.

Ballard C, O'Brien JT. Behavioural and psychological symptoms. In: Erkinjuntti T, Gauthier S, eds. *Vascular cognitive impairment*, London: Martin Dunitz, 2002; 237–52.

Ballard C, McKeith I, O'Brien J, *et al.*, Neuropathological substrates of dementia and depression in vascular dementia, with a particular focus on cases with small infarct volumes. *Dementia Geriatr Cogn Disord* 2000; **11**(2): 59–65.

Ballard C, Neill D, O'Brien J, McKeith IG, Ince P, Perry R. Anxiety, depression and psychosis in vascular dementia: prevalence and associations. *J Affect Dis* 2000a; **59**(2): 97–106.

Ballard C, Margallo-Lana M, Juszczak E, *et al.* Quetiapine and rivastigmine and cognitive decline in Alzheimer's disease: a randomised, placebo-controlled trial. *Br Med J* 2005; **330**(7496): 874.

Ballard CG, Patel A, Solis M, Lowe K, Wilcock G. A one-year follow-up study of depression in dementia sufferers. *Br J Psychiatry* 1996; **168**: 287–91.

Ballard C, O'Brien J, James I, Swann A. *Dementia: management of behavioral and psychological symptoms.* Oxford: Oxford University Press, 2001.

BNF, 2006.

BMJ Publishing Group, RPS Publishing, March 2006. British National Formulary

Brodaty H, Ames D, Snowdon J, *et al.* A randomized controlled trial of risperidone for the treatment of aggression, agitation, and psychosis of dementia. *J Clin Psychiatry* 2003; **64**: 134–43.

Burns A, Russell E, Stratton-Powell H, Tyrrell P, O'Neill P, Baldwin R. Sertraline in stroke-associated lability of mood. *Int J Geriat Psychiatry* 1999; **14**: 681–5.

Byrne J, Ballard C, Holmes C. Sensory stimulation in dementia. An effective option for managing behavioral problems. *Br Med J* 2002; **325**: 1312–13.

Cantillon M, Brunswick R, Molina D, *et al.*, Buspirone vs haloperidol: a double-blind trial for agitation in a nursing home population with Alzheimer's disease. *Am J Geriatr Psychiatry* 1996; **4**: 263–7.

Chan W, Lam LC, Choy CN, Leung VP, Li S, Chiu HF. A double-blind randomised comparison of risperidone and haloperidol in the treatment of behavioral and psychological symptoms in Chinese dementia patients. *Int J Geriatr Psychiatry* 2001; **16**: 1156–62.

Chiu E. Vascular burden and BPSD: a reconceptualization. *Int Psychogeriatrics* 2003; **15**(1): 183–6.

Chiu E, Yastrubetskaya O, Williams M. Pharmacotherapy of mood and behavior symptoms. In: Erkinjuntti T, Gauthier S, eds. *Vascular cognitive impairment.* London: Martin Dunitz, 2002.

Coccaro EF, Kramer E, Zemishlany Z, *et al.*, Pharmacological treatment of non-cognitive behavioral disturbances in elderly demented patients. *Am J Psychiatry* 1990; **147**: 1640–5.

Cohen D, Eisdorfer C, Gorelick P, *et al.* Psychopathology associated with Alzheimer's disease and related disorders. *J Gerontology* 1993; **8**(6): M255–60.

Cohen-Mansfield J, Billig N. Agitated behaviors in the elderly, I: a conceptual review. *J Am Geriatr Soc* 1986; **34**: 711–21.

Cohen-Mansfield J, Werner P, Marx MS. An observational study of agitation in nursing home residents. *Int Psychogeriatr* 1989; **1**: 153–65. Nonpharmacologic interventions for psychotic symptoms in dementia. *Psychiatry Neurol* 2003; **16**: 219–24.

Cooper JK, Mungas D. Risk factor and behavioral differences between vascular and Alzheimer's dementias: the pathway to end-stage disease. *J Geriatr Psychiatry Neurol* 1993; **1**: 29–33.

Cummings JL. A comparison of psychiatric symptoms in vascular dementia and Alzheimer's disease. *Am J Psychiatry* 1993; **150**: 1806–12.

Cummings JL, Mega M, Gray K, *et al.* The Neuropsychiatric Inventory: comprehensive assessment of psychopathology in dementia. *Neurology* 1994; **44**: 2308–14. Vascular subcortical dementias: clinical aspects. *Dementia* 1994; **5**: 177–80.

Cummings JL. Cholinesterase inhibitors: a new class of psychiatric compound. *Am J Psychiatry* 2000; **157**: 4–15.

DeDeyn PP, Rabheru K, Rasmussen A, *et al.* A randomised trial of risperidone, placebo, and haloperidol for behavioral symptoms of dementia. *Neurology* 1999; **53**: 946–55.

Devanand DP. Conventional neuroleptics in dementia. *Int Psychogeriatr* 2000; **12** (suppl 1): 253–61.

Donaldson C, Tarrier N, Burns A. The impact of the symptoms of dementia on caregivers. *Br J Psychiatry* 1997; **170**: 62–8.

Douglas S, James I, Ballard C. Non-pharmacological interventions in dementia. *Adv Psychiatric Treat* 2004; **10**: 171–9.

Erkinjuntti T, Gauthier S. *Vascular cognitive impairment.* London: Martin Dunitz, 2002.

Erkinjuntti T, Vataja R, Leppavuori A. Behavioural and psychological symptoms of dementia and vascular dementia. *Int Psychogeriatr* 2000; **12** (Suppl 1): 195–200.

Finkel S. Introduction to behavioral and psychological symptoms of dementia (BPSD). *Int J Geriatr Psychiatry* 2000; **15**: S2–4.

Finkel S, Silva CE, Cohen G, Miller S, Sartorius N. Behavioural and psychological signs and symptoms of dementia: a consensus statement on current knowledge and implications for research and treatment. *Int J Geriatr Psychiatry* 1997; **12**: 1060–1.

Fujikawa T, Takahashi T, Kinoshita A, *et al.* Quetiapine treatment for behavioral and psychological symptoms in patients with senile dementia of Alzheimer type. *Neuropsychobiology* 2004; **49**: 201–04.

Groves WC, Brandt J, Steinberg M, *et al.* Vascular dementia and Alzheimer's disease: is there a difference? A comparison of symptoms by disease duration. *J Neuropsychiatry Clin Neurosci* 2000; **12**: 305–15.

Hawkins JW, Tinklenberg JR, Sheikh JI, *et al.* A retrospective chart review of gabapentin for the treatment of aggressive and agitated behavior in patients with dementias. *Am J Geriar Psychiatry* 2000; **8**: 221–5.

Herrmann N. Valproic acid in the treatment of agitation in dementia. *Can J Psychiatry* 1998; **43**: 69–72.

Herrmann N. Recommendations for the management of behavioral and psychological symptoms of dementia. *Can J Neurol Sci* 2001, **28**: (Suppl 1): S96–107.

Holmberg SK. Evaluation of a clinical intervention for wanderers on a geriatric nursing unit. *Arch Psychiatric Nurs* 1997; **11**: 21–8.

Hope T, Keene J, Fairburn C, McShane R, Jacoby R. Behaviour changes in dementia 2: are there behavioral syndromes? *Int J Geriatr Psychiatry* 1997; **12**: 1074–8.

Howard R, Ballard C, O'Brien J, Burns A. Guidelines for the management of agitation in dementia. *Int J Geriatr Psychiatry* 2001; **16**: 714–17.

Jeste DV, Caliguiri MP, Paulsen JS, *et al.* Risk of tardive dyskinesia in older patients. A prospective longitudinal study of 266 outpatients. *Arch Gen Psychiatry* 1995; **52**: 756–65.

Katz IR, Jeste DV, Mintzer JE, *et al.* 1999. Comparison of risperidone and placebo for psychosis and behavioral disturbances associated with dementia: a randomized, double-blind trial (Risperidone study group). *J Clin Psychiatry* 1999; **60**: 107–15.

King AC, Oman RF, Brassington GS, Bliwise DL, Haskell WL. Moderate-intensity exercise and self-rated quality of sleep in older adults. A randomised controlled trial. *JAMA* 1997; **277**: 32–7.

Kozman MN, Wattis J, Curran S. Pharmacological management of behavioral and psychological disturbance in dementia. *Hum Psychopharmacol Clin Exp* 2006; **21**: 1–12.

Kunik ME, Huffman JC, Bharani MD, Hillman SL, Molinari VA, Orengo CA. Behavioural disturbance in geropsychiatric inpatients across dementia types. *J Geriatr Psychiatry Neurol* 2000; **13**: 49–52.

Lawlor B. Managing behavioral and psychological symptoms in dementia. *Br J Psychiatry* 2002; **181**: 463–5.

Lawlor B, Radcliffe J, Molchen SE, *et al.* A pilot placebo-controlled study of trazodone and buspirone in Alzheimer's dementia. *Int J Geriatr Psychiatry* 1994; **9**: 55–9.

Lavretsky H, Chui HC. Vascular dementia. In: Agronin ME, Maletta GJ, eds. *Principles and practice of geriatric psychiatry*. Balhimore MD: Lippincott Williams and Wilkins, 2006; 301–10.

Leroi I, Voulgari A, Breitner JCS, Lyketsos CG. The epidemiology of psychosis in dementia. *Am J Geriatr Psychiatry* 2003; **11**: 83–91.

Li Y-S, Meyer JS, Thornby J. Longitudinal follow-up of depressive symptoms among normal versus cognitively impaired elderly. *Int J Geriatr Psychiatry* 2001; **16**: 818–727.

Lind K, Edman A, Karlsson I, Sjogren M, Wallin A. Relationship between depressive symptomatology and the subcortical brain syndrome in dementia. *Int J Geriatr Psychiatry* 2002; **17**(8): 774–8.

Livingston G, Johnston K, Katona C, Paton J, Lyketsos CG, Old Age Task Force of the World Federation of Biological Psychiatry. Systematic review of psychological treatment approaches to the management of neuropsychiatric symptoms of dementia. *Am J Psychiatry* 2005; **162**: 1996–2021.

Lonergan E, Luxenberg J, Colford J, Birks J. Haloperidol for agitation in dementia. *Cochrane Database of Systematic Reviews*, 2002. Issue 2. Art No.: CD002852. DOI: 10.1002/14651858.CD002852.

Lyketsos CG, Lindell Veiel L, Baker A, Steele C. A randomized controlled trial of bright light therapy for agitated behaviors in dementia patients residing in long-term care. *Int J Geriatr Psychiatry* 1999; **14**(7): 520–5.

Lyketsos CG, Steinberg M, Tschanz JT, Norton MC, Steffens DC, Breitner JCS. Mental and behavioral disturbances in dementia: findings from the cache county study on memory in aging. *Am J Psychiatry* 2000; **157**: 708–14.

McKeith I. Galantamine for vascular dementia. *Lancet Neurol* 2002; **1**: 210.

McKeith I. Dementia with Lewy bodies. In: Agronin ME, Maletta GJ eds. *Principles and practice of geriatric psychiatry*. Baltimore, MD: Lippincott Williams and Wilkins, 2006; 311–18.

McManus DQ, Arvanitis LA, Kowalcyk BB. Quetiapine, a novel antipsychotic: experience in elderly patients with psychotic disorders. Seroquel trial 48 study group. *J Clin Psychiatry* 1999; **60**: 292–8.

McShane R, Keene J, Gedling K, *et al.* Do neuroleptic drugs hasten cognitive decline in dementia? Prospective study with necropsy follow up. *Br Med J* 1997; **314**: 266–70.

Mayer R, Darby SJ. Does a mirror deter wandering in demented older people? *Int J Geriatr Psychiatry* 1991; **6**: 607–09.

Miller LJ. Gabapentin for treatment of behavioral and psychological symptoms of dementia. *Ann Pharmacother* 2001; **35**: 427–31.

Moretti R, Torre P, Antonello RM, Cattaruzza T, Cazzato G. Olanzapine as a possible treatment of behavioral symptoms in vascular dementia: Risks of cerebrovascular events. *J Neurol* 2005; **252**: 1186–93.

Moretti R, Torre P, Antonello RM, Cazzato G. Behavioural alterations and vascular dementia. *The Neurologist* 2006; **12**(1): 43–7.

Namazi KH, Gwinnup PB, Zadorozny CA. A low intensity exercise/movement program for patients with Alzheimer's disease: the TEMP-AD protocol. *J Aging Phys Activity* 1994; **2**: 80–92.

National Institute for Health and Clinical Excellence, Social Care Institute for Excellence. Dementia: Supporting people with dementia and their carers in health and social care. NICE clinical guideline 42, November. National Collaborating Centre for Mental Health, 2006.

Newman SC. The prevalence of depression in Alzheimer's disease and vascular dementia in a population sample. *J Affect Dis* 1999; **52**: 169–76.

O'Brien JT, Erkinjuntti T, Reisberg B, *et al.* Vascular cognitive impairment. *Lancet Neurol* 2003; **2**(Feb): 89–98.

O'Brien J. Behaviours symptoms in vascular cognitive impairment and vascular dementia. *Int J Psychogeriatrics* 2003; **15**(1): 133–8.

O'Donnell BF, Drachman DA, Barnes HJ, *et al.* Incontinence and troublesome behaviors predict institutionalisation in dementia. *J Geriatr Psychiatry Neurol* 1992; **5**: 45–52.

Opie J, Rosewarne R, O'Connor DW. The efficacy of psychosocial approaches to behavior disorders in dementia: a systematic literature review. *Aust NZ Psychiatry* 1999; **33**: 789–99.

Overshott R, Burns A. Treatment of dementia. *J Neurol, Neurosurg Psychiatry* 2005; **76** (5): 53–9.

Perrin T. Lifted into a world of rhythm and melody. *J Dementia Care* 1998; **5**: 18–19.

Pinto C, Seethalakshmi R. Behavioural and psychological symptoms of dementia in an Indian population: Comparison between Alzheimer's disease and vascular dementia. *Int Psychogeriatrics* 2006; **18**(1): 87–93.

Porsteinsson AP, Tariot PN, Erb R, *et al.* Placebo-controlled study of divalproex sodium for agitation in dementia. *Am J Geriatr Psychiatry* 2001; **9**: 58–66.

Purandare N, Allen NHP, Burns A. Behavioural and psychological symptoms of dementia. *Rev Clin Gerontol* 2000; **10**: 245–60.

Reisberg B, Borenstein J, Salob SP, *et al.* Behavioural symptoms in Alzheimer's disease – phenomenology

and treatment. *J Clin Psychiatry* 1987; **48**(Suppl 5): 9–15.

Robert P. Understanding and managing behavioral symptoms in Alzheimer's disease and related dementias: Focus on rivastigmine. *Curr Med Res Opin* 2002; **18**(3): 156–71.

Rockwood K, Shea C. Behavioural and psychological symptoms in vascular cognitive impairment. In: Bowler JV, Hachinski V, eds. *Vascular cognitive impairment: preventable dementia*. Oxford: Oxford University Press, 2003.

Roman GC. Facts, myths, and controversies in vascular dementia. *J Neurol Sci* 2004; **226**: 49–52.

Roman GC. Rivastigmine for subcortical vascular dementia. *Expert Rev Neurotherapeutics* 2005; **5**(3): 309–13.

Rosler M. The efficacy of cholinesterase inhibitors in treating the behavioral symptoms of dementia. *Int J Clin Pract* 2002; Supplement 127 June: 20–36.

Sandborn WD, Bendfeldt F, Hamdy R. Valproic acid for physically aggressive behavior in geriatric patients. *Am J Geriatr Psychiatry* 1995; **3**: 239–42.

Schneider LS, Tariot PN, Dagerman KS *et al.* Effectiveness of atypical antipsychotic drugs in patients with Alzheimer's disease. *N Engl J Med* 2000; **335** (15): 1525–38.

Schneider LS, Dagerman KS, Insel P. Risk of death with atypical antipsychotic drug treatment for dementia. *JAMA* 2005; **294**: 1934–43.

Sival RC, Haffmans PMJ, Jansen PAF, Duursma SA, Eikelenboom P. Sodium valproate in the treatment of aggressive behavior in patients with dementia: A randomized placebo controlled clinical trial. *Int J Geriatr Psychiatry* 2002; **17**(6): 579–85.

Street J, Clark S, Gannon KS. Olanzapine treatment of psychotic and behavioral symptoms in patients with Alzheimer's disease in nursing care facilities: A double-blind, randomized, placebo-controlled trial. *Arch Gen Psychiatry* 2000; **57**: 968–77.

Sultzer DL, Levin HS, Mahler ME, High WM, Cummings JL. A comparison of psychiatric symptoms in vascular dementia and Alzheimer's disease. *Am J Psychiatry* 1993; **150**: 1806–12.

Swearer JM, Drachman DA, O'Donnell BF, Mitchell AL. Troublesome and disruptive behaviors in dementia. Relationships to disease severity. *J Am Geriatr Soc* 1988; **36**(9): 784–90.

Tariot P, Gaile SE, Castelli NA, Porsteinsson AP. Treatment of agitation in dementia. *New Direct Mental Hlth Serv* 1997; **76**: 109–23.

Tariot PN. Treatment of agitation in dementia. *J Clin Psychiatry* 1999; **60** (Suppl 8): 11–20.

Tariot PN, Erb R, Podgorski CA, *et al.* Efficacy and tolerability of carbamazepine for agitation and aggression in dementia. *Am J Psychiatry* 1998; **155**: 54–61.

Teri L, Logsdon RG, McCurry SM. Nonpharmacologic treatment of behavioral disturbance in dementia. *Med Clin N Am* 2002; **86**: 641–56.

Vataja R, Pohjasvaara T, Leppavuori A, *et al.* Magnetic resonance imaging correlates of depression after ischaemic stroke. *Arch Gen Psychiatry* 2001; **58**: 925–31.

Whall AL, Black ME, Groh CJ, Yankou DJ, Kupferschmid BJ, Foster NL. The effect of natural environments upon agitation and aggression in late-stage dementia patients. *Am J Alzheimer's Dis* 1997; **12**: 216–20.

Control of vascular risk factors

Deborah Gustafson and Ingmar Skoog

Introduction

The evidence base for the prevention of dementia and related brain pathologies is strongest for the control of vascular risk factors. A variety of vascular risk factors have been identified in relationship to Alzheimer's disease (AD) and other forms of dementia. As vascular factors are related to the leading causes of death during adulthood, such as cardiovascular disease and certain forms of cancer, the majority of data suggest that public health prevention messages relevant to these aforementioned disorders are also relevant for dementia if one lives to a high age.

Control of risk factors related to chronic diseases and the promotion of good health in human populations is an ultimate goal of epidemiologic and public health research. The World Health Organization reports a 223% expected increase from 1970 to 2025 of adults aged 60 and above, so that by 2025 there will be 1.2 billion people in this age group world-wide. Among those aged 65 and older in Western societies, the most rapidly growing group is age 85 and older. Dementia disorders, such as AD and vascular forms of dementia, are chronic diseases of aging that may be preventable. The incidence of dementia is around 1% at age 70–74, 2% by age 75–79, and approaches 10% by age 85 (Jorm *et al.*, 1987). Its prevalence is 1% by age 70, 30% at age 85 (Skoog *et al.*, 1993), and 50% at age 95

(Borjesson-Hanson *et al.*, 2004). These statistics are of the utmost importance as we witness an increasing lifespan and increasing prevalence of vascular risk factors for dementia, such as hypertension, obesity and other vascular morbidities. Clearly the control and prevention of vascular factors is necessary.

Effective control of vascular factors and facilitating prevention are challenges for implementation of public health programs. Overcoming this challenge can be facilitated via knowledge of individual risk. However, sadly, this is often lacking. In a large national study in the United States, lack of physician-based diagnoses has been reported among 22.9% with obesity, 11.3% with diabetes, 16.1% with hypertension, and 37.7% with hyperlipidemia (Diaz *et al.*, 2004). Being undiagnosed is even higher for certain high-risk groups, such as young, non-White, underinsured adults (Ayanian *et al.*, 2003; Diaz *et al.*, 2004). In addition, even after identification of a problem, there is often inadequate control; for example, 50% of hypertensives and 50% of hyperlipidemics have been observed to be poorly controlled (Qureshi *et al.*, 2001).

Successful prevention of disease depends on the ability to control and/or modify risk and protective factors. In the case of dementia, which is characterized by a potentially long latent period of pathological changes prior to clinical onset of disease, it is often not clear as to when the window of

Vascular Cognitive Impairment in Clinical Practice, ed. Lars-Olof Wahlund, Timo Erkinjuntti and Serge Gauthier. Published by Cambridge University Press. © Cambridge University Press 2009.

opportunity exists for implementation of adequate or even ultimate prevention and control efforts, but evidence continues to accumulate suggesting that a life course perspective is necessary in relationship to dementia. Discussion of the control of vascular factors will include hypertension, overweight and obesity, and hypercholesterolemia, with consideration for the overlapping syndromes they represent.

Hypertension

Hypertension is currently defined as systolic blood pressure (SBP) above 140 mmHg and/or diastolic blood pressure (DBP) above 90 mmHg. The threshold for hypertension has decreased during recent years, and new criteria have been established for pre-hypertensive stages, for example. Hypertension is a risk factor for stroke, ischemic white matter lesions (WMLS), silent infarcts, general atherosclerosis, myocardial infarction and cardiovascular morbidity and mortality. This risk increases with increasing blood pressure also at apparently healthy blood pressure ranges (Kannel, 2000). Treatment of hypertension reduces cardiovascular risk substantially, but a large proportion of individuals with hypertension are still not treated.

During the last decade, evidence has accumulated that hypertension may be a risk factor for cognitive decline and dementia, independent of the presence of cerebrovascular disease (CVD). Several longitudinal studies have suggested an association between AD and previous hypertension (Kivipelto et al., 2001; Launer et al., 2000; Qiu et al., 2003; Ruitenberg et al., 2001; Skoog et al., 1996; Wu et al., 2003), while some do not (Morris et al., 2007; Posner et al., 2002; Yoshitake et al., 1995). Some of these latter studies, however, reported associations with vascular dementia (Posner et al., 2002; Yoshitake et al., 1995). The use of antihypertensive drugs also appears to reduce the incidence of AD and dementia (Guo et al., 1996; 2001; Skoog et al., 1996). Other observational studies have been less con-

clusive, with non-significant odds ratios below 1.00 for risk of AD (in't Veld et al., 2001; Richards et al., 2000), although the former study showed a significant protective effect for overall dementia. It thus appears that treatment of hypertension might be one tool for prevention of dementia/cognitive decline.

Thus far, the following hypertension trials with dementia or cognitive function as secondary endpoints have been published: (1) the Systolic Hypertension in the Elderly Program (SHEP) ($N = 4736$) using chlorthalidon, a diuretic, as active treatment (Applegate et al., 1994; SHEP Cooperative Research Group, 1991); (2) Medical Research Council's (MRC) Treatment Trial of hypertension ($N = 4396$) using atenolol, a beta-blocker, or hydrochlorthiazide, a diuretic, as active treatments (Peart, 1987; Prince et al., 1996); (3) The Systolic Hypertension in Europe Study (Syst-Eur) ($N = 2418$) using nitrendipine, a calcium-channel blocker, as active treatment (Forette et al., 1998, 2002; Staessen et al., 1997); (4) The Study on Cognition and Prognosis in the Elderly (SCOPE) ($N = 4937$) using candersatan cilexetil, an angiotensin II type 1 (AT1) receptor blocker, as active treatment (Lithell et al., 2003); and (5) Perindopril Protection against Recurrent Stroke Study (PROGRESS) ($N = 6105$) using perindopril, an angiotensin-converting enzyme inhibitor, and indapamide, a diuretic, as active treatment (PROGRESS, 2001; Tzourio et al., 2003).

These studies found significant reductions of cardiovascular morbidity, but only Syst-Eur (Forette et al., 1998) reported a significantly reduced incidence of dementia in the treatment group. Interestingly, this effect remained during an open-label follow-up period (Forette et al., 2002). Regarding other cognitive outcomes, PROGRESS reported a significant 19% decreased incidence of "Significant cognitive decline", while SCOPE reported a non-significant 11% reduction. PROGRESS reported less decline in Mini-Mental State Examination (MMSE) in the active treatment group than in the placebo group, while MRC, SHEP, SCOPE, and Syst-Eur had no differences between the groups in mean change in cognitive testings. No study reported a higher risk for dementia or cognitive decline in the active treatment group. Some studies reported on some interesting sub-analyses. PROGRESS reported that dementia with recurrent stroke was reduced by 34%. SCOPE found that mean MMSE declined significantly less in the treatment group than in controls among those with mild cognitive dysfunction (defined as 28 points or less; Skoog, personal communication). In SHARE, active treatment reduced incidence of dementia if drop-outs were assigned a prevalence of 20–30% of dementia.

Overweight and obesity

There have been several prospective reports (Barrett-Connor *et al.*, 1996; Buchman *et al.*, 2005; Gustatson *et al.*, 2003; Kivipelto *et al.*, 2005; Nourhashemi *et al.*, 2003; Rosengren *et al.*, 2005; Stewart *et al.*, 2005; Whitmer *et al.*, 2005) evaluating BMI in relationship to dementia (Table 18.1). Most studies indicate that overweight (BMI 25–29.99 kg m^{-2}) and/or obesity (BMI $\geq$ 30 kg m^{-2}) increase dementia risk over long periods of follow-up (Gustafson *et al.*, 2003; Kivipelto *et al.*, 2005; Rosengren *et al.*, 2005; Whitmer *et al.*, 2005). In general, these studies evaluate BMI among those who have survived to approximately age 70, and therefore have not died due to other consequences of higher BMI levels and are now "at risk" for dementia. Traditionally, studies reporting that a low BMI or being underweight were risk factors for dementia (Faxen-Irving *et al.*, 2005; Hogan *et al.*, 1997; White *et al.*, 1996, 1998), and age-related brain changes, such as atrophy (Grundman *et al.*, 1996), were based on cross-sectional or case-control studies, and a prospective perspective was lacking. There are no published reports on the longitudinal BMI–dementia relationship considering the role of APOE *ε*4, the major susceptibility allele for dementia.

Numerous reports on cognitive performance related to BMI and other adiposity measures have also been published (Bagger *et al.*, 2004; Brubacher *et al.*, 2004; Elias *et al.*, 2005; Jeong *et al.*, 2005; Nourhashemi *et al.*, 2002; Patel *et al.*, 2004; Waldstein and Katzel, 2006), however, comparing these studies is difficult, as most are cross-sectional, have small sample sizes, measure cognitive function and adiposity in different ways, and define poor or low cognitive performance inconsistently. Many of these studies do not screen for other mental health outcomes, such as depression, or medication use, which may affect observed relationships. More research is needed in the area of adiposity and preclinical symptoms of dementia or cognitive impairment to determine at what point in the underlying biological pathway adiposity may be having an effect or when the influence of adiposity may change direction.

Metabolic or obesity syndromes may also be related to AD and dementia, as a high BMI rarely exists in isolation (Kalmijn *et al.*, 2000; Yaffe *et al.*, 2004). As many as one in five adults has a clinically characterized obesity syndrome (Ford *et al.*, 2002). Diabetes may also increase dementia risk (Akomolafe *et al.*, 2006; Leibson *et al.*, 1997; Martins *et al.*, 2006; Ott *et al.*, 1999; Pasquier *et al.*, 2006; Pilcher, 2006; Watson and Craft, 2006; Xu *et al.*, 2007). Memory impairment has been related to poor glycemic control (Greenwood *et al.*, 2003), and poorer cognition to insulin resistance (Greenwood and Winocur, 2005). However, the Framingham Heart Health Study showed that obesity, independent of diabetes status, was related to poorer cognitive performance among men (Elias *et al.*, 2005). Given the increasing occurrence of Type 2 diabetes among younger adults, and the role of insulin, insulin resistance, and related genes, diabetes may become increasingly important in dementia etiology. Syndromes in the periphery may be related to syndromes in the aging brain.

How high levels of adiposity may influence the health of the brain is complex. Adipose tissue is the largest endocrine organ in the human body, and secretes hormones, cytokines, and growth factors, which interact directly with blood vessels (DeMichele *et al.*, 2002; Williams *et al.*, 2002),

Table 18.1 Adult guidelines for vascular health parameters.

	Adult risk cut-offs (Association AH)
Blood pressure	<130/85 – optimal
	≥140/≥90 mm Hg (Han *et al.*, 2002)
Overweight and Obesity	≥25–29.99 kg m^{-2} – overweight
	≥30 – obese (NIH, 1998)
Waist circumference	Moderate risk: men, ≥94 cm, women, ≥80 cm
	High risk: men, ≥102 cm; women, ≥88 cm (Han *et al.*, 1995; NIH, 1998)
Blood cholesterol	<5.2 mM – optimal
	5.2 – 6.1 mM – borderline high risk
	≥6.2 mM – high risk
Triglycerides	>2.3 mM – borderline high or high
HDL	<1.0 mM – high risk
	>1.5 mM – optimal
LDL	<2.6 mM – optimal
	4.1 – 4.9 mM – high risk
	>4.9 mM – very high risk
Fasting glucose	5.6–6.9 mM – optimal
	>6.9 mM – diabetes
Fasting insulin	<10 IU/ml – optimal
Physical activity	Initial goal: moderate levels for 30 to 45 min, 3 to 5 days a week.
	Long-term goal: moderate-intensity at least 30 min or more on most, and preferably all, days of the week.

cross the blood–brain barrier (Lathe, 2001), and contribute to homeostasis. In addition, fat, as triglyceride, is also stored in non-adipose tissues such as the liver, pancreas and heart (McGavock *et al.*, 2006). That adipose tissue is important in elderly is illustrated by the classic example that adipose becomes the primary site of estrogen synthesis in post-menopausal women and is modulated by environmental factors (Gustafson and Kurzer, 1993). In terms of vascular effects, the relationship between BMI and dementia could be due to the effects of excess adiposity on blood pressure, blood lipids, cardiovascular disease, and general health of the vasculature. Obesity has been related to carotid artery wall thickening (DeMichele *et al.*, 2002);

vascular and coronary endothelial dysfunction (Brook *et al.*, 2001; Suwaidi *et al.*, 2001; Williams *et al.*, 2002); peripheral resistance; arterial stiffness; ventricular hypertrophy; and increased sympathetic activity, intravascular volume, cardiac output, and platelet aggregation (Yki-Järvinen and Westerbacka, 2000; Zhang and Reisin, 2000). In addition, adipose tissue secretes a variety of bioactive metabolites, such as sex hormones (estrogens, androgens, and progestins), insulin, insulin-like growth factor-I, transforming growth factor-beta, tumor necrosis factor-alpha, angiotensin II, leptin, neurotrophins, growth factors, cytokines, fatty acids and many other factors that may cross the blood–brain barrier (Hausman *et al.*,

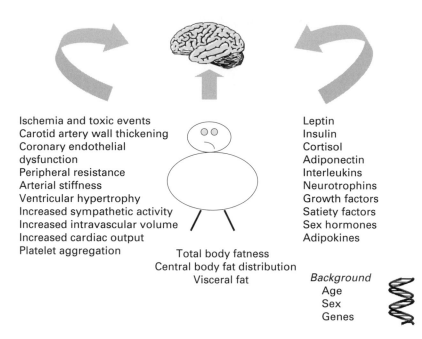

Ischemia and toxic events
Carotid artery wall thickening
Coronary endothelial
dysfunction
Peripheral resistance
Arterial stiffness
Ventricular hypertrophy
Increased sympathetic activity
Increased intravascular volume
Increased cardiac output
Platelet aggregation

Leptin
Insulin
Cortisol
Adiponectin
Interleukins
Neurotrophins
Growth factors
Satiety factors
Sex hormones
Adipokines

Total body fatness
Central body fat distribution
Visceral fat

Background
Age
Sex
Genes

Figure 18.1 The roles of adipose tissue in brain health and dementia processes may be described in relationship to its influence on health of the vasculature, as a source and influencer of the hormonal milieu, and in relationship to its physical location. Adipose tissue exerts its effects against a relatively fixed background of age, sex, and genes.

2001; Lathe, 2001) and affect brain health and subsequent dementia (see Figure 18.1). That these compounds are important is exemplified by published observations that a high BMI or more adiposity is independently related to dementia, even after adjustment for multiple vascular factors.

BMI and body fat distribution may also be associated with dementia via relationships with underlying brain pathologies associated with dementia, such as cerebral atrophy (Enzinger *et al.*, 2005; Gustafson *et al.*, 2004a; Jagust *et al.*, 2005; Ward *et al.*, 2005) and white matter lesions (Gustafson *et al.*, 2004b; Jagust *et al.*, 2005). This would implicate detrimental involvement of higher adiposity earlier on in dementing processes. In addition, blood–brain barrier disturbance is a common occurrence in those with dementia and vascular diseases (Blennow *et al.*, 1990), thus affecting transfer of adipose-derived compounds to the

brain. There have been no trials related to weight reduction or anti-obesity drugs and dementia.

Cholesterol

Cholesterol is important in AD, not only because of its relationship with cardiovascular disease, but due to its role in amyloid metabolism. Animal models have shown that hypercholesterolemia leads to the accumulation of intracellular amyloid (Sparks *et al.*, 1994). APOE, the major susceptibility gene for AD, is involved in lipid transport in the peripheral and central nervous systems, regulates cholesterol homeostasis in astrocytes and microglia, and is related to blood cholesterol levels. It has been shown that mutations in the APP gene up-regulate Aβ40 and Aβ42 production (Pangalos *et al.*, 2005). Aβ processing is sensitive to cholesterol levels and lipid trafficking, and brain cholesterol levels increase during AD progression (Höglund *et al.*, 2007). While there remain a number of questions regarding the amyloid hypothesis in relationship to AD, the potential link to cholesterol metabolism is noteworthy.

The human body contains about 100 g of cholesterol, most of which is made by the liver. Most of this cholesterol is incorporated into cell membranes, and myelin is especially rich in cholesterol. Cholesterol is a very important molecule as it is the parent compound of steroid hormones, such as estrogens and androgens, and it is the precursor of vitamin D. High levels of total and LDL cholesterol and low levels of HDL are well-established risk factors for cardiovascular disease. The association between blood cholesterol and stroke is less clear. Few studies have examined the relationship between blood cholesterol levels and vascular disease in late life, and there are few clinical trials of statins in the elderly. What do blood cholesterol levels mean for the brain? Brain cholesterol is synthesized in situ, and blood cholesterol does not cross the blood–brain barrier (BBB) unless it is converted to 24S-OH cholesterol first. There is no correlation between blood and CSF cholesterol, and the cellular basis for a link between Aβ generation and AD are poorly understood.

The epidemiology of blood cholesterol levels in relationship to AD and other forms of dementia are mixed. Some studies have shown that high blood cholesterol levels in mid-life may be risky (Kivipelto *et al.*, 2001, 2002; Notkola *et al.*, 1998), while others have shown no relationship between mid-life cholesterol levels and later dementia (Kalmijn *et al.*, 2000; Tan *et al.*, 2003) or incident dementia (Romas *et al.*, 1999; Yoshitake *et al.*, 1995). In contrast, there are reports of higher cholesterol levels being protective (Mielke *et al.*, 2005; Reitz *et al.*, 2004; Romas *et al.*, 1999). One recent report shows that blood cholesterol levels decline with cognitive impairment and may be reflective of dementia processes (Solomon *et al.*, 2007). Con-

sideration in the evaluation of epidemiologic studies are the changing levels of blood cholesterol over time, as well as the introduction of various types of cholesterol-lowering medications, such as statins. Statin use has not been consistently related to dementia risk in epidemiologic studies. Some major issues concerning statins are that they are not just HMGCoA reductase inhibitors. Statins have anti-inflammatory effects, may reduce the permeability of the BBB (lovastatin and simvastatin), and those that are highly lipophilic cross the BBB, whereas those that are not will not.

Prevention and control measures

Dementia prevention during adulthood is facilitated by individual knowledge of levels of blood pressure, BMI (and perhaps waist circumference), blood cholesterol, and fasting blood glucose and insulin (see Table 18.1). While control measures can be defined in general, on behalf of adults and based on studies of adults, guidelines for the elderly (age 70+) remain to be established and guidelines for children are in need of revision (e.g. lipids) (McCrindle *et al.*, 2007) or need to be established. The control of vascular risk in children is very important, as has been evidenced by cholesterol education programs since the 1970s (McCrindle *et al.*, 2007). As vascular disease is evidenced very early in life, it is never too early for vascular risk factor control. Of importance also in children, are co-existing conditions of obesity, hypertension, diabetes, and other metabolic syndromes. Due to the interrelatedness of all of these factors, weight control throughout life and the establishment of good lifestyle habits are critical. In addition, vascular factors should be considered against a background of dementia susceptibility factors, which include: age, female sex, family history of dementia and longevity, and educational attainment.

Simply stated, similar recommendations as have been ascribed for years for heart health, now may be applied for optimizing brain health. Recommendations stated by heart health organizations throughout the world include: (1) control blood pressure, (2) lose weight if you are overweight, (3) get regular physical activity, (4) avoid excessive alcohol, (5) stop smoking, (6) manage stress, (7) decrease sodium (salt) intake, (8) eat for heart health, (9) discuss the use of some medications with your doctor. (Association AH, 2007).

Other lifestyle factors and agents have shown potential protection for dementia, and are related to the Big 3 discussed here. Dietary intake of antioxidants and B vitamins, as well as dietary patterns that include fish and Mediterranean components, may foster brain health. Physical activity may be beneficial. Pharmacological agents include antihypertensive agents, statins, hormone replacement therapy (HRT), and non-steroidal anti-inflammatory drugs (NSAIDs), although double-blind, randomized controlled clinical trials have not been too informative in this regard (in't Veld et al., 2001; Zandi et al., 2002).

Maintaining a healthy weight and, for many, weight loss, is a cornerstone of the maintenance of vascular health. An expert panel, convened on behalf of the National Heart, Lung, and Blood Institute (National Institutes of Health, USA) (Expert Panel, 2005), formulated a variety of recommendations for the reduction of obesity and related vascular sequelae. Weight loss has been recommended to lower elevated blood pressure in overweight and obese persons with high blood pressure; to lower elevated levels of total cholesterol, LDL cholesterol, and triglycerides, to raise low levels of HDL cholesterol in overweight and obese persons with dyslipidemia; and to lower elevated blood glucose levels in overweight and obese persons with Type 2 diabetes. In addition, physical activity may decrease abdominal fat and help to maintain weight loss. Also, exercise psychologists recommend moderate intensity physical activity for best effects on mental health, also of attractive relevance for dementia prevention.

Types of prevention and considerations

There are three major forms of prevention – primary, secondary, and tertiary prevention – the definitions of which depend on when an intervention is initiated in relation to disease onset or its clinical symptoms. The aim of primary prevention is to intervene before clinical disease onset, either by promoting the initiation and maintenance of good health or by removing potential causes of disease, with the overall goal of reducing the incidence of disease (Last, 1988; Skoog et al., 1999). Primary prevention trials for clinical dementia could thus include individuals who possess one or more potential risk factors, such as hypertension, high cholesterol, or family history, or a demographic risk factor (such as high age).

Secondary prevention strategies are initiated after preclinical symptoms of a disease have become manifest. This is best accomplished through early detection efforts followed by definitive treatments. The goal in this case is to prevent preclincal forms of disease from progressing to manifest disease. In relationship to dementia, this would include intervening during a preclinical stage, such as mild cognitive impairment (MCI), or when memory complaints are mentioned, to prevent further progression to dementia (Skoog et al., 1999). In relationship to vascular factors, control of hypertension, a secondary prevention strategy for cardiovascular disease, becomes a primary prevention strategy for dementia. Tertiary prevention is to interfere with the progression of a disability, condition, or disorder so that it does not advance to stages beyond repair. The goal of tertiary prevention is to reduce the burden of the disease on society in terms of healthcare costs and numerous co-morbidities.

Placebo-controlled, randomized clinical trials are the gold standard for judging whether a specific factor or set of factors prevent disease or affect a disease outcome. Clinical trials are conducted in relation to all forms of prevention. Primary prevention trials are extremely expensive, as they require large sample sizes and a sufficient follow-up period during which monitoring must occur and effects be observed.

General methodological considerations

Research studies evaluating the efficacy of prevention and control measures for dementia must consider a number of factors, which are outlined below.

Age – Since age is the strongest predictor of dementia, the age of participants when an intervention is initiated and the age at which events are evaluated influences the interpretation of the results, and how they relate to disease pathogenesis. Trials to date have generally recruited participants in ages where dementia risk is low. Therefore, relatively small numbers of demented patients have been observed in several of these studies. The roles and relative influence of preventable risk factors in relationship to dementia may also differ, depending on whether they occur in early, mid-, or late life, or during critical stages of life change, such as the female menopause.

Healthy volunteer effect – It is well-known that individuals who take part in studies where risk and protective factors are identified are healthier than the general population, and this may have a multiple effects on observations from trials for dementia prevention. The incidence of dementia may not be as high among volunteers as in the general population since these healthy individuals practice lifestyle and healthcare habits that may reduce their risk. On the other hand, healthy volunteers theoretically live longer or survive, thus living to an age where they are more susceptible to dementia.

Selection of high-risk groups – In some intervention studies, participants are selected based on a risk factor, such as hypertension, hypercholesterolemia, or stroke. While this is advantageous from the standpoint of monitoring prevention and control of these related factors, generalizability is limited to individuals with these characteristics.

Cognitive function at baseline – Most population studies report that individuals with high baseline scores on simple cognitive tests, such as the Mini-Mental State Examination (MMSE), experience less cognitive decline and have a lower incidence of dementia during follow-up compared to those with lower scores (Aevarsson and Skoog, 2000). In most dementia prevention trials, participating volunteers have had fairly high cognitive function at baseline (Houx *et al.*, 2002), suggesting a rather low short-term risk of developing dementia. This may provide a rationale for recruiting high-risk groups (see above).

Sex – Since female sex is strongly associated with risk for dementia, and since men do not live as long as women, and since risk factors for dementia vary by sex in and of themselves and in relationship to dementia, the relative inclusion or exclusion of women and men in trials for dementia prevention is critical to interpretation of results. Results from trials in women, for example, may or may not be generalized as relevant for men.

Study design

(a) *Time of follow-up* – It is likely that prevention trials need a long time of follow-up to be able to detect a difference between placebo and active treatment. Time of follow-up in the large trials performed so far has been between 2 and 5 years. Thus, all trials measured relatively short-term effects of treatment. In contrast, epidemiologic studies reporting associations between hypertension or being overweight and obesity and AD reported that follow-ups had to be at least 5 years before dementia onset to detect differences between AD and controls or non-cases (Gustafson *et al.*, 2003; Kivipelto *et al.*, 2001; Launer *et al.*, 2000; Qiu *et al.*, 2003; Ruitenberg, 2000; Skoog *et al.*, 1996). Thus, time of follow-up might have been too short to detect an effect on the incidence of dementia in the trials conducted so far.

(b) *Timing* – The roles and relative influence of risk factors in relationship to dementia may differ, depending on their timing in relationship to disease onset. Perhaps the biggest lesson to be learned from clinical trials of preventive agents in dementia is how to address the question of timing. When is a potentially preventive agent maximally effective in retarding the onset of dementia? Also, when is it appropriate to intervene for any given individual? These are perhaps the most difficult questions to answer.

(c) *Selective attrition/missing data* – Selective attrition might affect the results of trials if missed assessments differed between the treatment group and placebo. For example, some studies have shown that those missing more cognitive assessments have also had more cardiovascular events during the study period (Di Bari *et al.*, 2001).

(d) *Factors related to outcome* – Cognitive endpoints in primary prevention trials may be dementia, significant cognitive decline, and/or change in cognitive function based on longitudinal performance on certain tests. Related outcomes may include biomarkers such as those observed via brain imaging, cerebrospinal fluid, or blood. If active treatment is related to change in cognitive function or certain biomarker levels, it may be an indication that the treatment has an effect on very early stages of dementia.

(e) *Dementia* – Consistent and valid diagnoses of dementia, which require comprehensive evaluations, are often difficult to standardize across studies and globally. Methods for detection of dementia vary among studies. Generally dementia diagnoses have been based on a combination of screening for the disease or the clinical impression from investigators, followed by a more formal investigation by local specialists and a central evaluation by an endpoint committee.

(f) *Rare outcomes* – As dementia is a rare event, prevention trials should not be conducted without sample size and power calculations.

(g) *Cognitive function* – Since dementia is a rare event, change in cognitive function based on psychometric tests, most often MMSE, is often used as a primary outcome measure. Interpretation of this type of end-point depends on several factors, including base-line performance (see above).

(h) *Practice and learning effect* – Repeated administrations of psychometric tests may result in higher scores at retesting, even after a period as long as one year, the so-called practice or learning effect (Di Bari *et al.*, 2002; Houx *et al.*, 2002). This may result from memorizing items or the development of better strategies in performing the tests. Trials using changes in cognitive test scores as primary end-points should be designed appropriately to estimate and minimize the consequences of a training effect in follow-up data.

(i) *Ceiling effect* – A ceiling effect refers to the phenomenon whereby a test may not be able to detect decline in cognitive function if most individuals score at or close to the maximum score (Houx *et al.*, 2002), especially when simple cognitive tests, such as MMSE (30-point scale), are used. In addition, increases in scores are not possible, which has often been observed in clinical trials, and may denote practice or learning effects.

(j) *Sensitivity to change* – As already alluded to, use of simple cognitive tests of global and cognitive function may not be sensitive enough to detect changes over time in unselected populations. Areas of cognitive function that tend to change with time include memory, attention and cognitive speed (Houx *et al.*, 2002).

(k) *Medications* – Medication use can influence performance during neuropsychiatric evaluations, and needs to be noted in any trial related to prevention and control.

(l) *Other medical conditions* – Other medical conditions, such as depression, can influence an individual's performance on cognitive tests, and if at all possible, should be queried about, if not formally evaluated.

Conclusions and directions to the future

The relationship between vascular factors and dementia is well-established and provides a springboard for the implementation of intervention and prevention efforts. Primary prevention trials related to lifestyle factors are greatly needed in relationship to dementia. Published clinical trials thus far have not given conclusive answers to whether dementia might be prevented through the use of pharmacologic agents. A more holistic or lifestyle approach to dementia prevention may provide complementary solutions to this burgeoning health concern of the twenty-first century.

ACKNOWLEDGMENTS

Dr. Gustafson is a Senior Researcher with the Swedish Research Council, and is also supported by grants from the National Institutes of Health/National Institutes on Aging 1R03AG026098–01A1 and the Swedish Brain Power Project.

REFERENCES

Aevarsson O, Skoog I. A longitudinal population study of the mini-mental state examination in the very old: Relation to dementia and education. *Dement Geriatr Cogn Disord* 2000; **11**(3): 166–75.

Akomolafe A, Beiser A, Meigs JB, *et al.* Diabetes mellitus and risk of developing Alzheimer disease: results from the Framingham Study. *Arch Neurol* 2006; **63**(11): 1551–5.

Applegate WB, Pressel S, Wittes J, *et al.* Impact of the treatment of isolated systolic hypertension on behavioral variables. Results from the Systolic Hypertension in the Elderly Program. *Arch Intern Med* 1994; **154**: 2154–60.

Association AH. Control your risk factors for high blood pressure. Available at: http://www.americanheart.org/presenter.jhtml?identifier=581, 2007.

Association AH. Metabolic syndrome. Available at: http://www.americanheart.org/presenter.jhtml?identifier=581.

Ayanian JZ, Zaslavsky AM, Weissman JS, Schneider EC, Ginsburg JA. Undiagnosed hypertension and hypercholesterolemia among uninsured and insured adults in the Third National Health and Nutrition Examination Survey. *Am J Public Health* 2003; **93**(12): 2051–4.

Bagger YZ, Tanko LB, Alexanderssen P, Qin G, Christiansen C. The implications of body fat mass and fat distribution for cognitive function in elderly women. *Obes Res* 2004; **12**: 1519–26.

Barrett-Connor E, Edelstein SL, Corey-Bloom J, Wiederholt WC. Weight loss precedes dementia in community-dwelling older adults. *J Am Geriatr Soc* 1996; **44**: 1147–52.

Blennow K, Wallin A, Fredman P, Karlsson I, Gottfries CG, Svennerholm L. Blood–brain barrier disturbance in patients with Alzheimer's disease is related to vascular factors. *Acta Neurol Scand* 1990; **81**(4): 323–6.

Borjesson-Hanson A, Edin E, Gislason T, Skoog I. The prevalence of dementia in 95 year olds. *Neurology* 2004; **63**(12): 2436–8.

Brook RD, Bard RL, Rubenfire M, Ridker PM, Rajagopalan S. Usefulness of visceral obesity (waist/hip ratio) in predicting vascular endothelial function in healthy overweight adults. *Am J Cardiol* 2001; **88**: 1264–9.

Brubacher D, Monsch AU, Stahelin HB. Weight change and cognitive performance. *Int J Obes Relat Metab Disord* 2004; **28**(9): 1163–7.

Buchman AS, Wilson RS, Bienias JL, Shah RC, Evans DA, Bennett DA. Change in body mass index and risk of incident Alzheimer disease. *Neurology* 2005; **65**(6): 892–7.

DeMichele M, Panico S, Iannuzzi A, *et al.* Association of obesity and central fat distribution with carotid artery wall thickening in middle-aged women. *Stroke* 2002; **33**(12): 2923–8.

Diaz VA, Mainous AG 3rd, Koopman RJ, Geesey ME. Undiagnosed obesity: implications for undiagnosed hypertension, diabetes, and hypercholesterolemia. *Fam Med* 2004; **36**(9): 639–44.

Di Bari M, Pahor M, Franse LV, *et al.* Dementia and disability outcomes in large hypertension trials: lessons learned from the systolic hypertension in the elderly program (SHEP) trial. *Am J Epidemiol* 2001; **153**(1): 72–8.

Di Bari M, Pahor M, Franse LV, *et al.* Evaluation and correction for a "training effect" in the cognitive assessment of older adults. *Neuroepidemiology* 2002; **21**(2): 87–92.

Di Bari M, Pahor M, Barnard M, *et al.* Evaluation and correction for a "training effect" in the cognitive assessment of older adults. *Neuroepidemiology* 2002; **21**(2): 87–92.

Elias MF, Elias PK, Sullivan LM, Wolf PA, D'Agostino RB. Obesity, diabetes and cognitive deficit: the

Framingham Heart Study. *Neurobiol Aging* 2005; **26** (Suppl.1): 11–16.

Enzinger C, Fazekas F, Matthews PM, *et al.* Risk factors for progression of brain atrophy in aging: Six-year follow-up of normal subjects. *Neurology* 2005; **64**(10): 1704–11.

Expert Panel on the Identification and Treatment of Overweight and Obesity in Adults. Aim for a Healthy Weight. Washington, DC: National Institutes of Health; 2005. 05–5213.

Faxen-Irving G, Basun H, Cederholm T. Nutritional and cognitive relationships and long-term mortality in patients with various dementia disorders. *Age Ageing* 2005; **34**(2): 136–41.

Ford ES, Giles WH, Dietz WH. Prevalence of the metabolic syndrome among US adults: Findings from the third National Health and Nutrition Examination Survey. *JAMA* 2002; **287**: 356–9.

Forette F, Seux ML, Staessen JA, *et al.* Prevention of dementia in randomised double-blind placebo-controlled Systolic Hypertension in Europe (Syst-Eur) trial. *Lancet* 1998; **352**(9137): 1347–51.

Forette F, Seux ML, Staessen JA, *et al.* The prevention of dementia with antihypertensive treatment: new evidence from the Systolic Hypertension in Europe (Syst-Eur) study. *Arch Intern Med* 2002; **162**(18): 2046–52.

Greenwood CE, Winocur G. High-fat diets, insulin resistance and declining cognitive function. *Neurobiol Aging* 2005; **26**(Suppl 1): 42–5.

Greenwood CE, Kaplan RJ, Hebblethwaite S, Jenkins DJ. Carbohydrate-induced memory impairment in adults with type 2 diabetes. *Diabetes Care* 2003; **26**(7): 1961–6.

Grundman M, Corey-Bloom J, Jernigan T, Archibald S, Thal LJ. Low body weight in Alzheimer's disease is associated with mesial temporal cortex atrophy. *Neurology* 1996; **46**(6): 1585–91.

Guo Z, Viitanen M, Fratiglioni L, Winblad B. Low blood pressure and dementia in elderly people: the Kungsholmen project. *Br Med J* 1996; **312**(7034): 805–08.

Guo Z, Qiu C, Viitanen M, Fastbom J, Winblad B, Fratiglioni L. Blood pressure and dementia in persons 75+ years old: 3-year follow-up results from the Kungsholmen Project. *J Alzheimer's Dis* 2001; **3**(6): 585–91.

Gustafson DRC, Kurzer MS. Flavonoid inhibition of aromatase enzyme activity in human preadipocytes. *J Steroid Biochem Mol Biol* 1993; **46**: 381–8.

Gustafson DRC, Rothenberg E, Blennow K, Steen B, Skoog I. An 18-year follow up of overweight and risk for

Alzheimer's disease. *Arch Intern Med* 2003; **163**: 1524–8.

Gustafson D, Lissner L, Bengtsson C, Björkelund C, Skoog I. A 24-year follow-up of body mass index and cerebral atrophy. *Neurology* 2004a; **63**: 1876–81.

Gustafson D, Steen B, Skoog I. Body mass index and white matter lesions in elderly women. An 18-year longitudinal study. *Int J Psychogeriatrics* 2004b; **16**: 327–36.

Han TS, van Leer EM, Seidell JC, Lean ME. Waist circumference action levels in the identification of cardiovascular risk factors: prevalence study in a random sample. *Br Med J* 1995; **311**(7017): 1401–5.

Han TS, Williams K, Sattar N, Hunt KJ, Lean ME, Haffner SM. Analysis of obesity and hyperinsulinemia in the development of metabolic syndrome: San Antonio Heart Study. *Obes Res* 2002; **10**(9): 923–31.

Hausman DB, DiGirolamo M, Bartness TJ, Hausman GJ, Martin RJ. The biology of white adipocyte proliferation. *Obesity Rev* 2001; **2**: 239–54.

Hogan DB, Ebly EM, Rockwood K. Weight, blood pressure, osmolarity, and glucose levels across various stages of Alzheimer's disease and vascular dementia. *Dement Geriatr Cogn Disord* 1997; **8**: 147–51.

Höglund K, Blennow K. Effect of HMG-CoA reductase inhibitors on beta-amyloid peptide levels: implications for Alzheimer's Disease. *CNS Drugs* 2007; **21**(6): 449–62.

Houx P, Shepherd J, Blauw G-J, *et al.* Testing cognitive function in elderly populations: the PROSPER study. *J Neurol Neurosurg Psychiatry* 2002; **73**: 385–9.

in't Veld BA, Ruitenberg A, Hofman A, Stricker BH, Breteler MM. Antihypertensive drugs and incidence of dementia: the Rotterdam Study. *Neurobiol Aging* 2001; **22**(3): 407–12.

Jagust W, Harvey D, Mungas D, Haan M. Central obesity and the aging brain. *Arch Neurol* 2005; **62**(10): 1545–8.

Jeong SK, Nam HS, Son MH, Son EJ, Cho KH. Interactive effect of obesity indexes on cognition. *Dement Geriatr Cogn Disord* 2005; **19**(2–3): 91–6.

Jorm AF, Korten AE, Henderson AS. The prevalence of dementia: a quantitative integration of the literature. *Acta Psychiatr Scand* 1987; **76**: 465–79.

Kalmijn S, Foley D, White L, *et al.* Metabolic cardiovascular syndrome and risk of dementia in Japanese-American elderly men. *Arterioscler Thromb Vasc Biol* 2000; **20**: 2255–60.

Kannel WB. Risk stratification in hypertension: New insights from the Framingham Study. *Am J Hypertens* 2000; **13**: 3S–10S.

Kivipelto M, Helkala EL, Laakso MP, *et al.* Midlife vascular risk factors and Alzheimer's disease in later life: longitudinal, population based study. *Br Med J* 2001; **322** (7300): 1447–51.

Kivipelto M, Helkala EL, Laakso MP, *et al.* Apolipoprotein E epsilon4 allele, elevated midlife total cholesterol level, and high midlife systolic blood pressure are independent risk factors for late-life Alzheimer disease. *Ann Intern Med* 2002; **137**(3): 149–55.

Kivipelto M, Ngandu T, Fratiglioni L, *et al.* Obesity and vascular risk factors at midlife and the risk of dementia and Alzheimer disease. *Arch Neurol* 2005; **62**(10): 1556–60.

Last J. *A Dictionary of Epidemiology.* Second edition. New York: Oxford University Press, 1988.

Lathe R. Hormones and the hippocampus. *J Endocrinol* 2001; **169**(2): 205–31.

Launer LJ, Ross GW, Petrovich H, *et al.* Midlife blood pressure and dementia: the Honolulu–Asia aging study. *Neurobiol Aging* 2000; **21**: 49–55.

Leibson CL, Rocca WA, Hanson VA, *et al.* Risk of dementia among persons with diabetes mellitus: a population-based cohort study. *Am J Epidemiol* 1997; **145**: 301–08.

Lithell H, Hansson L, Skoog I, *et al.* The Study on Cognition and Prognosis in the Elderly (SCOPE): principal results of a randomized double-blind intervention trial. *J Hypertens* 2003; **21**(5): 875–86.

Martins IJ, Hone E, Foster JK, *et al.* Apolipoprotein E, cholesterol metabolism, diabetes, and the convergence of risk factors for Alzheimer's disease and cardiovascular disease. *Mol Psychiatry* 2006; **11**(8): 721–36.

McCrindle BW, Urbina EM, Dennison BA, *et al.* Summary of the American Heart Association's scientific statement on drug therapy of high-risk lipid abnormalities in children and adolescents. *Arterioscler Thromb Vasc Biol* 2007; **27**(5): 982–5.

McGavock JM, Victor RG, Unger RH, Szczepaniak LS. Adiposity of the heart, revisited. *Ann Intern Med* 2006; **144**: 517–24.

Mielke MM, Zandi PP, Sjögren M, *et al.* Elevated total cholesterol levels in late-life associated with a reduced risk of dementia. *Neurology* 2005; **64**: 1689–95.

Morris MC, Scherr PA, Hebert LE, Glynn RJ, Bennett DA, Evans DA. Association of incident Alzheimer disease and blood pressure measured from 13 years before to 2 years after diagnosis in a large community study. *Arch Neurol* 2001; **58**(10): 1640–6.

National Institutes of Health NH, Lung and Blood Institute. Clinical guidelines on the identification, evaluation, and treatment of overweight and obesity in adults–the evidence report. Bethesda, MD: National Institutes of Health; 1998.

Notkola IL, Sulkava R, Pekkanen J, *et al.* Serum total cholesterol, apolipoprotein E epsilon 4 allele, and Alzheimer's disease. *Neuroepidemiology* 1998; **17**(1): 14–20.

Nourhashemi F, Andrieu S, Gillette-Guyonnet S, *et al.* Is there a relationship between fat-free soft tissue mass and low cognitive function? Results from a study of 7105 women. *J Am Geriatr Soc* 2002; **50**(11): 1796–801.

Nourhashemi F, Deschamps V, Larrieu S, Letenneur L, Dartigues JF, Barberger-Gateau P. Body mass index and incidence of dementia: the PAQUID study. *Neurology* 2003; **60**(1): 117–9.

Ott A, Stolk RP, van Harskamp F, Pols HA, Hofman A, Breteler MM. Diabetes mellitus and the risk of dementia: the Rotterdam Study. *Neurology* 1999; **53** (9): 1937–42.

Pangalos MN, Jacobsen SJ, Reinhart PH. Disease modifying strategies for the treatment of Alzheimer's disease targeted at modulating levels of the beta-amyloid peptide. *Biochem Soc Trans* 2005; **33**(Pt 4): 553–8.

Pasquier F, Boulogne A, Leys D, Fontaine P. Diabetes mellitus and dementia. *Diabetes Metab* 2006; **32**(5 Pt 1): 403–14.

Patel BN, Pang D, Stern Y, *et al.* Obesity enhances verbal memory in postmenopausal women with Down syndrome. *Neurobiol Aging* 2004; **25**(2): 159–66.

Peart S. Results of MRC (UK) trial of drug therapy for mild hypertension. *Clin Invest Med* 1987; **10**(6): 616–20.

Pilcher H. Alzheimer's disease could be "type 3 diabetes". *Lancet Neurol* 2006; **5**(5): 388–9.

Posner HB, Tang MX, Luchsinger J, Lantigua R, Stern Y, Mayeux R. The relationship of hypertension in the elderly to AD, vascular dementia, and cognitive function. *Neurology* 2002; **58**(8): 1175–81.

Prince MJ, Bird AS, Blizard RA, Mann AH. Is the cognitive function of older patients affected by antihypertensive treatment? Results from 54 months of the Medical Research Council's trial of hypertension in older adults. *Br Med J* 1996; **312**(7034): 801–05.

PROGRESS, Collaborative Group. Randomised trial of a perindopril-based blood-pressure-lowering regimen among 6105 individuals with previous stroke or transient ischemic attack. *Lancet* 2001; **358**: 1033–41.

Qiu C, von Strauss E, Fastbom J, Winblad B, Fratiglioni L. Low blood pressure and risk of dementia in the Kungsholmen project: a 6-year follow-up study. *Arch Neurol* 2003; **60**(2): 223–8.

Qureshi AI, Suri MF, Guterman LR, Hopkins LN. Ineffective secondary prevention in survivors of cardiovascular events in the US population: report from the Third National Health and Nutrition Examination Survey. *Arch Intern Med* 2001; **161**(13): 1621–8.

Reitz C, Tang MX, Luchsinger J, Mayeux R. Relation of plasma lipids to Alzheimer disease and vascular dementia. *Arch Neurol* 2004; **61**(5): 705–14.

Richards SS, Emsley CL, Roberts J, *et al.* The association between vascular risk factor-mediating medications and cognition and dementia diagnosis in a community-based sample of African-Americans. *J Am Geriatr Soc* 2000; **48**(9): 1035–41.

Romas SN, Tang MX, Berglund L, Mayeux R. APOE genotype, plasma lipids, lipoproteins, and AD in community elderly. *Neurology* 1999; **53**(3): 517–21.

Rosengren A, Skoog I, Gustafson D, Wilhelmsen L. Body mass index, other cardiovascular risk factors, and hospitalization for dementia. *Arch Intern Med* 2005; **165**(3): 321–6.

Ruitenberg A. *Vascular factors in dementia. Observations in the Rotterdam Study.* Rotterdam: Erasmus University, 2000.

Ruitenberg A, Skoog I, Ott A, *et al.* Blood pressure and risk of dementia: results from the Rotterdam Study and the Gothenburg H-70 Study. *Dement Geriatr Cogn Disord* 2001; **12**(1): 33–9.

SHEP Cooperative Research Group. Prevention of stroke by antihypertensive drug treatment in older persons with isolated systolic hypertension: final results of the systolic hypertension in the elderly program. *JAMA* 1991; **265**: 3255–64.

Skoog I, Nilsson L, Palmertz B, Andreasson L-A, Svanborg A. A population-based study of dementia in 85-year-olds. *N Engl J Med* 1993; **328**: 153–8.

Skoog I, Lernfelt B, Landahl S, *et al.* 15-year longitudinal study of blood pressure and dementia. *Lancet* 1996; **347**: 1141–5.

Skoog I, Kalaria RN, Breteler MM. Vascular factors and Alzheimer disease. *Alzheimer Dis Assoc Disord* 1999; **13** (Suppl 3): S106–14.

Solomon A, Kareholt I, Ngandu T, *et al.* Serum cholesterol changes after midlife and late-life cognition: twenty-one-year follow-up study. *Neurology* 2007; **68**(10): 751–6.

Sparks DL, Scheff SW, Hunsaker JC 3rd, Liu H, Landers T, Gross DR. Induction of Alzheimer-like beta-amyloid immunoreactivity in the brains of rabbits with dietary cholesterol. *Exp Neurol* 1994; **126**(1): 88–94.

Staessen JA, Fagard R, Thijs L, *et al.* Randomised double-blind comparison of placebo and active treatment for older patients with isolated systolic hypertension. *Lancet* 1997; **350**: 757–64.

Stewart R, Masaki K, Xue QL, *et al.* A 32-year prospective study of change in body weight and incident dementia: the Honolulu–Asia Aging Study. *Arch Neurol* 2005; **62**(1): 55–60.

Suwaidi JA, Higano ST, Holmes DR, Lennon R, Lerman A. Obesity is independently associated with coronary endothelial dysfunction in patients with normal or mildly diseased coronary arteries. *J Am Coll Cardiol* 2001; **37**: 1523–8.

Tan ZS, Seshadri S, Beiser A, *et al.* Plasma total cholesterol level as a risk factor for Alzheimer disease: the Framingham Study. *Arch Intern Med* 2003; **163**(9): 1053–7.

Tzourio C, Anderson C, Chapman N, *et al.* Effects of blood pressure lowering with perindopril and indapamide therapy on dementia and cognitive decline in patients with cerebrovascular disease. *Arch Intern Med* 2003; **163**: 1069–75.

Waldstein SR, Katzel LI. Interactive relations of central versus total obesity and blood pressure to cognitive function. *Int J Obes (Lond)* 2006; **30**(1): 201–07.

Ward MA, Carlsson CM, Trivedi MA, Sager MA, Johnson SC. The effect of body mass index on global brain volume in middle-aged adults: a cross sectional study. *BMC Neurol* 2005; **5**: 23.

Watson GS, Craft S. Insulin resistance, inflammation, and cognition in Alzheimer's Disease: Lessons for multiple sclerosis. *J Neurol Sci* 2006; **245**(1–2): 21–33.

White H, Pieper C, Schmader K, Fillenbaum G. Weight change in Alzheimer's disease. *J Am Geriatr Soc* 1996; **44**: 265–72.

White H, Pieper C, Schmader K. The association of weight change in Alzheimer's Disease with severity of disease and mortality: a longitudinal analysis. *J Am Geriatr Soc* 1998; **46**: 1223–7.

Whitmer RA, Gunderson EP, Barrett-Connor E, Quesenberry CP, Jr., Yaffe K. Obesity in middle age and future risk of dementia: a 27 year longitudinal population based study. *Br Med J* 2005; **330**(7504): 1360.

Williams IL, Wheatcroft SB, Shah AM, Kearney MT. Obesity, atherosclerosis and the vascular endothelium: mechanisms of reduced nitric oxide bioavailability in obese humans. *Int J Obes Relat Metab Disord* 2002; **26**(6): 754–64.

Wu C, Zhou D, Wen C, Zhang L, Como P, Qiao Y. Relationship between blood pressure and Alzheimer's disease in Linxian County, China. *Life Sci* 2003; **72** (10): 1125–33.

Xu W, Qiu C, Winblad B, Fratiglioni L. The effect of borderline diabetes on the risk of dementia and Alzheimer's disease. *Diabetes* 2007; **56**(1): 211–6.

Yaffe K, Kanaya A, Lindquist K, *et al*. The metabolic syndrome, inflammation, and risk of cognitive decline. *JAMA* 2004; **292**(18): 2237–42.

Yki-Järvinen H, Westerbacka J. Vascular actions of insulin in obesity. *Int J Obes Relat Metab Disord* 2000; **24**: S25–8.

Yoshitake T, Kiyohara Y, Kato I, *et al*. Incidence and risk factors of vascular dementia and Alzheimer's disease in a defined elderly Japanese population: the Hisayama Study. *Neurology* 1995; **45**(6): 1161–8.

Zandi P, Breitner J, Anthony J. Is pharmacological prevention of Alzheimer's a realistic goal? *Expert Opin Pharmacother* 2002; **3**: 365–80.

Zhang R, Reisin E. Obesity–hypertension: the effects on cardiovascular and renal systems. *J Hypertension* 2000; **13**: 1308–14.

Websites with information on the control of vascular risk factors.

Topic	Web address
blood pressure/ hypertension	http://www.nhlbi.nih.gov/ health/public/heart
blood cholesterol/ hypercholesterolemia	http://www.nhlbi.nih.gov/ health/public/heart http://www.american-heart.org
overweight/obesity	http://www.nhlbi.nih.gov/ health/public/heart http://www.dh.gov.uk/ PolicyAndGuidance/ HealthAndSocialCareTopics/Obesity

Index